KT-119-350

Human Walking

Human Walking

THIRD EDITION

EDITED BY

Jessica Rose, PhD

Assistant Professor, Department of Orthopaedic Surgery
Stanford University School of Medicine
Director, Motion & Gait Analysis Laboratory
Lucile Packard Children's Hospital
Palo Alto, California

James G. Gamble, MD, PhD

Professor, Department of Orthopaedic Surgery
Stanford University School of Medicine
Medical Director, Motion & Gait Analysis Laboratory
Lucile Packard Children's Hospital
Palo Alto, California

LIPPINCOTT WILLIAMS & WILKINS
A **Wolters Kluwer** Company
Philadelphia • Baltimore • New York • London
Buenos Aires • Hong Kong • Sydney • Tokyo

Acquisitions Editor: Robert Hurley
Managing Editor: Michelle LaPlante
Production Manager: Bridgett Dougherty
Senior Manufacturing Manager: Benjamin Rivera
Marketing Director: Sharon Zinner
Design Coordinator: Holly McLaughlin
Production Services: Techbooks
Printer: Edward Brothers

© 2006 by LIPPINCOTT WILLIAMS & WILKINS
530 Walnut Street
Philadelphia, PA 19106 USA
LWW.com

All rights reserved. This book is protected by copyright. No part of this book may be reproduced in any form or by any means, including photocopying, or utilized by any information storage and retrieval system without written permission from the copyright owner, except for brief quotations embodied in critical articles and reviews. Materials appearing in this book prepared by individuals as part of their official duties as U.S. government employees are not covered by the above-mentioned copyright.

Printed in the USA

Library of Congress Cataloging-in-Publication Data

Human walking / [edited by] Jessica Rose, James G. Gamble.— 3rd ed.
    p.   ; cm.
  Includes bibliographical references and index.
  ISBN 0-7817-5954-4
  1. Walking. I. Rose, Jessica. II. Gamble, James Gibson.
  [DNLM: 1. Locomotion—physiology. 2. Walking—physiology. 3. Biomechanics.
 4. Gait—physiology. WE 103 H918855 2006]
  QP310.W3H85 2006
  612.7′6—dc22

                                          2005022885

Care has been taken to confirm the accuracy of the information presented and to describe generally accepted practices. However, the authors, editors, and publisher are not responsible for errors or omissions or for any consequences from application of the information in this book and make no warranty, expressed or implied, with respect to the currency, completeness, or accuracy of the contents of the publication. Application of this information in a particular situation remains the professional responsibility of the practitioner.

The authors, editors, and publisher have exerted every effort to ensure that drug selection and dosage set forth in this text are in accordance with current recommendations and practice at the time of publication. However, in view of ongoing research, changes in government regulations, and the constant flow of information relating to drug therapy and drug reactions, the reader is urged to check the package insert for each drug for any change in indications and dosage and for added warnings and precautions. This is particularly important when the recommended agent is a new or infrequently employed drug.

Some drugs and medical devices presented in this publication have Food and Drug Administration (FDA) clearance for limited use in restricted research settings. It is the responsibility of the health care provider to ascertain the FDA status of each drug or device planned for use in their clinical practice.

To purchase additional copies of this book, call our customer service department at (800) 638-3030 or fax orders to (301) 223-2320. International customers should call (301) 223-2300.

Visit Lippincott Williams & Wilkins on the Internet: at LWW.com. Lippincott Williams & Wilkins customer service representatives are available from 8:30 am to 6 pm, EST.

10 9 8 7 6 5 4 3 2 1

To Will, Thomas, Jamie, Justin, Laura, Jeffrey, Jayson, Jared and all the other children of the world.

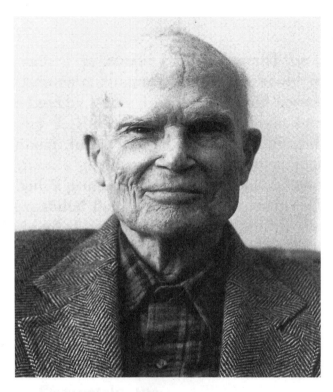

Henry J. Ralston, PhD
1906–1993

Henry J. Ralston, Professor of Physiology, University of California School of Medicine, San Francisco, co-authored the 1st edition of *Human Walking*. Dr. Ralston was an internationally renowned investigator in the physiology and biophysics of human locomotion. Dr. Ralston was also a talented teacher, educating several generations of neuromuscular physiology students as part of the Physical Therapy and Medicine Departments at the University of California at San Francisco as well as teaching general physiology for nearly three decades.

Known to his friends, family, and colleagues as "Bip," a name given to him as an infant, Ralston was a descendant of a family that came to San Francisco from Scotland in the early 1860s; the family started an iron works company that survived until the Depression. Ralston worked his way through the University of California at Berkeley as a newspaper writer and initiated the first regular column in San Francisco reviewing and critiquing radio programs. His PhD thesis concerned the biological effects of ionizing radiation.

Just after World War II, Dr. Ralston began the collaboration with Dr. Verne T. Inman that would result in a series of major contributions to the field of human locomotion. Supported by funding from various federal agencies, Inman and Ralston began the Lower Extremity Amputee Research Laboratory, which soon evolved into the Biomechanics Laboratory. With colleagues in bioengineering at the University of California at Berkeley, as well as with physicians and scientists at the University of California at San Francisco, the laboratory pioneered work that revolutionized the design of lower limb prosthetic devices. His physiological investigations focused on neuromuscular physiology and the energetics of walking and led to improved surgical approaches to lower limb repair and enhanced design of prostheses. *Human Walking* was a culmination of Dr. Ralston's ground breaking research and his collaboration with Dr. Inman.

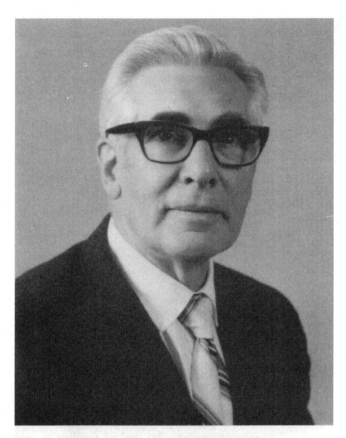

Verne T. Inman, MD, PhD
1905–1980

Verne T. Inman, Professor Emeritus and former Chairman of the Department of Orthopaedic Surgery, University of California School of Medicine, San Francisco, co-edited the 1st edition of *Human Walking.*

Dr. Inman was born in San Jose, California, November 6, 1905. He received both his medical education and formal training in human anatomy at the University of California.

Dr. Inman's primary research interest since his student days may be best described as functional anatomy. His studies on the actions of the shoulder joint, the clavicle, the abductor muscles of the hip, and the ankle are classics in the field. He was one of the pioneers in the use of electromyography to analyze muscle function.

Shortly after World War II, Dr. Inman, along with colleagues in engineering and physiology, became involved in lower limb prosthetics research. This led to the formation of the Biomechanics Laboratory at the University of California at San Francisco and Berkeley, of which he was director from 1957 to 1973 and consultant until his death.

Dr. Inman had long expressed the wish to prepare a book summarizing the research studies on human walking in the Biomechanics Laboratory, and *Human Walking* is the culmination of that wish.

CONTENTS

CONTRIBUTORS

Janet M. Adams, PT, MS, DPT
Professor and Chair, Department of Physical Therapy
California State University, Northridge
Northridge, California

Frank C. Anderson, PhD
Engineering Research Associate
Division of Biomechanical Engineering
Stanford University
Stanford, California

Allison S. Arnold, PhD
Physical Science Research Associate
Division of Biomechanical Engineering
Stanford University
Stanford, California

Jennette L. Boakes, MD
Clinical Associate Professor of Orthopaedic Surgery
UC Davis School of Medicine
Pediatric Orthopaedic Surgeon
Shriners Hospitals for Children
Sacramento, California

Erin E. Butler, MS
Biomechanical Engineer
Motion & Gait Analysis Laboratory
Lucile Packard Children's Hospital
Palo Alto, California

Dudley S. Childress, PhD
Professor (Emeritus)
Biomedical Engineering and Physical
*   Medicine & Rehabilitation*
Northwestern University
Chicago, Illinois

Roy B. Davis, PhD
Director, Motion Analysis Laboratory
Shriners Hospitals for Children
Greenville, South Carolina

Scott L. Delp, PhD
Professor and Chair
Bioengineering Department
Stanford University
Stanford, California

Maurice Druzin, MD
Professor, Department of Obstetrics and Gynecology
Division of Maternal & Fetal Medicine
Stanford University School of Medicine
Stanford, California

James G. Gamble, MD, PhD
Professor, Department of Orthopaedic Surgery
Stanford University School of Medicine
Medical Director, Motion & Gait Analysis Laboratory
Lucile Packard Children's Hospital
Palo Alto, California

Steven A. Gard, PhD
Director, Northwestern University Prosthetics
*   Research Laboratory & Rehabilitation*
*   Engineering Research Program*
Research Associate Professor, Physical Medicine & Rehabilitation,
Northwestern University
Research Health Scientist, Jesse Brown VA Medical Center
Chicago, Illinois

Saryn R. Goldberg, PhD
Clinical Research Scientist
Physical Disabilities Branch of the
*   National Institutes of Health*
Bethesda, Maryland

William L. Haskell, PhD
Professor Emeritus, Department of Medicine
Stanford Prevention Research Center
Stanford University School of Medicine
Stanford, California

Verne T. Inman, MD, PhD[†]
Professor Emeritus and Former Chairman of the
*   Department of Orthopaedic Surgery*
University of California School of Medicine
San Francisco, California

M. Elise Johanson, PT, MS
Research Health Scientist
VA Palo Alto Health Care System
Rehabilitation Research & Development Center
*   and Motion & Gait Analysis Laboratory*
Lucile Packard Children's Hospital
Palo Alto, California

Kenton R. Kaufman, PhD
Director, Orthopaedic Biomechanics Laboratory
Professor, Biomedical Engineering
Mayo Clinic
Rochester, Minnesota

Rosanne Kermoian, PhD
Senior Research Scientist, Department of Orthopaedic Surgery
Stanford University School of Medicine
Motion & Gait Analysis Laboratory
Lucile Packard Children's Hospital
Palo Alto, California

Richard G. Klein, PhD
Professor, Department of Anthropological Sciences
Program in Human Biology
Stanford University
Stanford, California

Rudi Kobetic, MS
Motion Study Laboratory
L. Stokes Cleveland VA Medical Center
Cleveland, Ohio

[†]Deceased

John W. Michael, MEd, CPO
President, CPO Services, Inc.
Portage, Indiana
Adjunct Faculty
School of Applied Physiology
Georgia Institute of Technology
Atlanta, Georgia

Don W. Morgan, PhD
Professor, Department of Health and Human Performance
Middle Tennessee State University
Murfreesboro, Tennessee

Marcus G. Pandy, PhD
Professor, Department of Biomedical Engineering
The University of Texas at Austin
Austin, Texas

Jacquelin Perry, MD
Professor Emeritus, Department of Orthopaedics
*   and Department of Biokinesiology & Physical Therapy*
University of Southern California
Los Angeles, California

George T. Rab, MD
Professor and Chair, Department of Orthopaedic Surgery
UC Davis School of Medicine
Sacramento, California

Henry J. Ralston, PhD[†]
Professor of Physiology
University of California School of Medicine
San Francisco, California

Jessica Rose, PhD
Assistant Professor, Department of Orthopaedic Surgery
Stanford University School of Medicine
Director, Motion & Gait Analysis Laboratory
Lucile Packard Children's Hospital
Palo Alto, California

Stephen Skinner, MD
Clinical Professor, Department of Orthopedic Surgery
UC Davis School of Medicine
Chief of Orthopaedics
Shriners Hospitals for Children
Sacramento, California

Edith V. Sullivan, PhD
Professor, Department of Psychiatry & Behavioral Sciences and
*   Neurosciences Program*
Stanford University School of Medicine
Stanford, California

David H. Sutherland, MD
Professor Emeritus,
*   Department of Orthopaedic Surgery*
University of California, San Diego
Motion Analysis Laboratory
San Diego Children's Hospital
San Diego, California

Frank Todd, BA
Berkeley, CA

Leslie Torburn, PT, MS
Physical Therapist
Motion & Gait Analysis Laboratory
Lucile Packard Children's Hospital
Palo Alto, California

Ronald J. Triolo, PhD
Associate Professor of Orthopaedics &
*   Biomedical Engineering*
Case Western Reserve University
VA Rehabilitation Research Career Scientist
Cleveland, Ohio

Timothy D. Weaver, PhD
Department of Human Evolution
Max Planck Institute for Evolutionary Anthropology
Leipzig, Germany

[†]Deceased

PREFACE

The third edition of *Human Walking* embraces the multidisciplinary approach and pragmatic spirit that was a major theme of the first and second editions. The increased breadth and depth of material for the third edition reflects the expanding nature of the field. Our understanding of human walking and the information available has increased exponentially over the past decade. New areas of knowledge have developed over the last several years in fields such as physical anthropology, neuromotor development, and biomechanics, with groundbreaking advances in biomechanical modeling and artificial walking. Increasingly precise measurement techniques have made it possible to study the neuromuscular activation and intricate biomechanics of human walking and have deepened our understanding of the neurological and musculoskeletal mechanisms underlying walking disorders. The third edition summarizes and integrates this new information with our classical understanding of human walking.

The first edition of *Human Walking*, published in 1981, was written by an interdisciplinary team of investigators, composed of Verne T. Inman, an orthopedic surgeon, Henry J. Ralston, a physiologist, and Frank Todd, an engineer. In the years following the publication of the first edition, a generation of students and researchers used *Human Walking* as both a primary text and a reference as they expanded the available knowledge in the field of motion analysis. In the second edition, we chose to preserve the multidisciplinary approach as well as the pragmatism of the previous edition, while extending the scope and the scale of the book. We invited a diverse group of distinguished contributors to share their ideas, information, and expertise. The third edition expands on this theme. We have preserved the classic and original chapter "Human Locomotion" written by Verne T. Inman, Henry J. Ralston, and Frank Todd, and added commentary on the determinants of gait that integrates new information. There are updated chapters on Kinematics of Normal Walking, Kinetics of Normal Walking, Energetics of Walking, Muscle Activity During Walking, Development of

Gait, Clinical Gait Analysis, Lower Limb Prostheses and Restoring Walking After Paralysis. Furthermore, we have expanded the multidisciplinary approach to include new chapters on rapidly developing fields such as The Evolution of Human Walking, Gait Adaptations in Adulthood, Walking for Health, and Simulation of Walking. It was clear a decade ago that biomechanical modeling would make interesting contributions to our understanding of human walking. However, it was not certain how rapidly these contributions would come and how important they would ultimately be for identifying the sources of pathological gait. Chapter 12, "Simulation of Walking," shows just how valuable biomechanical modeling can be and provides a fresh understanding of the scientific basis for the treatment of patients with walking disorders. Biomechanical modeling is now used in the clinical setting to plan such surgical procedures as tendon transfers, tendon lengthenings, and osteotomies. The final chapter, "Six Take-Home Lessons," summarizes some of the essential elements of human walking for students who are new to the field.

Human walking is an extremely complex activity whose apparent simplicity disappears when one attempts a quantitative or even qualitative description of the process. Fortunately, the theories and techniques of modern motion analysis have markedly improved our ability to describe and understand normal and pathological ambulation. Much of the current success is a result of the wide interest in human walking as demonstrated by a diverse group of clinicians and scientists currently working in the field, including orthopaedic surgeons, physical therapists, bioengineers, physiatrists, neurologists, orthotists, prosthetists and exercise physiologists. The third edition of *Human Walking* is geared to this diverse group of students, researchers, and clinicians, and continues the pragmatic tradition of providing useful information from a broad spectrum of expertise while offering a springboard for future advances in the field by the next generation.

Jessica Rose
James G. Gamble
September 2005

Human Locomotion

Verne T. Inman, Henry J. Ralston, and Frank Todd
Commentary by Dudley S. Childress and Steven A. Gard

Locomotion, a characteristic of animals, is the process by which the animal moves itself from one geographic position to another. Locomotion includes starting, stopping, changes in speed, alterations in direction, and modifications for changes in slope. These events, however, are transitory activities that are superimposed on a basic pattern. In walking and running animals, this pattern can be defined as a rhythmic displacement of body parts that maintains the animal in constant forward progression.

The majority of mammals are quadripedal. When walking slowly, quadrupeds tend to coordinate their four limbs so that three of their feet are on the ground. A crawling infant uses its limbs in a sequence that is essentially quadripedal, only advancing one while the other three support its body on the floor. This provides the stability of a tripod. This stability is lost when the animal becomes bipedal, and while bipedal locomotion seems simpler, it requires greater neural control. The mastering of the erect bipedal type of locomotion is a relatively prolonged affair and appears to be a combination of instinct and learning.

If walking is a learned activity, it is not surprising that each of us displays certain personal peculiarities superimposed on the basic pattern of bipedal locomotion. Physical anthropologists have studied the differences between races and measured the variations in skeletal parts. Anatomists are aware of the presence of individual variations. All of us are aware that individuals walk differently; one can often recognize an acquaintance by his manner of walking even when seen at a distance. Tall, slender people walk differently from short, stocky people. People alter their manner of walking when wearing shoes with different heel heights. A person walks differently when exhilarated than when mentally depressed. With these ideas in mind, one may legitimately question the usefulness of anthropometric data and averages in furthering our understanding of human walking.

Certainly everyone has his own idiosyncratic way of walking, and there is no such thing as an average person. However, most of us do walk with reasonable facility and, as will be shown later, with surprising efficiency. A conclusion that seems inescapable is that each of us learns to integrate the numerous variables that nature has bestowed on our individual neuromusculoskeletal systems into a smoothly functioning whole. Obviously, our bipedal plantigrade type of progression imposes gross similarities on our manner of walking. These are easily identified. We must oscillate our legs, and as we do our bodies rise and fall with each step. The movements parallel to the plane of progression are large, and the individual variations in relation to the size of the total angular displacements are relatively small. When these aspects of human walking are considered, the use of average values helps to develop a general understanding of the basic relationships that exist between the major segments of the lower limb. Upon these basic activities are superimposed numerous less obvious movements of individual parts of the body. These small movements occur in planes closer to the coronal and transverse planes of the body, and in these small movements, the individual variations are much greater.

Furthermore, when the locations of axes of movement are determined and ranges of motion measured both in the cadaver and in the living, marked individual differences are disclosed. The differences in these small movements bestow on each of us a distinctive manner of walking. Here, the use of average values can hinder the recognition of certain interrelationships that must exist between the participating joints. This is particularly true when one is trying to understand the functional behavior of the joints of the ankle and foot.

A hypothesis is easily formulated that seems to explain most observations, including the peculiar behavior of the major segments of the body during walking. This hypothesis states that the human body will integrate the motions of the various segments and control the activity of the muscles so that the metabolic energy required for a given distance walked is minimized. In later sections, it will be shown that any interference with normal relationships between various segments of the body invariably increases the metabolic cost of walking.

PROCESS OF WALKING

The term *walking* is nonspecific. Its connotation is that of a cyclic pattern of body movements that are repeated over and over, step after step. Consequently, descriptions of walking customarily deal with what happens in the course of just one cycle, with the assumption that successive cycles are all about the same. Although this assumption is not strictly true, it is a reasonable approximation. Apart from the multiple variations that may occur between different individuals or within the same individual as a result of changes in the speed of walking, or such factors as alterations in footwear, there are certain observable events that are shared by all.

Human walking is a process of locomotion in which the erect, moving body is supported by first one leg and then the other. As the moving body passes over the supporting leg, the other leg swings forward in preparation for its next support phase. One foot or the other is always on the ground, and during that period when the support of the body is transferred from the trailing to the leading leg there is a brief period when both feet are on the ground. As a person walks faster, these periods of double support become smaller fractions of the walking cycle until, eventually, as a person starts to run, they disappear altogether and are replaced by brief periods when neither foot is on the ground. The cyclic alternations of the support function of each leg and the existence of a transfer period when both feet are on the ground are essential features of the locomotion process known as walking.

In the act of walking there are two basic requisites: (1) continuing ground reaction forces that support the body, and (2) periodic movement of each foot from one position of support to the next in the direction of progression. These elements are necessary for any form of bipedal walking no matter how distorted by physical disability. They are equally necessary when prosthetic or orthotic devices are used.

These two basic requisites of walking give rise to specific body motions that are universally observable during walking. As the body passes over the weight-bearing limb, three different deviations occur from uniform progression in a straight line. With each step, the body speeds up and slows down slightly, it rises and falls a few centimeters, and it weaves slightly from side to side. These motions are related to one another in a systematic fashion.

The body must slow down and then speed up again during each step because the support provided by the legs does not remain directly under the body at all times. A supporting foot starts out ahead of the body where it tends to slow the body down, and then it passes under the body and to the rear, where it tends to speed the body up again. This motion is difficult to see, but easy to sense when a person carries a shallow pan of water. It is almost impossible to prevent the water from surging backward and forward as a result of the alternating accelerations and decelerations of the body.

As the body passes over the supporting leg, it rises until the foot is directly underneath and then descends again as the foot passes behind. The highest point in elevation occurs when the speed is lowest, and the lowest point in elevation occurs when the speed is highest.

During the period of single support, the body also tends to shift laterally over the support limb. The pelvis achieves its maximal lateral displacement somewhat after midstance and then starts back toward the other side. The amount of lateral sway increases when the tread width is increased. While individual variations in the measured magnitudes of these motions will always be observed in any group of people, the motions will be present to some degree in everyone. Normally there is symmetry in the movement, and the patterns repeat themselves with each successive cycle.

Although the displacements of the entire body through space may be described as translational, this translation is achieved by the angular displacements of various segments of the body about axes that lie in the proximity of joints. A principal task in describing human locomotion is to measure the angular displacements of the various segments during the translational movement of the body as a whole. Because the translational movements are the final product of the angular displacements of the individual segments, and these are easily discernible and measurable, they may be used as one set of parameters for the description of the walking cycle. However, a description that deals solely with movement and ignores the forces that produce these motions constitutes only a small part of the entire story of human walking.

MAJOR DISPLACEMENTS OF THE BODY DURING WALKING

Synchronous movements of nearly all the major parts of the body occur during walking at moderate speeds. The pelvis lists, rotates, and undulates as it moves forward. The segments of the lower limb show displacements in all three planes of space, while the shoulders rotate and the arms swing out of phase with the displacements of the pelvis and legs. It seems reasonable to begin the description of walking with a discussion of the translation of the body as a whole through space. To do this, the concept of the pathway of the center of mass of the body will be used. The center of mass of any body is a point such that if any plane is passed through it, the mass moments on one side of the plane are equal to the mass moments on the other. If the body is suspended at this center of mass, it will not tend to tip in any direction. During walking, the center of mass of the body, although not remaining in an absolutely fixed position, tends to remain within the pelvis. This is

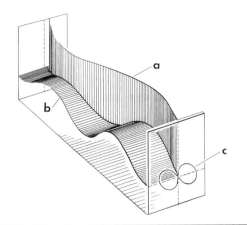

FIGURE 1-1. Displacements of center of mass in three planes of space during single stride (cycle). The actual displacements have been greatly exaggerated. (**A**), Lateral displacement in a horizontal plane; (**B**), vertical displacement. Combined displacements of **A** and **B** as projected onto a plane perpendicular to the plane of progression are shown in **C**.

phase. The center of mass falls to its lowest level during the middle of double weightbearing, when both feet are in contact with the ground. The curve is remarkably smooth and is found to fluctuate evenly between maxima and minima of displacements, with few irregularities. It is interesting to note that at their maximal vertical displacement, the head and the center of mass are slightly lower than when the subject is standing on both feet. In other words, in a smooth walk, a person is slightly shorter than when he is standing, so that if he were to walk through a tunnel the height of which corresponded exactly to his standing height he could do so without fear of bumping his head.

The center of mass of the body is also displaced laterally in the horizontal plane. In this plane, too, it describes a sinusoidal curve, the maximal values of which alternately pass to the right and to the left in association with the support of the weight-bearing limb. The curve is sinusoidal, at one-half the frequency of the vertical displacement.

When viewed from the back, the body is seen to undulate up and down and swing from side to side during each cycle. If the vertical and lateral displacements are considered as pure sine waves, with the frequency of the vertical displacements being precisely twice that of the lateral displacements and the peaks being achieved at the same time, then the curve of displacement of the center of mass, as projected onto a plane at right angles to the line of progression, is in the form of a "U." At higher speeds of walking, this situation is approximated; at lower speeds, however, the peak of the curve for vertical displacement is reached slightly before the peak of lateral displacement. This causes the curve of movement of the center of mass as projected on a coronal plane (a vertical plane at a right angle to the line of progression) to resemble a slightly distorted lazy 8 (Fig. 1-2).

convenient for two reasons. Measurements of the movements of the pelvis in the three planes of space are readily made, and the pelvis becomes a suitable structure to separate the body into upper and lower parts, which behave differently during walking.

In normal level walking, the center of mass describes a smooth sinusoidal curve when projected on the plane of progression (Fig. 1-1). The total amount of vertical displacement in normal adult men is typically about 5 cm at the usual speeds of walking. The summits of these oscillations appear at about the middle of the stance (foot on ground) phase of the supporting limb. The opposite limb is at this time in the middle of its swing (foot off ground)

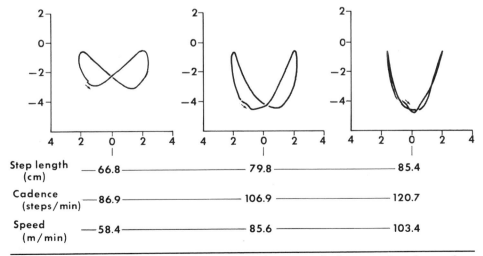

Step length (cm)	66.8	79.8	85.4
Cadence (steps/min)	86.9	106.9	120.7
Speed (m/min)	58.4	85.6	103.4

FIGURE 1-2. Effect of variations in speed on displacement of pelvis as projected onto plane perpendicular to plane of progression (see Fig. 1-1**C**).

For the sake of simplicity, a series of models will be employed to illustrate how the smooth sinusoidal displacement pathway is achieved in bipedal locomotion (5,6). The first model will show the body as consisting solely of a bar representing the pelvis, with the center of mass depicted as a small block lying midway between the two hips (Fig. 1-3). The legs will be represented as rigid levers without foot, ankle, or knee mechanisms, articulated only at the hip joints, which will permit flexion and extension only. Such a system of quasilocomotion would produce something analogous to the process of stepping off distances with a pair of compasses or dividers, the pathway of the center of mass of such a system being a series of intersecting arcs.

The radius of each arc would be equal to the length of the limbs, and with each step, the extent of flexion and extension of the hip joint would be the same. Locomotion of this type might be imitated, but imperfectly, by walking on one's heels with the knees fixed in extension. Such a type of locomotion would require that the center of mass be elevated to a height equal to the height of the center of mass in the standing person; it would also result in a severe jolt at the point of intersection of each two arcs, where there is an abrupt change in the direction of movement of the center of mass. Decreasing the total elevation, depressing the center of mass, and smoothing the series of interrupted arcs require coordinated movements involving all the joints of the lower limb. These individual movements can be considered as elements that contribute to the total process of walking. A qualitative description of the principal elements is presented in the following paragraphs to provide a basis for the quantitative descriptions in later chapters.

Pelvic Rotation

In normal level walking, the pelvis rotates about a vertical axis alternately to the right and to the left, relative to the line of progression. At the customary cadence and stride of typical people, the magnitude of this rotation is approximately 4 degrees on either side of the central axis, or a total of some 8 degrees. This value usually increases markedly when speed is increased. Because the pelvis is a rigid structure, the rotations occur alternately at each hip joint and require a deviation from pure flexion and extension of the hips.

The significance of pelvic rotation can best be appreciated by a study of the theoretical model (Fig. 1-4). The effects of pelvic rotation are to flatten somewhat the arc of the passage of the center of mass in compass gait by elevating the ends of that arc. In consequence, the angles at the intersections of successive arcs are rendered less abrupt and, at the same time, are elevated in relation to the summits. In this way, the severity of the impact at floor contact is reduced. The force required to change the direction of

the center of mass in the succeeding arc of translation is less, and the angular displacement at the hip in flexion and extension is reduced.

Pelvic List

In normal walking, the pelvis lists downward in the coronal plane on the side opposite to that of the weight-bearing limb (positive Trendelenburg). At moderate speeds, the alternate angular displacement is about 5 degrees. The displacement occurs at the hip joint, producing an equivalent relative adduction of the supporting limb and relative abduction of the other limb, which is in the swing phase of the cycle. To permit pelvic list, the knee joint of the non–weight-bearing limb must flex to allow clearance for the swing-through of that member.

The effects of pelvic list on the pathway of the center of mass are evident in the experimental model (Fig. 1-5). As the lateral list occurs while the body is passing over the vertical supporting member in early stance phase, the center of mass is lowered. Thus, the summit of the arc is lowered, further flattening the pathway. In addition and perhaps more importantly, pelvic list contributes to the effectiveness of the abductor mechanism of the hip (the abductor muscles and iliotibial tract). The latter effect will be discussed in greater detail in the section on the phasic action of muscles (see Chapter 6).

Knee Flexion in Stance Phase

A characteristic of walking at moderate and fast speeds is knee flexion of the supporting limb as the body passes over it. This supporting member enters stance phase at heel strike with the knee joint in nearly full extension. Thereafter, the knee joint begins to flex and continues to do so until the foot is flat on the ground. A typical magnitude of this flexion is 15 degrees. Just before the middle of the period of full weight bearing, the knee joint once more passes into extension, which is immediately followed by the terminal flexion of the knee. This begins simultaneously with heel rise, as the limb is carried into swing phase. During this period of stance phase, occupying about 40% of the cycle, the knee is first extended, then flexed, and again extended before its final flexion.

During the beginning and end of the stance phase, knee flexion contributes to smoothing the abrupt changes at the intersections of the arcs of translation of the center of mass (Fig. 1-6).

These three elements of gait—pelvic rotation, pelvic list, and knee flexion during early stance phase, all act in the same direction by flattening the arc through which the center of mass of the body is translated. The first (pelvic rotation) elevates the ends of the arc, and the second and third (pelvic list and knee flexion) depress its summit. The net

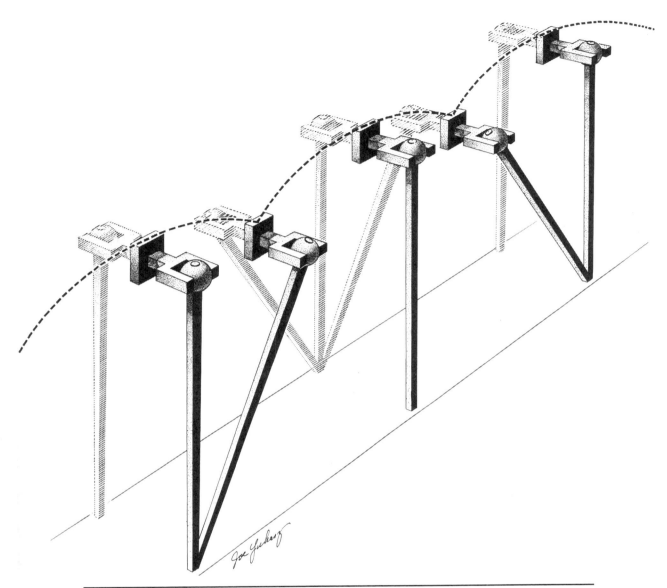

FIGURE 1-3. Simplified model depicting bipedal locomotion. The pelvis is a double-forked bar articulating with spheres depicting the hip joints and carrying a small block that represents the center of mass of the body. The legs are straight members without knee, ankle, or foot components. Note that the pathway of the center of mass is through a series of intersecting arcs. (From Saunders JB, Inman VT, Eberhart HD. The major determinants in normal and pathological gait. *J Bone Joint Surg* 1953; 35–A:543.)

effect is the passage of the center of mass through a segment of a circle, the radius of which is about 2.2 times longer than the length of the lower limb. The effective lengthening of the limbs reduces materially the range of flexion and extension at the hip joint required to maintain the same length of stride.

The three elements so far discussed (pelvic rotation, pelvic list, and knee flexion) act to decrease the magnitude of the vertical displacement of the center of mass of the body. However, if no additional elements were active, the pathway of the center of mass would still consist of a series of arcs, and at their intersections the center of mass would be subject to a sudden change in vertical displacement. This would result in a jarring effect on the body. Thus, an additional mechanism must be active that smooths the pathway of the center of mass by a gradual change in the vertical displacement of the center of mass from a downward to an upward direction, converting what would be a

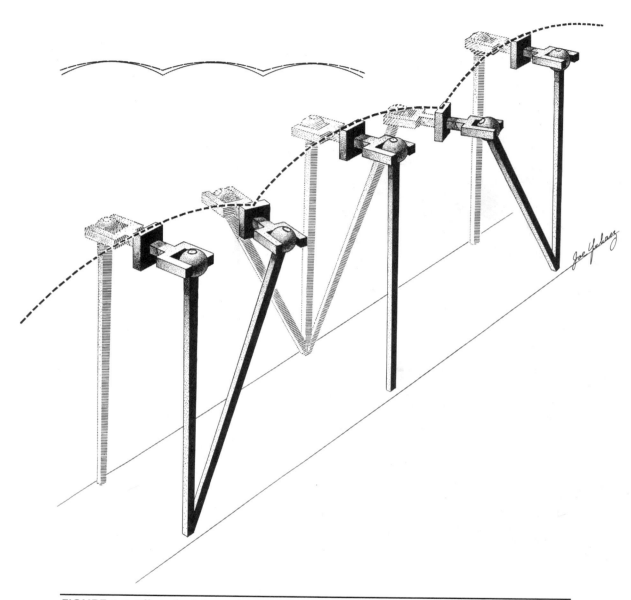

FIGURE 1-4. Effect of pelvic rotation. By permitting the pelvis to rotate in a horizontal plane during locomotion, the center of mass is prevented from falling as far during the phase of double weight bearing as was shown in Figure 1-3. The solid line at the top represents the curve shown Figure 1-3. (Adapted from Saunders JB, Inman VT, Eberhart HD. The major determinants in normal and pathological gait. *J Bone Joint Surg* 1953;35–A:543.)

series of intersecting arcs into a sinusoidal path. This is accomplished by certain movements in the knee, ankle, and foot.

The single most important factor in achieving the conversion of the pathway of the center of mass from a series of intersecting arcs to a smooth curve is the presence of a foot attached to the distal end of the limb. Through its action, the foot enables the pathway of displacement of the knee to remain relatively horizontal during the entire stance phase. This in turn allows the initial knee flexion to act more effectively in smoothing the pathway of the hip. To understand the mechanics involved, a series of simple drawings may be helpful. In Figure 1-7, the actual pathway of the knee joint during stance phase is shown. Except for an initial rise, the pathway is relatively flat. In Figure 1-8, three other situations are shown. If no foot is attached to the shank, the pathway of the knee is an arc whose radius is the distance from the floor to the knee. By simply

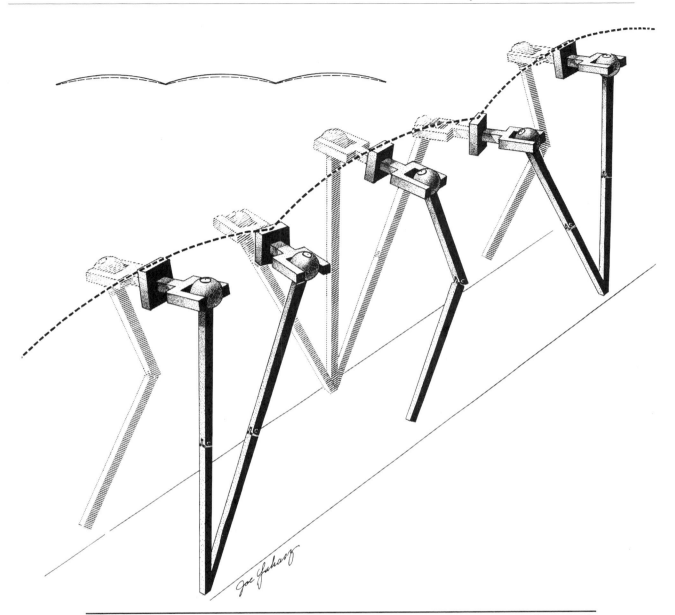

FIGURE 1-5. Effect of pelvic list. Normally the pelvis drops slightly on the non–weight-bearing side during walking (positive Trendelenburg). The result is that the center of mass need not be elevated as much when the body passes over the weight-bearing leg during midstance. Because of the pelvic list, the swinging leg becomes relatively too long to clear the floor during the midswing phase. Flexion of the knee allows for this clearance. The solid line at the top represents the curve shown in Figure 1-4. (Adapted from Saunders JB, Inman VT, Eberhart HD. The major determinants in normal and pathological gait. *J Bone Joint Surg* 1953;35–A:543.)

adding a foot rigidly fixed to the shank (no ankle), the pathway, although it is composed of two arcs, approaches more closely the normal course. Provision of a flail ankle results in a pattern resembling the pathway of the knee without any foot. Provision of a normal ankle, however (Fig. 1-9), with proper phasing of the extensor and flexor muscles and only a minor amount of motion occurring in the ankle

joint, results in achievement of the normal pathway of the knee joint.

At the time of heel strike, the center of mass of the body is falling. This downward movement is decelerated by slight flexion of the knee against the resistance of the quadriceps. After heel strike, the foot is plantar flexed against the resisting tibialis anterior muscle. This plantar

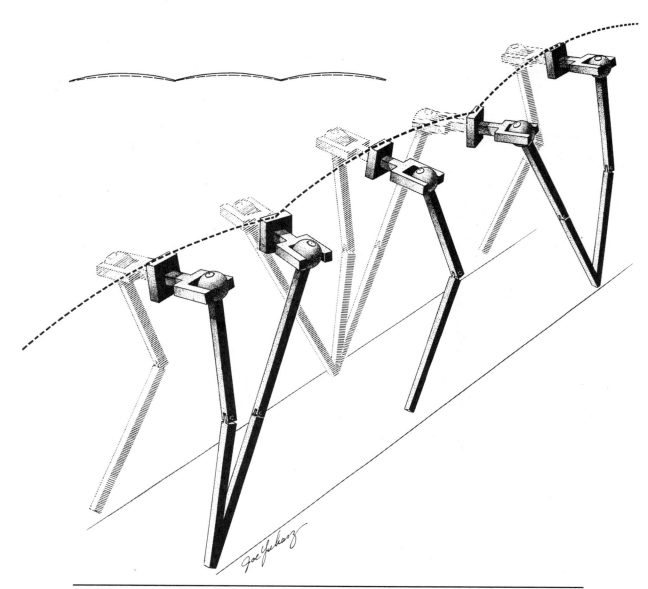

FIGURE 1-6. Knee flexion during stance. Except at very low speeds of walking, the knee undergoes approximately 15 degrees of flexion immediately after heel strike and continues to remain flexed until the center of mass has passed over the weight-bearing leg. The effect of this knee flexion is twofold. Initially, it absorbs part of the impact of the body at heel strike and later it decreases the amount that the center of mass must be elevated as it passes over the weight-bearing leg. The solid line at the top represents the curve shown in Figure 1-5. (Adapted from Saunders JB, Inman VT, Eberhart HD. The major determinants in normal and pathological gait. *J Bone Joint Surg* 1953;35–A:543.)

flexion of the foot occurs about a point where the heel contacts the floor. Rotation about this point causes the leg to undergo relative shortening and the ankle to be carried slightly forward in the direction of progression until the foot is flat. Contraction of the quadriceps acting on the knee and the tibialis anterior muscle on the foot causes these movements to be slowed, and the downward motion of the center of mass of the body is smoothly decelerated. In addition, as the foot receives the weight of the body dur-

ing midstance, it pronates to a varying degree. Although this pronation contributes only a few millimeters to the further relative shortening of the leg, the elastic components in the plantar region of the foot assist in absorbing the shock of impact.

The center of mass begins its upward movement immediately after it has passed in front of the weightbearing foot, as the forward momentum of the body carries the body up and over the weight-bearing leg. After the center

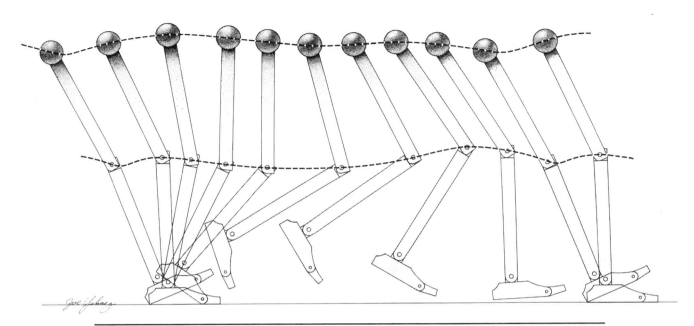

FIGURE 1-7. Pathway of knee in walking at moderate speed. Note that there is a slight elevation immediately after heel strike, but for the remainder of stance phase the pathway is relatively straight and shows only a slight declination from the horizontal. (Reproduced from Saunders JB, Inman VT, Eberhart HD. The major determinants in normal and pathological gait. *J Bone Joint Surg* 1953;35–A:543.)

of mass has passed over and in front of the foot, its immediate fall is delayed by relative elongation of the weight-bearing leg through extension of the knee, plantar flexion at the ankle, and supination of the foot. All these elements acting in proper relationships lead to the smoothing of the passage of the center of mass into an approximately sinusoidal pathway (Figs. 1-10, 1-11, and 1-12).

Lateral Displacement of Body

As mentioned previously, the body is shifted slightly over the weight-bearing leg with each step; there is a total lateral displacement of the body from side to side of approximately 4 to 5 cm with each complete stride. This lateral displacement can be increased by walking with the feet

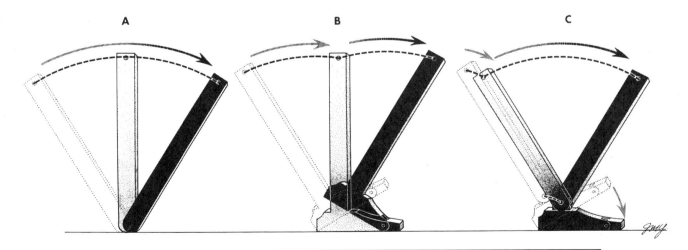

FIGURE 1-8. Effect of foot on pathway of knee. (**A**) Arch described when there is no foot. (**B**) Effect of foot without ankle. Note that the pathway now comprises two intersecting arcs. However, it does not fall abruptly at the end of stance and begins to resemble the normal pathway. (**C**) Effect of foot and flail ankle. (Reproduced from Saunders JB, Inman VT, Eberhart HD. The major determinants in normal and pathological gait. *J Bone Joint Surg* 1953;35–A:543.)

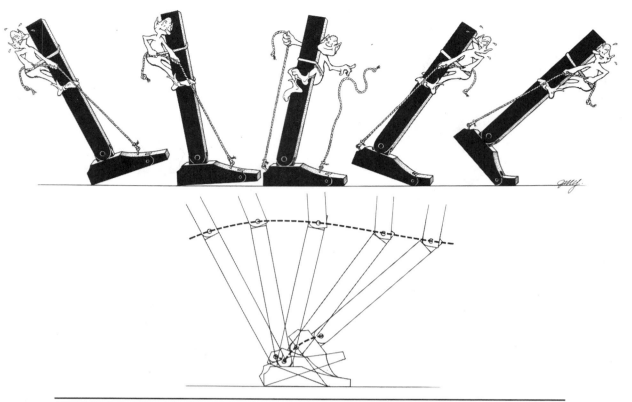

FIGURE 1-9. Effect of ankle motion, controlled by muscle action, on pathway of knee. The smooth and flattened pathway of the knee during stance phase is achieved by forces acting from the leg on the foot. Foot slap is restrained during initial lowering of the foot; afterward, the plantar flexors raise the heel.

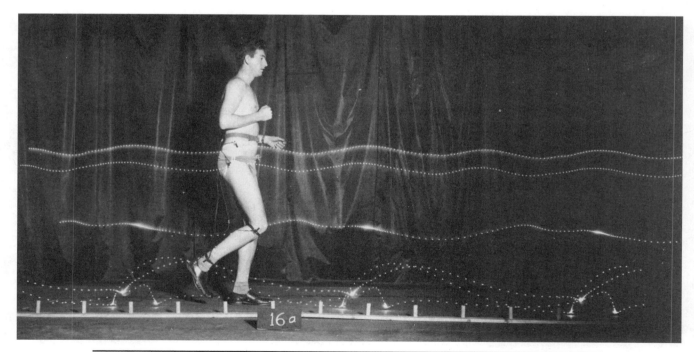

FIGURE 1-10. Interrupted light studies. The photograph was obtained by having a subject walk in front of the open lens of a camera while carrying small light bulbs located at the hip, knee, ankle, and foot. A slotted disc was rotated in front of the camera producing a series of white dots at equal time intervals. Note that the curve of displacement at the hip is a smooth curve but is not sinusoidal. This is due to the differences in phase of the two legs. (From Eberhard HD, Inman VT. An evaluation of experimental procedures used in a fundamental study of human locomotion. *Ann N Y Acad Sci* 1951;51:1213.)

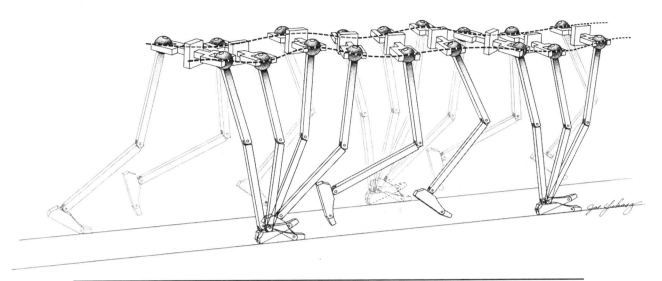

FIGURE 1-11. Vertical displacements of hip joints. Although the pathways of the hip joints are smooth curves, they are not sinusoidal and they are 180° out of phase. (From Saunders JB, Inman VT, Eberhart HD. The major determinants in normal and pathological gait. *J Bone Joint Surg* 1953;35–A:543.)

more widely separated (Fig. 1-13) and decreased by keeping the feet close to the plane of progression (Fig. 1-14). Normally, the presence of the tibiofemoral angle (slight genu valgum) permits the tibia to remain essentially vertical and the feet close together, while the femurs diverge to articulate with the pelvis.

Rotations in Transverse Plane

Reference has already been made to the transverse rotations of the pelvis that occur during walking. These rotations are easily seen when attention is called to them. There are also other transverse rotations, involving the parts of the body above and below the pelvis that merit attention.

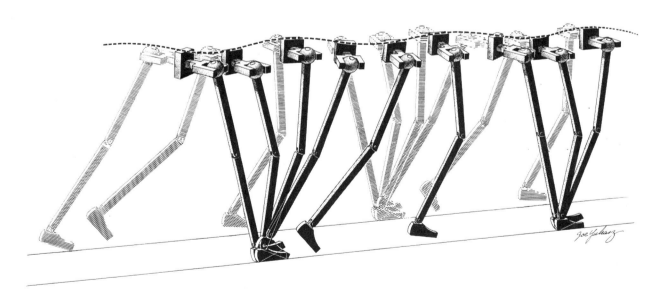

FIGURE 1-12. Sinusoidal pathway of center of mass. The center of mass, which lies between the hip joints, is equally affected by the displacements of each hip. The combined effect is a sinusoidal curve of low amplitude. (From Saunders JB, Inman VT, Eberhart HD. The major determinants in normal and pathological gait. *J Bone Joint Surg* 1953;35–A:543.)

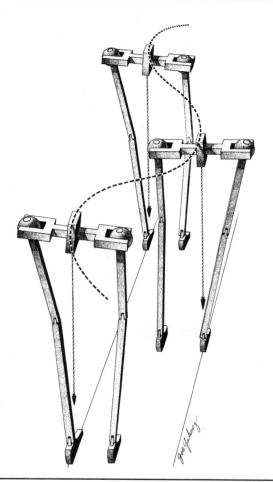

FIGURE 1-13. Lateral displacement of center of mass. During each step, the body is displaced over the weight-bearing leg. With a wide walking base (stride width) the amplitude is large. (From Saunders JB, Inman VT, Eberhart HD. The major determinants in normal and pathological gait. *J Bone Joint Surg* 1953;35–A:543.)

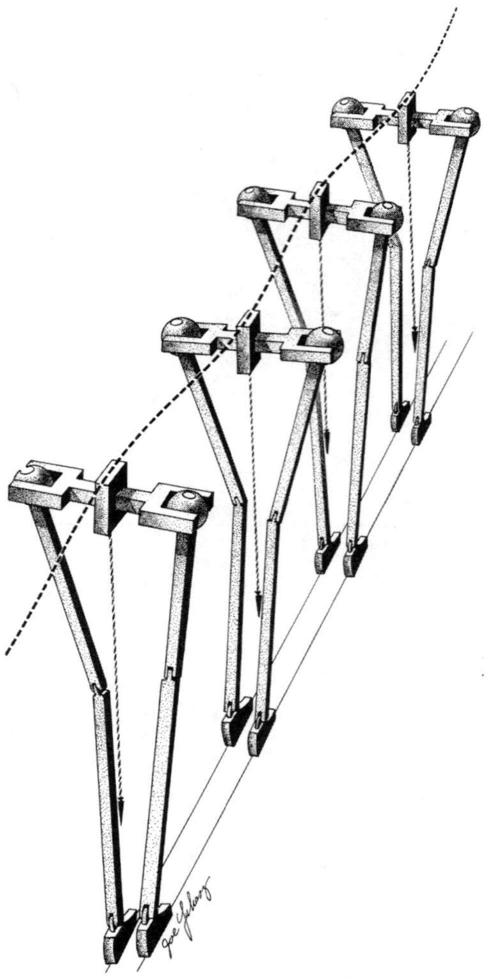

FIGURE 1-14. Effect of narrow walking base. By providing the model with a degree of genu valgum, the walking base is narrowed and the amplitude of lateral displacement is decreased while the shank remains vertical. (From Saunders JB, Inman VT, Eberhart HD. The major determinants in normal and pathological gait. *J Bone Joint Surg* 1953;35–A:543.)

Rotations of Thorax and Shoulders

That the thorax and shoulders rotate during walking is easily seen. Interestingly, at moderate speeds of walking, these rotations are approximately 180° out of phase with the pelvic rotation. The rotation of the shoulders produces arm swing, and even the casual observer recognizes that the forward swing of one leg is accompanied by a forward swing of the arm on the opposite side. This opposite rotation of the pelvis as compared with the shoulders appears to provide a balancing effect that smooths the forward progression of the body as a whole. Its suppression leads to inability to progress in a straight line at higher speeds of walking and, as will be shown, to increased energy expenditure through greater muscular effort.

Rotations of Thigh and Leg (Shank)

Less obvious but still considerable are the transverse rotations of the thigh and shank (4). In contrast to the shoulders, the rotations of the thigh and shank are in phase with the pelvic rotation. The interesting fact is that their rotatory displacements increase progressively from pelvis to thigh to shank. Thus, the shank on the average rotates approximately 3 times as much in a transverse plane as does the pelvis. These rotations, however, show marked differences and constitute one of the factors that provide distinctive characteristics to each individual's appearance when walking.

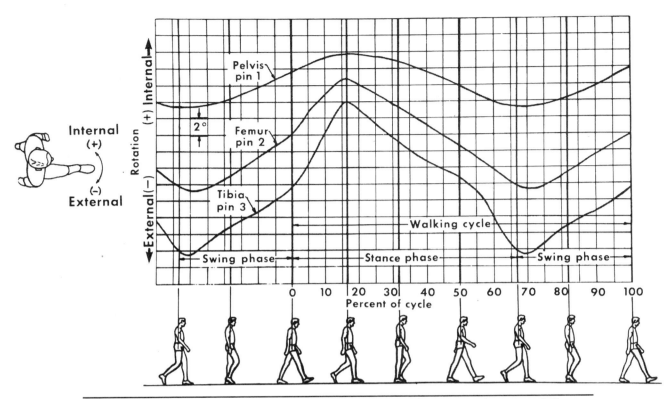

FIGURE 1-15. Rotations of pelvis, femur, and tibia in transverse plane: composite curves of 19 young male adults. (Adapted from Levens AS, Inman VT, Blosser JA. Transverse rotation of the segments of the lower extremity in locomotion. *J Bone Joint Surg* 1948;30–A:859.)

In general, the pelvis, thigh, and leg begin to rotate internally toward the weight-bearing leg at the beginning of its swing phase. This rotation is continued during the double weight-bearing phase and into midstance. At midstance, there is an abrupt change, and the leg begins to rotate externally and continues to do so until the beginning of its next swing phase (Fig. 1-15).

Rotations in the Ankle and Foot

During the swing phase of walking, the segments of the lower limb (including the foot) are free in space and can rotate internally without restriction (Fig. 1-16A). During the stance phase, the foot is on the floor and external rotation of the leg occurs because mechanisms exist in the ankle and foot that permit the leg to rotate externally while the foot remains stationary. If such mechanisms did not exist, the foot would have to slip as shown in Figure 1-16B.

There is an interesting interrelationship between the ankle and the hindfoot. Both the ankle and subtalar joints are capable to varying degrees of absorbing the transverse rotations of the shank during the stance phase of walking.

The axis of the ankle joint has been found to vary in obliquity in the coronal plane from 2 degrees to 23 degrees (3). The ability of the ankle to participate in the absorption of the rotations of the shank depends on the obliquity of the ankle axis and the range of flexion and extension used. The effect of an oblique axis on the foot during the swing phase and on the shank during the stance phase is clearly shown in Figures 1-17 and 1-18. During the swing phase, with the foot free, the foot toes outward on dorsiflexion and inward on plantar flexion (Fig. 1-17). During stance, with the foot fixed to the floor, relative dorsiflexion produces internal rotation of the shank, and relative plantar flexion causes external rotation of the shank (Fig. 1-18). Therefore, the ankle joint, in proportion to the obliquity of its axis and the amount of dorsiflexion, may participate in the absorption of the transverse rotations of the shank during the stance phase.

However, the structure that is principally involved is the subtalar joint. Its ability to permit transverse rotation of the leg without slippage of the foot on the ground is clearly shown in the following figures. The subtalar joint is a single-axis joint whose axis is inclined approximately 45 degrees to the foot (horizontal) and shank (vertical) in the standing position. It functions essentially as a mitered

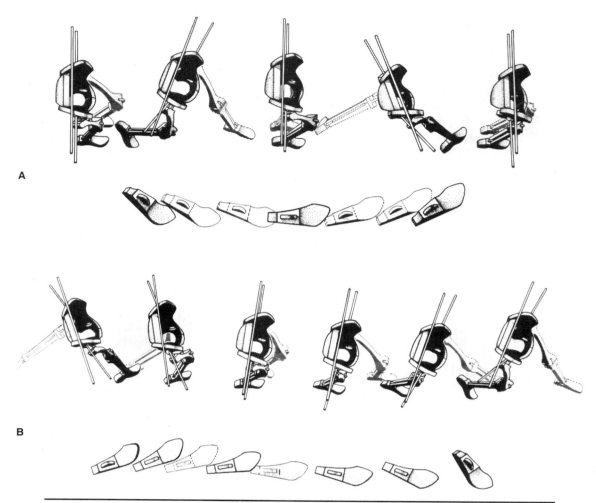

FIGURE 1-16. Transverse rotations of pelvis, leg, and foot. A model of the pelvis and lower limb is viewed from above. Small sticks have been attached to the pelvis and femurs to reveal more clearly that the leg rotates through a greater range than the pelvis. The transverse rotations are readily seen. The actual angular displacements have been exaggerated approximately threefold for emphasis. Note that in (**A**) the swinging leg is free to rotate internally from toe-off to heel strike. In (**B**) the leg is in stance phase and must rotate externally through the same amount. On a slippery surface, the foot would have to slip as shown in the figure.

hinge; the basic mechanism is shown in Figures 1-19 and 1-20. In the living, the relationship between internal and external rotation of the leg and pronation and supination of the foot may be easily demonstrated by affixing targets on the leg and midfoot (Fig. 1-21). The interaction between the ankle and subtalar joints during a single stride in a young adult male is shown in Figure 1-22.

The changing of the foot from a mobile structure during the first part of the stance phase into a rigid lever at push-off is a complicated and not completely understood mechanism. That such a mechanism exists is readily demonstrated in a normal foot. If the forefoot is grasped by the examiner and firmly held, as would occur if the forefoot were supporting the body weight on the walking surface, eversion of the heel produces what is in essence a pronated foot (Fig. 1-23). In this situation, two interesting observations may be made. The degree of plantar flexion and dorsiflexion that is possible in the midfoot is maximal. The amount of dorsiflexion appears to be limited by the plantar aponeurosis, which becomes taut when the forefoot is forcibly dorsiflexed against the everted heel. With the foot in this position, dorsiflexion of the great toe produces additional tension on the plantar aponeurosis, and the arch rises (Hicks' windlass action) (2). Support of the longitudinal arch in the pronated foot seems to depend predominantly on the plantar fasciae and the aponeurosis. If the heel is inverted while the forefoot is fixed, the longitudinal arch is seen to rise, the plantar aponeurosis

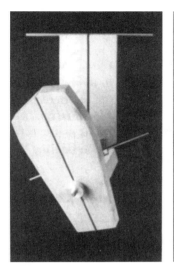
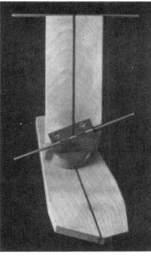

FIGURE 1-17. Simple wooden model of shank and foot with hinge representing ankle joint. The axis has been inclined 25 degrees to the floor. The shank is fixed and the foot is free to move. Note that on dorsiflexion, the foot toes outward and on plantar flexion toes inward. (From Inman VT. *The Joints of the Ankle.* Baltimore: Williams & Wilkins, 1976.)

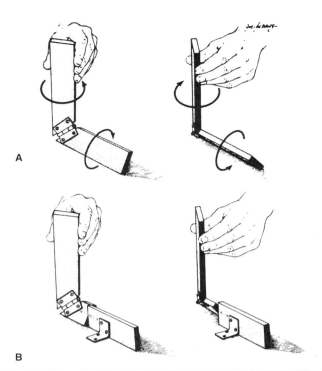

FIGURE 1-19. Action of subtalar joint. Two pieces of wood have been connected by a hinge whose axis is positioned between the vertical member (shank) and the horizontal member (foot) at 45 degrees. Note that in **A,** internal and external rotation of the shank around a vertical axis causes the foot to rotate around a horizontal axis. In **B,** a pivot joint has been inserted in the foot to represent the transverse tarsal joint, thus permitting the forefoot to remain in a fixed position. (From Inman VT, Mann RA. Biomechanics of the foot and ankle. In: Mann RA, ed. DuVries' *Surgery of the Foot,* 4th ed. St. Louis: The C. V. Mosby Co., 1978.)

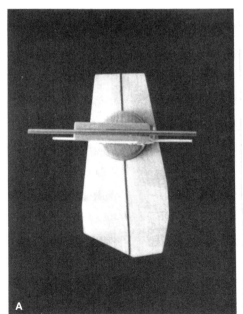
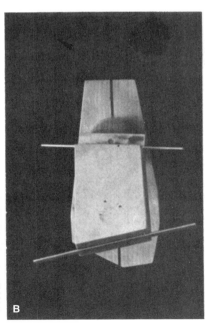
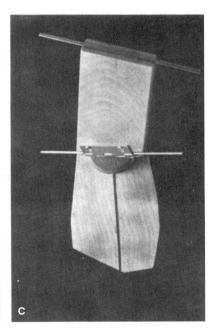

FIGURE 1-18. Same model as in Figure 1-17. The foot is fixed and the shank is moved from its neutral position (**A**) to a position of relative dorsiflexion (**B**). Note that internal rotation of the shank has occurred. In **C,** the shank has been moved to a position of relative plantar flexion in relation to the foot. Note that the shank has rotated externally. (From Inman VT. *The Joints of the Ankle.* Baltimore: Williams & Wilkins, 1976.)

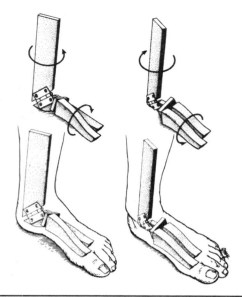

FIGURE 1-20. Action of subtalar joint, represented as hinge located at angle of 45 degrees to shank and foot. The forefoot has been divided into two segments. The medial segment represents the three medial rays articulating with the hindfoot through the talonavicular joint. The lateral segment represents the two lateral rays articulating with the hindfoot through the calcaneocuboid joint. Note that rotation of the shank is accompanied by supination and pronation of the foot. (From Inman VT, Mann RA. *DuVries' Surgery of the Foot*. St Louis: Mosby, 1978.)

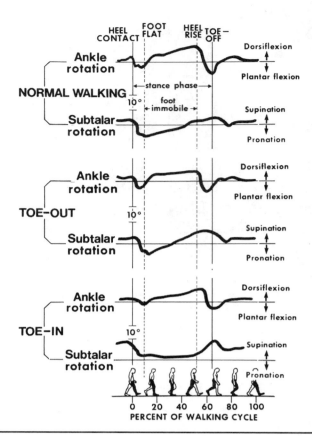

FIGURE 1-22. Synchronous motion in ankle and subtalar joints. Note that variations in the degree of toe-out and toe-in cause variations in the magnitude, phasic action, and angular movements of both ankle and subtalar joints. (From Wright DB, Desai SM, Henderson WH. Action of the subtalar and ankle-joint complex during the stance phase of walking. *Bone Joint Surg* 46–A:361, 1964.)

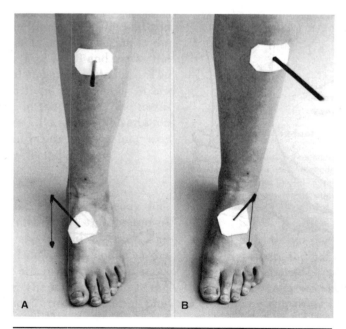

FIGURE 1-21. Rotation of leg accompanied by pronation and supination of foot. (**A**) Internal rotation of leg causing foot to pronate. (**B**) External rotation of leg causing foot to supinate. (From Inman VT. *The Joints of the Ankle*. Baltimore: Williams & Wilkins, 1976.)

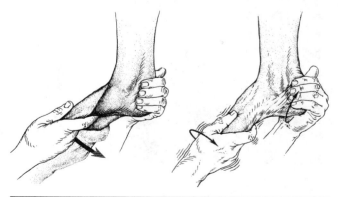

FIGURE 1-23. Change from mobile to rigid foot. With heel everted, maximal midfoot motion is permitted; with heel inverted and forefoot fixed, the foot becomes rigid.

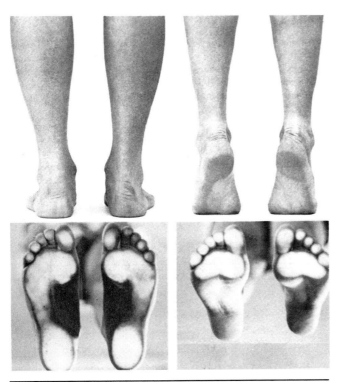

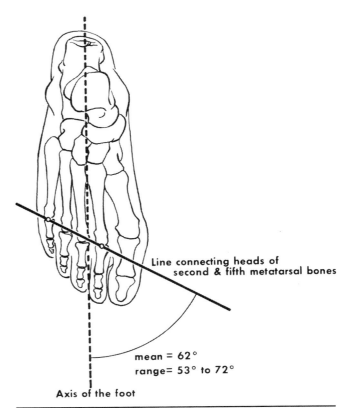

FIGURE 1-24. Rising on toes. Note that as the body weight is transferred to the forefoot, the heels invert, the legs rotate externally, and the longitudinal arches rise. The barograph records the distribution of weight (*white areas*) between all the metatarsal heads and the toes. (From Inman VT, Mann RA. *DuVries' Surgery of the Foot*. St. Louis: The C.V. Mosby Co., 1978.)

FIGURE 1-26. Angle of metatarsal heads: the angle between the long axis of the foot and a line connecting the heads of the second and fifth metatarsals, measured in 100 randomly selected x-rays. (Data from Moskowitz PS. Anthropometric studies of the human metatarsus as seen on x-ray. I. Normal feet. [Thesis]. Unpublished, 1967.)

becomes lax, and the Hicks' windlass action is suppressed. However, something occurs in the transverse tarsal articulations that results in a rigid foot. No fully adequate explanation for this phenomenon has been published, and a review of the literature reveals that only a few studies have been undertaken (1).

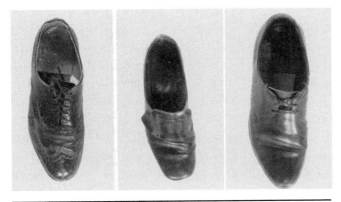

FIGURE 1-25. Crease between cap and vamp in well-worn shoes.

Inversion of the heel occurs when a standing person transfers the body weight from the heel to the forefoot and rises onto the metatarsal heads and toes (Fig. 1-24). This results in an attempt to supinate the foot, with raising of the longitudinal arch on the medial side and depressing of the arch on the lateral side. With this movement, the body weight is shifted to the lateral side of the foot. Fortunately, the presence of shorter metatarsals on the lateral side of the foot permits this supination to occur and results in the lateral metatarsals and toes participating to a greater degree in bearing the body weight.

To distribute the weight between all metatarsal heads, the foot must deviate laterally at push-off. That this occurs normally in walking is confirmed by the inspection of any well-worn shoe. A crease in the leather is evident in the region of the juncture of the cap and vamp of the shoe. This crease is always oblique to the longitudinal axis of the shoe (Fig. 1-25) and marks the position of the metatarsophalangeal articulations. The crease shows individual variations in obliquity in accordance with the variations in the angle of the metatarsophalangeal break. Figure 1-26 shows the variation in the angle of the metatarsal heads and the long axis of the foot in 100 randomly selected x-rays.

REFERENCES

1. Elftman H. The transverse tarsal joint and its control. *Clin Orthop* 1960;16:41.
2. Hicks JH. The mechanics of the foot. II. The plantar aponeurosis and the arch. *J Anat* 1954;88:25.
3. Inman VT. *The Joints of the Ankle*. Baltimore: Williams & Wilkins, 1976:29–44.
4. Levens AS, Inman VT, Blosser JA. Transverse rotation of the segments of the lower extremity in locomotion. *J Bone Joint Surg* 1948;30–A:859.
5. Saunders JB, Inman VT, Eberhart HD. The major determinants in normal and pathological gait. *J Bone Joint Surg* 1953;35–A:543.
6. Inman VT. Special Article: Human locomotion. *Can Med Assoc J* 1966;94:1047–1054.

Commentary on the Six Determinants of Gait

Dudley S. Childress and Steven A. Gard

The original material by Inman, Ralston and Todd in Chapter 1 is an overall perspective of walking, providing a three-dimensional qualitative description of major angular displacements of the body during gait. The determinants that are described originate from two early papers associated with Inman, "Major Determinants in Normal and Pathological Gait" (1) and "Human Locomotion" (2). The 1953 paper "Major Determinants in Normal and Pathological Gait" is considered to be a landmark document in the human gait field. The two papers, along with Chapter 1 (3), are widely known and frequently referenced. For example, the determinants are discussed extensively in *Muscles, Reflexes, and Locomotion* (4) where McMahon presents them as useful because of their simplicity and completeness. Whittle (5) suggests that the six determinants of gait combine together so that the trajectory of the COM is smooth and has a reasonably large radius of curvature, thereby reducing energy expenditure (according to Inman). In the third edition of his book, Whittle (6) acknowledges that the determinants may be questioned. Perry (7) mentions the six determinants only briefly.

The concept of the six determinants of gait was an original idea that has been appealing to clinicians, investigators and educators. Part of the broad general appeal may have been the beautifully rendered drawings associated with the early papers and with the book *Human Walking*. Inman and his colleagues are to be commended for proposing an innovative and forward-thinking theory and for illustrating the concepts so well graphically. Unfortunately, no empirical data supporting the theory were presented in the original paper, nor were the determinants ever objectively tested or evaluated. The accuracy of stance phase knee flexion in some of the attractive walking illustrations can be questioned. Anyway, at least in the United States, the six determinants of gait became pervasive in clinical, research, and educational fields involved with gait. The six determinants have been taught to prosthetists, orthotists, physical therapists, medical students, kinesiologists, and other persons involved in analysis and study of human walking. Bowker (8) in the *Atlas of Limb Prosthetics* illustrates how the determinants have been explained for educational purposes through the years.

The basic concept proposed was that the first three determinants—pelvic rotation [first], pelvic list [second] and knee flexion in stance phase [third]—all presumably act to flatten the trajectory of the body center of mass (BCOM) and thereby reduce the vertical translation of the body during able-bodied walking. The thought behind this concept was that energy is saved if the vertical translation is reduced by each determinant. The fourth and fifth determinants—foot mechanism [fourth] and ankle mechanism [fifth]—were claimed to smooth the trajectory of the BCOM, particularly where the trajectories of each step intersect. The sixth determinant is basically the lateral displacement of the BCOM, which typically needs to be kept narrow for good ambulation. It should be noted that some authors (4,5,6) describe the action of the six determinants in slightly different ways than Inman does (1,3).

Because of increased understanding of normal walking, a number of investigators are convinced that several of the original six determinants of gait probably serve functions other than those originally claimed. The purpose of the six determinants of gait has been called into question by several studies that have critically evaluated their effect in normal walking (9–11). Pelvic rotation, the first determinant, may be used to increase step length, especially at faster walking speeds, but it reportedly has little effect on the vertical displacement of the body's center of mass (12). Similarly, pelvic obliquity and stance-phase knee flexion, the second and third determinants of gait, respectively, appear to have virtually no effect on the vertical excursion of the body during able-bodied walking (9,10). These results have been supported by an investigation of Quesada and Rash (13). Inman's own data (2) shows one reason why this is true: pelvic list and stance-phase knee flexion both occur at the wrong time to have much influence in flattening the trajectory of the BCOM.

Vertical motion of the body's center of mass appears to be reduced by foot and ankle rocker mechanisms (14), which serve to effectively lengthen the leg, and not by the first three determinants as claimed. Inman et al. (3) observed that during single support the body appears to move along the arc of a circle that has a radius about 2.2 times longer than the length of the leg. Furthermore, they allude to the important role of foot and ankle rocker mechanisms and their effect on flattening the trajectory of the knee joint center.

ALTERNATIVE MODELS

Perry (7) has detailed the foot/ankle mechanisms, suggesting that the three foot rocker mechanisms—heel, ankle, and forefoot—can facilitate forward progression. It is believed that these three foot rocker mechanisms are integrated during walking to create a single, smooth "roll-over shape" for the foot/ankle system that facilitates progression of the center of pressure (COP) distally along the plantar surface of the foot; this effectively lengthens the leg and flattens the trajectory of the body center of mass (14). Using a rocker-based inverted pendulum model (Figure 1A-1), the vertical displacement of the body can be accounted for by the geometrical constraints imposed by the legs and the roll-over shape of the foot (Figure 1A-2). The flatter trajectory of the BCOM is actually a section of a prolate cycloid brought about by the circular rocker and the attached mass. The results (14) show that the effective leg length is approximately 1.5 to 1.8 times as long as the actual leg length, compared with the 2.2 value of Inman (3). Inman was one of the first investigators to suggest the concept of effective leg length or virtual leg length.

Hansen et al. (15) have shown that the human foot/ankle provides a roll-over shape that is approximately circular with a radius of about one-third of the anatomical leg length. They have further shown that the roll-over shape of the physiologic foot-ankle tends to be relatively invariant to changes in walking speed, heel height, and added weight.

The model of Figure 1A-2 is only an approximation of reality (e.g. the legs are completely straight, the BCOM location is fixed, etc.). Nevertheless, it turns out to be predic-

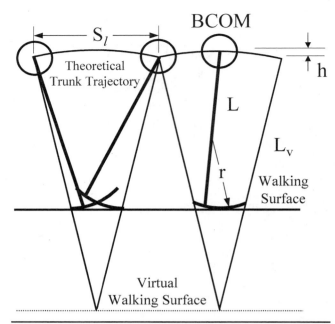

FIGURE 1A-2 In a rocker-based inverted pendulum model, the foot rocker (with radius r) effectively lengthens the anatomical leg (L) to create an effective leg length (L_v) that flattens the vertical displacement of the body (h) for a given step length (S_l).

tive over typical walking speeds, provides some results in closed mathematical form, yet is simple enough to be held together for thinking purposes. For example, it predicts that the vertical movement "h" is inversely proportional to the virtual leg length and proportional to the step length squared (14). It can also be shown that to an approximation, "h" is linearly related to the speed of walking.

The heel-rise characteristic observed by Kerrigan et al. (16) can be accounted for using the model of Figure 1A-2 (see the position of the heel near toe-off). The model suggests that heel rise is a natural consequence of the geometry of the system and not causal. It is conjectured that differences between the general results of Croce et al. (11) and those of Gard and Childress (14) may be more related to differences in language usage and interpretations than to differences in fact.

CONCLUSIONS

Data suggest that the first three determinants do not reduce the vertical displacement of the BCOM during able-bodied gait. The second and third determinants appear to provide shock absorption. The shock absorption determinants (second and third) seem likely to smooth the discontinuities associated with heel contact (create sinusoidal trajectories). The fourth and fifth determinants are associated with the foot and ankle complex, which is believed to create a nearly circular rocker to assist with forward progression and to create a BCOM trajectory that is a section of a prolate cycloid (the BCOM is outside the circle

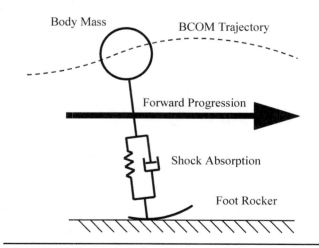

FIGURE 1A-1 Conceptual walking model that incorporates several of the functional aspects of able-bodied gait.

of rotation of the rocker). The prolate cycloid trajectories appear to provide most of the observed flattening of the trajectories, rather than the first three determinants.

It should be noted that the mechanisms of healthy human walking never try to make the trajectory of the BCOM a straight line parallel to the walking surface in the direction of progression. Humans do not roll like a ball. The human walking structure is somewhat similar to an inverted pendulum, and walking is often described as falling from one foot and leg and being caught by the opposite foot and leg. Going up and down is not necessarily inefficient for a walker if the motion can be utilized for storing and returning mechanical energy. As an example, it has been suggested (17) that walking is somewhat similar to a hard boiled egg rolling end over end on a rigid surface. The center of mass of the egg goes up and down as the egg rolls but energy loss is quite small (theoretically zero). The energy is exchanged between kinetic and potential forms.

There is a scientific aphorism that says, "It had been seen many times before but never observed." Over the years since the paper of Saunders et al. (1) the six determinants have been seen often but never closely observed. It appears that close observation of the six determinants over the last decade has been productive and that further study and reconciliation may continue to produce surprising findings.

REFERENCES FOR COMMENTARY

1. Saunders JB, Inman VT, Eberhart HD. The Major Determinants in Normal and Pathological Gait. *JBJS* 1953;35-A(3):543–58.
2. Inman VT. Special Article: Human Locomotion. *Can Med Assoc J* 1966;94:1047–54.
3. Inman, VT, Ralston, HJ, Todd, F. *Human Walking*. Williams and Wilkins, 1st edition, p. 6–14, 1981.
4. McMahon, TA. *Muscles, Reflexes, and Locomotion*. Princeton University Press, p. 192–198, 1984.
5. Whittle, MW. *Gait Analysis: An Introduction*. 1st edition, Butterworth Heinemann, p. 74–77, 1991.
6. Whittle, MW. *Gait Analysis: An Introduction*, 3rd edition, Butterworth Heinemann, p. 77–81, 2002.
7. Perry, J. *Gait Analysis: Normal and Pathological Function*. Thorofare N.J.: SLACK Inc., p. 40–42, 1992.
8. Bowker JH. Kinesiology and Functional Characteristics of the Lower Limb. Chapter 18. In: American Academy of Orthopaedic Surgeons, editors. *The Atlas of Limb Prosthetics: Surgical and Prosthetic Principles*. St. Louis: C.V. Mosby Company, 1981; 261–71.
9. Gard SA, Childress DS. The Effect of Pelvic List on the Vertical Displacement of the Trunk During Normal Walking. *Gait Posture*. 1997;5:233–8.
10. Gard SA, Childress DS. The Influence of Stance-Phase Knee Flexion on the Vertical Displacement of the Trunk During Normal Walking. *Arch Phys Med Rehabil*. 1999;80(1):26–32.
11. Croce UD, Riley PO, Lelas JL, Kerrigan DC. A Refined View of the Determinants of Gait. *Gait Posture* 2001;14(2):79–84.
12. Kerrigan DC, Riley PO, Lelas JL, Croce UD. Quantification of Pelvic Rotation as a Determinant of Gait. *Arch Phys Med Rehabil* 2001;82:217–20.
13. Quesada, PM, Rash GS. Simulation of Walking Without Stance Phase Knee Flexion. *Gait and Posture* 1998;7(2):151, 152. [Abstracts of the 3rd Annual North American Society of Gait and Clinical Movement Analysis].
14. Gard SA, Childress DS. What Determines the Vertical Displacement of the Body During Normal Walking? *J Prosthet Orthot.* 2001;13(3):64–67.
15. Hansen AH, Childress DS, Knox E. Roll-over Shapes of Human Locomotor Systems: Effects of Walking Speed. *Clinical Biomechanics* 2004;19(4):407–414.
16. Kerrigan D, Croce, UD, Marciello M., Riley PO. A Refined View of the Determinants of Gait: Significance of Heel Rise. *Arch Phys Med Rehabil* 2000;81:1077–1080.
17. Margaria, R. *Biomechanics and Energetics of Muscular Exercise*, Oxford University Press, Chapter 3, "Biomechanics of human locomotion", p. 86, 1976.

Chapter 2

The Evolution of Human Walking

Timothy D. Weaver and Richard G. Klein

The other chapters in this volume focus on how the human musculoskeletal system is integrated to produce human walking, which we will refer to as human bipedalism. Our focus in this chapter is similar, except that we proceed from an evolutionary perspective, building on the fossil evidence for bipedalism, which spans more than 4 million years. Because the evolution of bipedalism cannot be understood in isolation, we examine its place within the broader sweep of human evolution, and we consider some of the theory behind the behavioral reconstructions we make from fossils. Our goal is to summarize both what we think occurred in human evolution and why we think so.

Bipedalism intrigues paleoanthropologists (that is, specialists in human evolution) not simply for the anatomy that allows it, but also because it appears to be the characteristic that first distinguished humans from apes. Long before there was a significant fossil record, Charles Darwin and his key ally, Thomas Huxley, proposed that humans originated in Africa, because it was home to our closest living relatives, the chimpanzees and the gorilla. The degree of genetic difference between humans and the African apes suggests that they last shared a common ancestor between 8 and 5 million years ago, and the oldest known human fossils now amply confirm Darwin's and Huxley's prescience that this ancestor lived in Africa. The fossil record before 5 million years ago is too meager to clearly illuminate the split, but abundant human fossils that date from slightly before 4 million years ago and later confirm it. The fossils reveal a variety of human (that is, bipedal) species that all appear to share a recent common ancestor (Fig. 2-1). Thus far, there is no basis for assuming that the bipedal adaptation arose more than once, although prudence demands that we leave the possibility open, pending the accumulation of many more fossils from before 4 million years ago.

The central place of bipedalism in human origins has not always been apparent (79). When the fossil evidence was much more poorly known, some specialists believed that bipedalism evolved concurrently with other human novelties, such as brains that are large both absolutely and relative to body mass, small canine teeth that do not differ substantially in size between the sexes, extended childhoods, long life-spans, and an advanced capacity for culture. Other authorities suggested that brain expansion came first and that it was then the catalyst for other distinctive traits, including bipedalism. However, fossil discoveries that are made almost yearly in Africa now abundantly demonstrate the temporal primacy of bipedalism. The earliest well-known bipedal ancestors of 4 to 3 million years ago retained small, apelike brains and many other apelike characteristics of the head and upper body (46,85). The spotty fossil record from before 4 million years ago implies that yet earlier humans were even more apelike (12,26–28,40,50,66,83). In short, the fossil record demonstrates conclusively that bipedalism evolved millions of years before large brains and other human specializations.

The credit for discovering that the first bipedal species was otherwise apelike belongs to Raymond Dart, an anatomist at the University of the Witwatersrand Medical School in Johannesburg, South Africa. In 1925, Dart described a child's skull that had been found in 1924 in ancient cave deposits at Taung, about 320 km southwest of Johannesburg (19). The skull showed that even in adulthood the child's brain would have been scarcely larger than a chimpanzee's, but the inferred orientation of the large basal aperture (foramen magnum) through which connections pass from the brain to the spinal column suggested to Dart that the skull had been balanced above an upright spinal column in the typically human (bipedal) manner. He assigned the skull to the new genus and species, *Australopithecus africanus*, and he concluded that it represented "an extinct link between man and his simian ancestor." From the late 1930s onwards, when other fossils that broadly resembled the "Taung child" were found in Africa, paleoanthropologists have commonly grouped them in the "australopithecines," or "australopiths" for short. Most specialists now recognize at least two genera (*Australopithecus* and *Paranthropus*) and multiple species of australopiths, and they believe that one of the known species, or perhaps a yet-to-be-discovered close relative, gave rise to the first member of our own genus, *Homo* (see Fig. 2-1). Some

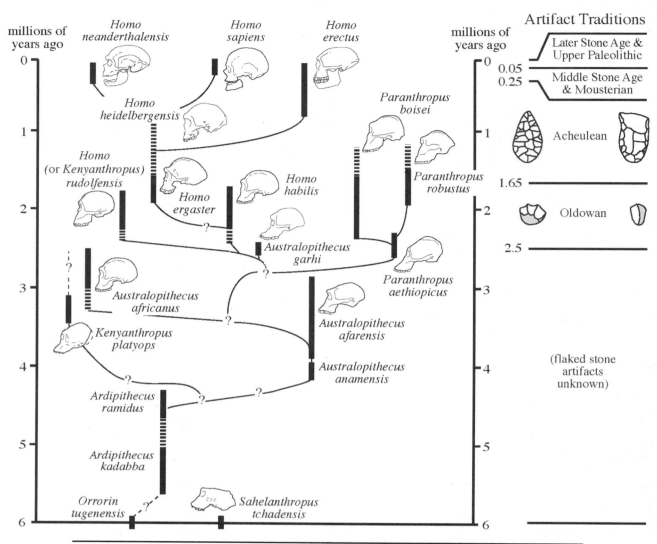

FIGURE 2-1. A simplified phylogeny of hominins, illustrating the evolutionary relationships among the species mentioned in the text.

australopith species persisted after *Homo* had emerged, but the last became extinct by 1 million years ago (see (36) for further discussion).

Traditionally, the australopiths and *Homo* have been lumped in the zoological family Hominidae (hominids in the vernacular), and the chimpanzees (two species), gorilla, and orangutan have been assigned to a separate family, the Pongidae (or pongids). However, it is now clear that the chimpanzees and gorilla are more closely related to humans than they are to the orangutan, and many authorities thus prefer a scheme that includes the chimpanzees and the gorilla in the Hominidae. In this scheme, which we accept here, the australopiths and *Homo* are separated from great apes at the tribal level, as the Hominini or hominins.

The australopiths were similar to apes in many important anatomic respects, including small absolute and relative brain size, large, forwardly projecting faces, relatively long arms and short legs, curved finger and toe bones, and at least in some species, a conically-shaped ribcage, which expanded conspicuously towards the waist. They contrasted with apes in the smaller size of their canine teeth and in the larger size and thicker enamel of their premolars and molars. However, their most striking difference from apes was in the lower body. Australopith pelves, legs, and feet were all similarly shaped to those of later humans because they were constructed for habitual bipedalism (46,85). The australopith mix of apelike and human features is readily apparent in three-way comparisons of the skull and pelvis (Fig. 2-2): australopith skulls more closely resemble chimpanzee ones, but their pelves are conspicuously more like those of living humans. The striking features that distinguish

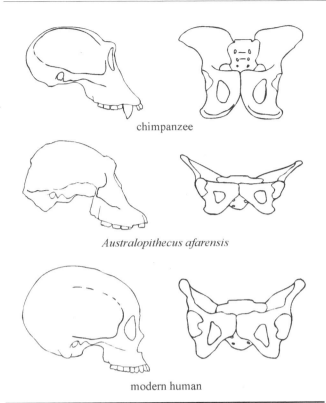

FIGURE 2-2. Chimpanzee, australopith, and modern human skulls (**left**) and pelves (**right**) [pelves redrawn after (72)]. Note that the australopith skull more closely resembles the chimpanzee one, while the australopith pelvis looks more like the modern human one.

people from apes in the head and upper body began to appear only after 2 million years ago in the genus *Homo*.

AN OVERVIEW OF HUMAN EVOLUTION

Our purpose here is to place the evolution of human walking within the broader framework of human evolution. We proceed in rough chronological order, from the oldest known hominin species to the most recent. Our focus is on the anatomical evidence for bipedalism, but we also summarize change in other anatomical regions, particularly the brain, that must have impacted bipedalism, and we touch on the natural selective forces, especially changes in climate, which probably drove large-scale anatomical change. We conclude with a summary of some differences among living human populations in the anatomy for walking.

In the introduction, we noted that genetic differences, or more precisely, the inferred rate at which such differences accrued, place the last shared ancestor of people and the African apes between 8 and 5 million years ago.

Molecular genetics shows that humans, chimpanzees, and gorillas are so closely related that depending on the genetic region, chimpanzees may appear more like humans or more like gorillas (49). However, the large majority of regions link chimpanzees most closely to humans, and it now appears that the gorilla line separated 8 to 6 million years ago and that the chimpanzee and human lines split 2 to 1 million years later (15). An estimate of roughly 6 million years for the human-chimpanzee split is consistent with the geologic ages of the oldest putative hominin species (12,27,28,64,66,75,84). We emphasize putative, because so far, there is no unambiguous skeletal evidence that any 6 to 5 million-year-old species was bipedal. The strongest case is for the species *Orrorin tugenensis*, which among other parts is represented by a nearly complete proximal femur with many features that imply bipedalism. These include a femoral neck with a groove on the rear for the obturator externus tendon, indicating full hip extension, and cortical bone that is thicker on the inferior margin than the superior one, indicating the action of human-like hip abductors during the one-legged stance phase of walking (26,50). The hominin status of the other species depends mainly on tantalizing characters in their skulls, jaws, or teeth, along with some ambiguous features of the lower body (12,27,28). Even with a wider range of fossils, however, it may be difficult to distinguish the earliest hominin from its ancestors and contemporaries, because the anatomical differences were probably subtle.

Before molecular genetics demonstrated the especially close relationship between chimpanzees and humans, anatomical analyses tended to link chimpanzees more closely to gorillas. The apparent contradiction between the data sets means either that chimpanzees and gorillas evolved many detailed anatomical similarities independently, or more likely, that the last shared ancestor of chimpanzees, gorillas, and humans resembled chimpanzees and gorillas far more closely than it did humans. Fossil ape species generally support this inference, because they tend to possess most of the features that unite chimpanzees and gorillas to the exclusion of humans (78). Many of the striking anatomical similarities between chimpanzees and gorillas are thus probably primitive features that were lost in humans after the human and chimpanzee lineages diverged.

Like the living apes, the last shared ancestor of humans and chimpanzees was probably constructed for arm-over-arm climbing and under-branch hanging in the trees (56). Its posture in the trees would thus have been orthograde like that of bipedal humans, with the spinal column perpendicular to the ground. In this regard, it would have contrasted sharply with tree-living monkeys, which tend to walk quadrupedally on the surfaces of branches, with the spinal column parallel to the ground in the manner of strictly terrestrial quadrupeds. On the ground, the last shared ancestor would have been quadrupedal, and it could have walked the way that chimpanzees and gorillas do, with the forelimbs resting on the knuckles and the hind limbs on the soles of the feet (17,53,79). Chimpanzees and gorillas routinely move from place to place on the ground, and "knuckle-walking" clearly meets their needs. So far, there is no unequivocal evidence that hominins descend from a knuckle-walking ancestor, but if new fossil finds show that they did, hypotheses for the origins of bipedalism would have to explain why there was a shift from one form of specialized terrestrial walking to another. On the other hand, if future finds suggest that the last shared ancestor of chimpanzees and people probably spent little time on the ground, we would have to explain only why hominins adopted bipedalism rather than knuckle-walking or some other form of terrestrial locomotion.

We will briefly address hypotheses for the origins of bipedalism near the end of this chapter. Here, we stress that the immediate impetus for bipedalism may always be difficult to establish, but the effects of global climate change on regional environments almost certainly provide the ultimate cause. In the interval between 8 and 5 million years ago, when the human, chimpanzee, and gorilla lineages diverged, ice sheets expanded, sea level fell, atmospheric levels of CO_2 decreased, global temperatures declined, and aridity increased at low latitudes (52). In equatorial Africa, where the hominins emerged, once continuous forests became fragmented into islands separated by stretches of woodland and grassland. Many mammal species that were adapted to tropical forests became extinct, and species that were better suited to more open, grassier habitats burgeoned. Ape species were among the losers, and for the first time, monkey species came to outnumber them, reflecting the greater ability of many monkeys to exploit more open settings (14). Hominins presumably derive from an ape that likewise found a way to benefit from more open vegetation. Contrasts between early hominin and chimpanzee teeth suggest that to begin with, a major difference between the human and chimpanzee lineages may have been dietary—early hominins may have focused on hard, brittle food items found mainly on or near the ground, while their earliest ancestors, like living chimpanzees, probably concentrated on relatively soft fruits found in trees (73). This difference in dietary preference could have produced ecological and geographic separation that promoted genetic separation and the formation of new species. Fresh fossil discoveries are required to determine if this scenario is correct, and if so, to illuminate it in greater detail.

By at least 4 million years ago, the australopiths had evolved indisputable anatomical adaptations for bipedalism, but they also preserved numerous apelike characteristics that were lost in later people (70). The most conspicuous retained trait was a combination of relatively long arms and short legs. To some extent, the shortness of aus-

tralopith legs may reflect their generally short stature, because in living humans, taller individuals tend to have relatively longer legs. Australopith males averaged less than five feet tall, and females may have been much shorter (16,45). The most complete australopith skeletons are from especially small individuals, and this may enhance the impression that australopiths were especially short legged (24). Still, there is some unequivocal anatomical evidence (see below) that the australopith gait was kinematically different from that of later humans, and short legs may have made long-distance travel energetically expensive and/or time consuming (35,71). Short legs would probably also have forced the transition from walking to running to occur at a fairly low velocity (37,38). These energetic, time, and velocity constraints may mean that australopith dependence on bipedalism was more limited than for later hominins or at least that their home ranges were smaller. Arguably, long arms and other apelike upper body retentions imply that the australopiths continued to rely on trees for food and refuge and that they used bipedalism mainly to travel short distances between tree patches. Plant or animal fossils that accompany australopith fossils at some sites show that trees often remained plentiful nearby (51). Longer legs in an australopith species dated to around 2.5 million years ago (7) may anticipate a shift to the more complete investment in bipedalism that indisputably marks *Homo* after 2 million years ago.

Sparse fossils indicate that *Homo* emerged between 2.5 and 2 million years ago, but it is well known only after 2 million years ago. The oldest widely recognized species is *Homo habilis*, but variation in skull and tooth size in specimens dated to around 1.9 million years ago suggests that *H. habilis* could comprise two species—a smaller version that would be narrowly understood (*H. habilis*) and a larger one for which the name *H. rudolfensis* has been proposed. *H. habilis/rudolfensis* was unquestionably bipedal, but the details of its bipedalism cannot be established, for lack of sufficiently complete limb bones that are directly associated with diagnostic skulls or jaws.

One or both variants of *Homo habilis* is presumed to have produced the oldest known flaked stone tools, dated to about 2.5 million years ago. The tools occur in clusters that mark the oldest known archaeological sites and they are often accompanied by fragmentary animal bones that provide the oldest direct evidence for human carnivory (36).

About 1.8 million years ago *Homo habilis* was supplanted by the more advanced species *Homo ergaster* (also sometimes called early African *Homo erectus*). Specialists generally assume that *H. ergaster* evolved from *H. habilis* (or one of its constituents), but it may actually represent a parallel development that originated before 2 million years ago. The more important point is that it is known not only from skulls, jaws, and isolated limb bones, but also from the nearly complete skeleton of an 8- to 11-year-old boy

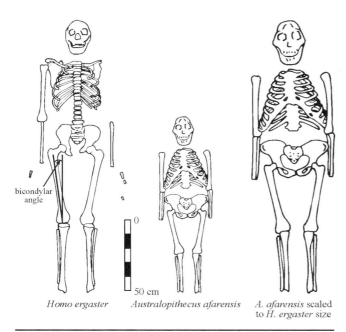

bicondylar
angle

0

50 cm

Homo ergaster   *Australopithecus afarensis*   *A. afarensis* scaled
to *H. ergaster* size

FIGURE 2-3. Differences in body size and proportions between *Australopithecus afarensis* and *Homo ergaster* [redrawn from (61)]. In both species, the brain was significantly smaller than in living humans.

who died in northern Kenya about 1.6 million years ago (76). Together with less complete specimens, the skeleton shows that *H. ergaster* had lost the apelike features that arguably facilitated tree climbing in the australopiths. In all major respects, including relatively short arms and long legs, stature and body mass approximating that of living equatorial Africans, a barrel- (vs. cone-) shaped ribcage and relatively small premolars and molars, it contrasted with the australopiths in essentially the same way that living humans do (Fig. 2-3) (16,44). The leg bones differ in small details from those of living humans, but none of the differences indicate a significant difference in bipedalism. The change in thorax shape could imply a reduction in gut size that was probably tied to a diet of higher quality foods (5). Either meat or subterranean tubers would fit the bill, and even cooking could be implied, although the archaeological record provides no evidence for fire until after 500,000 years ago. The skeletal changes that mark *H. ergaster*, together with archaeological indications that it was the first human species to occupy tree-poor environments, suggest a transformation in thermoregulation (including the loss of body hair to enhance sweating) and possibly the development of foraging patterns, group sizes, and social relations foreshadowing those of historic hunter-gatherers (4,23,25).

Homo ergaster contrasted most conspicuously with living humans in its much smaller brain and in the low ratio of brain size to body mass, in which it hardly differed from earlier species (46). From an obstetrical per-

spective, the small brain had a distinct advantage, because full-term fetuses with smaller heads could pass more easily through the pelvic inlet, mid-plane, and outlet (birth canal) and they were thus less likely to cause infant and/or maternal mortality (57,58). Compared to pelvic shape in living humans then, shape in *H. ergaster* was less subject to tension between obstetrical requirements and the demands of bipedalism, and it is thus possible that *H. ergaster* was a more efficient biped. The human brain appears to have remained absolutely and relatively small until about 600,000 years ago, after which it expanded rapidly to approximate the modern average (46,59). Brain expansion probably affected the anatomy of the pelvis and femur, but many more fossils are required to document the pattern of change after *H. ergaster* and to determine if there were implications for bipedalism.

By 500,000 years ago, *Homo ergaster* had given rise to at least three geographically distinct evolutionary lineages that culminated in three separate species: *Homo neanderthalensis* (the Neandertals) in Europe, *Homo sapiens* (modern humans and their immediate ancestors) in Africa, and *Homo erectus* (the relatively poorly known nonmodern contemporaries of the Neandertals and early modern humans) in eastern Asia (Fig. 2-1). Beginning roughly 50,000 years ago, *H. sapiens* spread from Africa to replace the last representatives of *H. neanderthalensis* and *H. erectus*. More advanced cultural behavior, perhaps grounded in a neurologic change, underlay the spread (36), and there is no reason to suppose it was assisted by differences in human walking. The skeletal anatomy of the Neandertals is particularly well known, and despite some detailed differences in pelvis and femur shape, Neandertals probably walked in exactly the same way as modern humans (80). However, Neandertal legs were shorter than those of their modern European successors (and of most living humans) (31), and the Neandertals may thus have expended more energy per unit of walking distance (71).

Large-scale or macroevolutionary change in the human form ceased after 40,000 to 30,000 years ago, when modern humans had established themselves everywhere, but small-scale, or microevolutionary, change continued. Some of the change reflects random genetic drift (chance changes in gene frequencies that are particularly likely to occur in small populations), but some was adaptive and reflects the natural selective effects of climate differences.

Average body size and shape varies with latitude in most widespread mammalian species and humans are no exception (8,30,48,63,81). The reason is that differences in latitude correlate closely with differences in temperature and humidity, and humans like other animals have evolved different body shapes in response. Thus, people whose ancestry traces to equatorial latitudes tend to have especially slim trunks with long limbs, while people who come from arctic or subarctic latitudes tend to have much stockier trunks with short limbs. Average male trunk breadth, as reflected in hip breadth (the maximum distance between the iliac crests of the pelvis), varies from 23 to 30 cm among living human populations (63), and the variation in average leg length is similar. The narrow hipped, long-legged equatorial body form facilitates heat dissipation in settings where this is obviously desirable, while the broader hipped, shorter legged arctic form retards heat loss in settings where heat retention is crucial.

To the extent that climatic differences impact pelvic breadth and leg length, they also affect the precise implementation of bipedalism in different populations. The wide range in modern body form shows that the modern skeleton is not optimized for bipedalism, but represents a compromise between the demands of bipedalism and other constraints like climate and of course obstetrics.

THE THEORETICAL BASIS FOR BEHAVIORAL RECONSTRUCTION

Reconstructing the locomotor behavior of an extinct species is complicated by the possibility that some anatomical features represent nonfunctional ancestral retentions. Thus, in the previous section, we noted that the long arms and other apelike characteristics of the australopiths may indicate an apelike ability to climb trees, when they may mean only that the australopiths were directly descended from a tree-climbing ape. To illustrate how evolutionary history or phylogeny can complicate behavioral interpretations, we consider how we would reconstruct the locomotor behavior of modern humans if all we knew were skeletal anatomy.

The modern human skeleton has many obvious anatomical adaptations for bipedal locomotion. The key traits include a short pelvis that brings the sacrum very close to the hip joints, laterally facing iliac blades, a complexly curved vertebral column, an angle between the femur and tibia at the knee (the bicondylar angle), and a foot that has a well-developed longitudinal arch with a big toe that is aligned parallel to the others. However, modern humans also have laterally facing and extremely mobile shoulder joints, which in apes are clearly adaptations for arm-over-arm climbing and under-branch suspension. Given anatomy alone then, there would be no reason to suppose that modern humans were more committed to bipedalism than to arm-swinging through the trees. We know differently mainly because we can observe living humans directly.

We might also avoid a false conclusion if we distinguished anatomical features that are primitive (that is, ones that were present in the last shared ancestor of a species group) from ones that are derived or advanced (that is, ones that developed after various species had diverged from a shared ancestor). Derived features imply a shift in anatomy, and it is therefore reasonable to conclude

that they reflect actual behaviors. In contrast, primitive features might reflect behaviors that are no longer being performed. Of course, the distinction between primitive and derived features requires a knowledge of evolutionary history, and behavioral reconstructions that proceed without such knowledge will always be questionable. In the modern human case, the fossil record shows that adaptations for tree climbing are primitive, while adaptations for bipedalism are derived. Even in the absence of eyewitness accounts then, it could be concluded that bipedalism is important to us, while tree climbing might not be.

For the purpose of behavioral reconstruction, it is further important to distinguish between genetically determined and behaviorally plastic skeletal traits. Plastic traits, as we use the term, are ones that change in response to activities during an individual's lifetime, and they are therefore not meaningfully characterized as primitive or derived. The simple presence of a plastic feature shows that a particular behavior was being performed (78).

The human bicondylar angle exemplifies a behaviorally plastic skeletal feature that unambiguously implies bipedalism, and a fossil femur is sufficient to determine if the angle was present. The bicondylar angle is defined as the angle between the shaft of the femur and a line perpendicular to a plane surface (Fig. 2-3, left), when the femur is placed with the (distal) condyles flat against this surface. In adult humans, the angle is usually around 9 to 10 degrees, while in adult chimpanzees it is generally close to 0 degrees (meaning that chimpanzees lack a conspicuous bicondylar angle). The substantial angle in humans helps to center the body over one leg while the other is in swing phase, and without it, bipedal locomotion would be energetically expensive to employ over long distances. However, human infants start out like adult chimpanzees with no observable bicondylar angle, and the angle appears only after children begin to walk. Biomechanical studies demonstrate that the adult human bicondylar angle is a direct consequence of the forces that bipedalism imposes during development (67), and this makes it the best available skeletal indicator of habitual bipedalism. With this and our more general theoretical framework in mind, we now consider the fossils that document the evolution of human walking.

THE FOSSIL EVIDENCE FOR EARLY HUMAN WALKING

The oldest-known hominin species for which bipedalism has been unambiguously inferred is *Australopithecus anamensis*, dated to between 4.2 and 3.9 million years ago in northern Kenya (40). The fossil sample of this species includes not only the usual jaws and teeth that tend to dominate the fossil record, but also a fragmentary tibia that preserves numerous indications of bipedalism. The most important indication is the approximate angle between the shaft and the articular surface for the talus, or astragalus, at the distal (ankle) end (40,78). In chimpanzees, the shaft slopes away laterally from this surface, and the contrast reflects a difference in the position of the knee, which lies directly above the ankle in humans and lateral to it in apes. In the last section, we stressed that the bicondylar angle is the least ambiguous skeletal indicator of bipedalism in humans, and the right angle between the tibia and the distal articular surface indirectly indicates it. The bipedal status of *A. anamensis* is thus secure.

The fossil samples for most geologically younger australopiths include a wider range of skeletal parts that bear upon walking, and they uniformly imply bipedalism. Perhaps most importantly, the femora always exhibit a typically human bicondylar angle, and the pelvis presents oft-cited modifications for bipedal walking, including the positioning of the sacrum close to the hip joints and the lateral orientation of the iliac blades (34,42,54). In these features and others, the australopiths were unmistakably derived away from the apes in the direction of living humans.

However, along with the derived features that demonstrate bipedalism, the australopiths exhibited primitive traits that are usually associated with tree climbing and also some unique traits that are unknown in either apes or later humans. We noted previously that the traits associated with climbing are often interpreted to mean that the australopiths depended on trees for food and refuge. Some researchers have also proposed that these traits and the ones that are unique to the australopiths imply a posturally and kinematically unique form of bipedalism (1–3,9,62,69,70).

The most widely discussed proposal stems from the assessment of a partial skeleton and other bones of *Australopithecus afarensis*, which lived in eastern Africa between roughly 3.9 and 2.9 million years ago. According to this analysis, individuals of *A. afarensis* lacked the modern human ability to extend the hip and the knee, and they thus walked with a bent-hip, bent-knee gait (69,70). Critics have disputed the anatomical features behind this conclusion and some have also noted that walking with flexed hip and knee joints would inhibit the pendular transfer of kinetic and potential energy that typifies human walking. Without this energy transfer, walking would be energetically far more expensive (13,18,77), and studies of living humans show that less hip and knee extension would also increase the energetic costs of running (47). However, most primates already walk with a compliant gait (65), so bipedalism employing partially flexed hip and knee joints may have been energetically no less efficient than the locomotion of the last shared ancestor of humans and apes. If this is accepted, then an energetically expensive gait in australopiths could represent a primitive retention.

In living humans, the promontory angle of the sacrum (that is, the angle between the ventral and superior sur-faces of the first sacral vertebra) is generally acute, but in the best preserved sacrum of *Australopithecus afarensis*, it is closer to 90 degrees (2). This suggests that the vertebral column was oriented less vertically in *A. afarensis*, however, the promontory angle varies substantially in living humans (78). An angle near 90 degrees has also been found in at least one Neandertal (80). Thus, on present evidence, the promontory angle found in *A. afarensis* does not necessarily imply a different posture from later humans.

A quasi-static equilibrium biomechanical model founded on observations of living humans and applied to the partial skeleton of *Australopithecus afarensis* referred to above suggests that by comparison to living humans, *A. afarensis* should have had an enlarged femoral head and increased mediolateral buttressing of the femoral shaft and ilium (62). It does not, and the implication could be that *A. afarensis* walked with an elevated hip on the nonsupport side to minimize abductor and hip joint reaction forces and mediolateral bending of the femoral shaft of the stance leg. However, the fit between predicted hip joint reaction force and femoral head size is loose in living humans. Women, for example, have wide biacetabular breadths and short femoral necks relative to men, but they do not have disproportionately large femoral heads (11).

The idea that australopiths retained an apelike ability to climb is more compelling than suggestions that their bipedalism was posturally and kinematically unique. The anatomical features that support special climbing ability include relatively long arms and short legs, many features of the hand and shoulder that reflect well developed musculature for under-branch grasping and hanging, indications of longer hamstring moment arms, and a deep peroneal groove on the fibula. Anatomical details of the hip, knee, and ankle joints imply increased mobility (70). Arguably, the dramatic shift in body size and shape that marked the emergence of *Homo ergaster* about 1.8 million years ago is also pertinent. The shift is difficult to explain if the australopith locomotor repertoire differed little from that of later humans. Even if the long legs of *H. ergaster* were an adaptation only to longer range foraging and do not mean that tree climbing had become less important, the reason that *H. ergaster* had lost so many other primitive features is inexplicable, unless *H. ergaster* signals a significant behavioral shift towards greater reliance on bipedalism and less dependence on tree climbing.

The problem remains that the supposed australopith tree-climbing adaptations are almost all primitive, and they could represent nonfunctional retentions inherited from the last shared human and ape ancestor (39). Additionally, some of the anatomical differences from living humans could reflect different obstetrical and visceral constraints, given that australopith brains were much smaller relative to body mass and that their intestines may have been relatively larger (5,41,72). In the absence of unequivocally derived adaptations or behaviorally plastic traits that indicate tree climbing, it may always be difficult to show that tree climbing was a significant component of australopith behavior.

The locomotor skeleton of *Homo ergaster* closely resembled that of living humans, but it was not identical. Most notably, compared to the femora of living humans, those of *H. ergaster* tended to have longer, anteroposteriorly flatter necks with lower angles between the neck and the shaft and more mediolaterally reinforced shafts with thicker cortical bone (22,74,76). There are no complete pelves, but the femoral characteristics may mean that the pelvis was exceptionally broad from side to side and flat from front to back (platypelloid). If so, this would be a feature that *H. ergaster* retained from its australopith ancestry. Such a pelvis may require long femoral necks to keep the hip abductors in an advantageous position for opposing large body weight moments during one-legged stance, and mediolaterally thick femoral shafts may be required to resist the large bending moments that result from long femoral necks and an extremely platypelloid pelvis (60).

It was probably much later in human evolution, after brain size had more closely approached the modern average, that the pelvis achieved its present configuration. The oldest evidence for such a pelvis comes from the Sima de los Huesos site in northern Spain, dated to about 400,000 years ago (6,10). The associated cranial remains indicate that the Sima people were on or near the evolutionary line to the classic Neandertals. The Sima pelvis is large, most likely that of a male, but it is not markedly broad and flat, and its inlet exhibits a typically human shape. The implication is that once absolute and relative brain size approximated the values in living humans, basic pelvic form was fixed, and there were probably no further anatomical changes that significantly affected bipedalism.

HYPOTHESES FOR THE ORIGINS OF BIPEDALISM

In closing, we return to an issue that we deliberately skirted before—an explanation for why bipedalism evolved. The initial selective advantages may have included; (a) the ability to carry meat or other food items to trees, other refuges, or other group members (29,43); (b) an enhanced facility to gather small-diameter fruits from short trees (32); (c) a reduction in the amount of skin surface exposed to direct sunlight at midday, thus reducing the danger of heat stress, particularly on the brain (82); (d) the freeing of the hands for tool use (20), or for carrying the young long distances (68); (e) a decrease in the energy required to walk at low speeds (85); (f) the ability to see more clearly or farther during passage from place to place (21); (g) or the enhancement of threat displays that reduced violent conflicts over scarce resources (33).

The various alternatives are difficult to falsify, and one or more of them could have operated in concert. However, it may be possible to narrow the choices somewhat by considering the developmental mechanisms that underlie bipedalism. For example, as we noted previously, the adult human bicondylar angle develops only in response to the mechanical forces that bipedalism produces during development. Thus, the presence of a human bicondylar angle implies that juveniles were habitually walking bipedally. This means that a viable explanation for the origins of human bipedalism must consider bipedal locomotion not just in adults, but also in juveniles, and any explanation that focuses tightly on adult behavior is unlikely.

SUMMARY

Genetic evidence indicates that the human and chimpanzee lineages diverged about 6 million years ago. It is widely assumed that the earliest humans walked bipedally, but the oldest indisputable fossil evidence for bipedalism is only slightly more than 4 million years old. Bipedalism is well documented in all human species after 4 million years ago, including both the australopiths, which dominate the record before 2 million years ago and members of the genus *Homo*, the earliest of which appeared between 2.5 and 2 million years ago. Anatomical differences between the australopiths and later *Homo* suggest that the australopiths may have employed a kinematically unique bipedal gait and that they remained proficient tree climbers, but the case remains debatable.

Homo ergaster, which appeared in eastern Africa about 1.8 million years ago, is the oldest known human species to lack the apelike features that the australopiths retained and also the oldest that unquestionably walked in the fully modern way. Minor differences between *H. ergaster* and later humans in locomotor anatomy may reflect the relatively small size of the *H. ergaster* brain, which placed more limited constraints on the pelvic inlet (birth canal). Between 600,000 and 300,000 years ago, brain size expanded to near the modern average, and the pelvis was modified to its present form. This is essentially a compromise between the demands of obstetrics and those of bipedalism. After 50,000 years ago, when modern humans spread from Africa to predominately replace nonmodern humans in Eurasia, differences in climate selected for differences in body shape and proportions, which affected human locomotion in minor ways.

ACKNOWLEDGMENTS

We are grateful to the curators who generously allowed us to study comparative and fossil material under their care, to David DeGusta and Teresa Steele for commenting on drafts of this chapter, and to Kathryn Cruz-Uribe for help with the illustrations. The L.S.B. Leakey Foundation, the Morrison Institute for Population and Resource Studies at Stanford University, the A.W. Mellon Foundation, the Department of Anthropological Sciences at Stanford University, and a Michael Guyer Postdoctoral Fellowship from the University of Wisconsin-Madison provided financial support for research by TW reported in this chapter.

REFERENCES

1. Abitbol MM. Evolution of the lumbosacral angle. *Am J Phys Anthropol* 1987;72:361–372.
2. Abitbol MM. Lateral view of *Australopithecus afarensis:* primitive aspects of bipedal positional behavior in the earliest hominids. *J Hum Evol* 1995;28:211–229.
3. Abitbol MM. Reconstruction of the STS 14 (*Australopithecus africanus*) pelvis. *Am J Phys Anthropol* 1995;96:143–158.
4. Aiello LC, Key C. Energetic consequences of being a *Homo erectus* female. *Am J Hum Biol* 2002;14:551–565.
5. Aiello LC, Wheeler P. The expensive-tissue hypothesis. *Curr Anthropol* 1995;36:199–221.
6. Arsuaga J-L, Lorenzo C, Carretero J-M, Gracia A, Martínez I, García N, et al. A complete human pelvis from the Middle Pleistocene of Spain. *Nature* 1999;399:255–258.
7. Asfaw B, White TD, Lovejoy CO, Latimer BM, Simpson S, Suwa G. *Australopithecus garhi:* a new species of early hominid from Ethiopia. *Science* 1999;284:629–636.
8. Ashton KG, Tracy MC, de Queiroz A. Is Bergmann's rule valid for mammals? *American Naturalist* 2000;156:390–415.
9. Berge C. How did the australopithecines walk? A biomechanical study of the hip and thigh of *Australopithecus afarensis. J Hum Evol* 1994;26:259–273.
10. Bischoff JL, Shamp DD, Aramburu A, et al. The Sima de los Huesos hominids date to beyond U/Th equilibrium (>350 kyr) and perhaps to 400–500 kyr: New radiometric dates. *J Archaeol Sci* 2003;30:275–280.
11. Brinckmann P, Hoefert H, Jongen HT. Sex differences in the skeletal geometry of the human pelvis and hip joint. *J Biomech* 1981;14:427–430.
12. Brunet M, Guy F, Pilbeam D, et al. A new hominid from the Upper Miocene of Chad, central Africa. *Nature* 2002;418:145–151.
13. Cavagna GA, Heglund NC, Taylor CR. Mechanical work in terrestrial locomotion: two basic mechanisms for minimizing energy expenditure. *Am J Physiol* 1977;233(5):R243–R261.
14. Cerling TE, Harris JM, MacFadden BJ, et al. Global vegetation change through the Miocene/Pliocene boundary. *Nature* 1997;389:153–158.
15. Chen F-C, Li W-H. Genomic divergences between humans and other hominoids and the effective population size of the common ancestor of humans and chimpanzees. *Am J Hum Genet* 2001;68:444–456.
16. Collard M. Grades and transitions in human evolution. In: Crow TJ, ed. *The Speciation of Modern Homo sapiens.* Oxford: Oxford University Press; 2002:61–100.
17. Corruccini RS, McHenry HM. Knuckle-walking hominid ancestors. *J Hum Evol* 2001;40:507–511.
18. Crompton RH, Yu L, Weijie W, Günther M, Savage R. The mechanical effectiveness of erect and "bent-hip, bent-knee" bipedal walking in *Australopithecus afarensis. J Hum Evol* 1998;35:55–74.
19. Dart RA. *Australopithecus africanus:* The man-ape of South Africa. *Nature* 1925;115:195–197.
20. Darwin C. *The Descent of Man and Selection in Relation to Sex.* London: John Murray and Sons; 1871.
21. Day MH. Bipedalism: pressures, origins and modes. In: Wood BA, Martin L, Andrews P, eds. *Major Topics in Primate and Human Evolution.* Cambridge: Cambridge University Press; 1986:188–202.
22. Day MH. Postcranial remains of *Homo erectus* from Bed IV, Olduvai Gorge, Tanzania. *Nature* 1971;232:383–387.
23. Foley RA. *Another Unique Species: Patterns in Human Evolutionary Ecology.* Essex: Longman Scientific & Technical; 1987.
24. Franciscus RG, Holliday TW. Hindlimb skeletal allometry in Plio-Pleistocene hominids with special reference to AL-288-1 ("Lucy"). *Bulletins et Mémoires de la Société d'Anthropologie de Paris* 1992;4(1–2):5–20.
25. Franciscus RG, Trinkaus E. Nasal morphology and the emergence of *Homo erectus. Am J Phys Anthropol* 1988;75:517–527.
26. Galik K, Senut B, Pickford M, et al. External and internal morphology of the BAR 1002'00 *Orrorin tugenensis* femur. *Science* 2004;305:1450–1453.
27. Haile-Selassie Y, Suwa G, White TD. Late Miocene teeth from Middle Awash, Ethiopia, and early hominid dental evolution. *Science* 2004;303:1503–1505.
28. Haile-Selassie Y. Late Miocene hominids from the Middle Awash, Ethiopia. *Nature* 2001;412:178–181.
29. Hewes GW. Food transport and the origin of hominid bipedalism. *Amer Anthropol* 1961;63:687–710.
30. Holliday TW. Body proportions in Late Pleistocene Europe and modern human origins. *J Hum Evol* 1997;32:423–447.
31. Holliday TW. Brachial and crural indices of European late Upper Paleolithic and Mesolithic humans. *J Hum Evol* 1999;36:549–566.
32. Hunt KD. Ecological morphology of *Australopithecus afarensis:* traveling terrestrially, eating arboreally. In: Strasser E, Fleagle JG, McHenry HM, et al., eds. *Primate Locomotion: Recent Advances.* New York: Plenum Press; 1998:397–418.
33. Jablonski NG, Chaplin G. Origin of habitual terrestrial bipedalism in the ancestor of the Hominidae. *J Hum Evol* 1993;24:259–280.
34. Johanson DC, Lovejoy CO, Kimbel WH, et al. Morphology of the Pliocene partial hominid skeleton (A.L. 288-1) from the Hadar Formation, Ethiopia. *Am J Phys Anthropol* 1982;57:403–451.
35. Jungers WL. Lucy's limbs: skeletal allometry and locomotion in *Australopithecus afarensis. Nature* 1982;297:676–678.
36. Klein RG, Edgar B. *The Dawn of Human Culture.* New York: John Wiley and Sons; 2002.
37. Kramer PA, Eck GG. Locomotor energetics and leg length in hominid bipedality. *J Hum Evol* 2000;38:651–666.
38. Kramer PA. Modeling the locomotor energetics of extinct hominids. *J Exp Biol* 1999;202:2807–2818.
39. Latimer BM. Locomotor adaptations in *Australopithecus afarensis:* the issue of arboreality. In: Coppens Y, Senut B, eds. *Origine(s) de la Bipédie chez les Hominidés.* Paris: CNRS; 1991:169–176.
40. Leakey MG, Feibel CS, McDougall I, Walker A. New four-million-year-old hominid species from Kanapoi and Allia Bay, Kenya. *Nature* 1995;376:565–571.
41. Lovejoy CO, Heiple KG, Burstein AH. The gait of *Australopithecus. Am J Phys Anthropol* 1973;38(3):757–779.
42. Lovejoy CO. Evolution of human walking. *Sci Am* 1988;259:118–125.
43. Lovejoy CO. The origin of man. *Science* 1981;211:341–350.
44. McHenry HM, Coffing K. *Australopithecus to Homo:* transformations in body and mind. *Ann Rev Anthropol* 2000;29:125–146.
45. McHenry HM. How big were the early hominids? *Evol Anthro* 1992;1:15–20.
46. McHenry HM. Tempo and mode in human evolution. *Proc Nat Acad Sci USA* 1994;91:6780–6786.
47. McMahon TA, Valiant G, Frederick E. Groucho running. *J Appl Physiol* 1987;62(6):2326–2337.
48. Meiri S, Dayan T. On the validity of Bergmann's rule. *J Biogeograph* 2003;30:331–351.
49. Pääbo S. The mosaic that is our genome. *Nature* 2003;42:409–412.
50. Pickford M, Senut B, Gommery D, Treil J. Bipedalism in *Orrorin tugenensis* revealed by its femora. *Comptes Rendus Palevol* 2002;1:191–203.
51. Reed KE. Early hominid evolution and ecological change through the African Plio-Pleistocene. *J Hum Evol* 1997;32:289–322.
52. Retallack GJ. Cenozoic expansion of grasslands and climatic cooling. *J Geol* 2001;109:407–426.
53. Richmond BG, Begun DR, Strait DS. Origin of human bipedalism: the knuckle-walking hypothesis revisited. *Yearbook of Physical Anthropology* 2001;44:70–105.

54. Robinson JT. *Early Hominid Posture and Locomotion*. Chicago: University of Chicago Press; 1972.
55. Rodman PS, McHenry HM. Energetics and the origin of hominid bipedalism. *Am J Phys Anthropol* 1980;52:103–106.
56. Rose MD. The process of bipedalization in hominids. In: Coppens Y, Senut B, eds. *Origine(s) de la Bipédie chez les Hominidés*. Paris: CNRS; 1991:37–48.
57. Rosenberg KR. Reply to Baskerville. *Curr Anthropol* 1989;30:486–488.
58. Rosenberg KR. The evolution of modern human childbirth. *Yearbook of Physical Anthropology* 1992;35:89–124.
59. Ruff CB, Trinkaus E, Holliday TW. Body mass and encephalization in Pleistocene *Homo*. *Nature* 1997;387:173–176.
60. Ruff CB. Biomechanics of the hip and birth in early *Homo*. *Am J Phys Anthropol* 1995;98:527–574.
61. Ruff CB. Climatic adaptation in hominid evolution: the thermoregulatory imperative. *Evol Anthropol* 1993;2:53–60.
62. Ruff CB. Evolution of the hominid hip. In: Strasser E, Fleagle JG, McHenry HM, et al., eds. *Primate Locomotion: Recent Advances*. New York: Plenum Press; 1998:449–469.
63. Ruff CB. Morphological adaptation to climate in modern and fossil hominids. *Yearbook of Physical Anthropology* 1994;37:65–107.
64. Sawada Y, Pickford M, Senut B, et al. The age of *Orrorin tugenensis*, an early hominid from the Tugen Hills, Kenya. *Comptes Rendus Palevol* 2002;1:293–303.
65. Schmitt D. Insights into the evolution of human bipedalism from experimental studies of humans and other primates. *J Exp Biol* 2003;206:1437–1448.
66. Senut B, Pickford M, Gommery D, et al. First hominid from the Miocene (Lukeino formation, Kenya). *Comptes Rendus de L'Academie des Sciences. Serie II, Fascicule A-Sciences de la Terre et des Planetes* 2001;322(2):137–144.
67. Shefelbine SJ, Tardieu C, Carter DR. Development of the femoral bicondylar angle in hominid bipedalism. *Bone* 2002;30:765–770.
68. Sinclair ARE, Leakey MD, Norton-Griffiths M. Migration and hominid bipedalism. *Nature* 1986;324:307–308.
69. Stern JT, Susman RL. The locomotor anatomy of *Australopithecus afarensis*. *Am J Phys Anthropol* 1983;60:279–317.
70. Stern JT. Climbing to the top: a personal memoir of *Australopithecus afarensis*. *Evol Anthropol* 2000;9(3):113–133.
71. Steudel-Numbers KL, Tilkens MJ. The effect of lower limb length on the energetic cost of locomotion: implications for fossil hominins. *J Hum Evol* 2004;47:95–109.
72. Tague RG, Lovejoy CO. The obstetric pelvis of A.L. 288-1 (Lucy). *J Hum Evol* 1986;15:237–255.
73. Teaford MF, Ungar PS. Diet and the evolution of the earliest human ancestors. *Proc Natl Acad Sci USA* 2000;97:13506–13511.
74. Trinkaus E. Femoral neck-shaft angles of the Qafzeh-Skhul early modern humans, and activity levels among immature Near Eastern Paleolithic hominids. *J Hum Evol* 1993;25:393–416.
75. Vignaud P, Duringer P, Taïsso Mackaye H, et al. Geology and palaeontology of the Upper Miocene Toros-Menalla hominid locality, Chad. *Nature* 2002;418:152–155.
76. Walker A, Leakey R, eds. The Nariokotome Homo erectus Skeleton. Cambridge: Harvard University Press; 1993.
77. Wang WJ, Crompton RH, Li Y, Gunther MM. Energy transformation during erect and 'bent-hip, bent-knee' walking by humans with implications for the evolution of bipedalism. *J Hum Evol* 2003;44:563–579.
78. Ward CV. Interpreting the posture and locomotion of *Australopithecus afarensis*: where do we stand? *Yearbook of Physical Anthropology* 2002;45:185–215.
79. Washburn SL. Human evolution after Raymond Dart. In: Tobias PV, ed. *Hominid Evolution Past, Present, and Future*. New York: Alan R. Liss; 1985:3–18.
80. Weaver TD. A multi-causal functional analysis of hominid hip morphology [Ph.D.]. Stanford: Stanford University; 2002.
81. Weaver TD. The shape of the Neandertal femur is primarily the consequence of a hyperpolar body form. *Proc Natl Acad Sci USA* 2003;100:6926–6929.
82. Wheeler PE. The thermoregulatory advantages of hominid bipedalism in open equatorial environments: the contribution of increased convective heat loss and cutaneous evaporative cooling. *J Hum Evol* 1991;21:107–115.
83. White TD, Suwa G, Asfaw B. *Australopithecus ramidus*, a new species of early hominid from Aramis, Ethiopia. *Nature* 1994;371:306–312.
84. WoldeGabriel G, Haile-Selassie Y, Renne PR, et al. Geology and paleontology of the Late Miocene Middle Awash valley, Afar rift, Ethiopia. *Nature* 2001;412:175–177.
85. Wood B, Richmond BG. Human evolution: taxonomy and paleobiology. *J Anat* 2000;196:19–60.

Chapter 3

Kinematics of Normal Human Walking

Kenton R. Kaufman and David H. Sutherland

OVERVIEW

A principle of science, and of medicine in particular, is that one must understand the normal or natural history of a studied phenomenon before attempting to describe and study the pathological or abnormal. It was just such desire that launched the University of California San Francisco/Berkeley Laboratory investigations into the kinematics of normal human walking. Through an unfortunate accident, Professor Howard D. Eberhart, an engineer, became an amputee and was astounded that limb prosthetics had never been adequately studied scientifically and was still basically an art form. When he questioned Dr. Inman, he was invited to join a collaborative effort to study normal human walking so that prosthetic research could benefit from a solid background of engineering. A decade of intense, multidisciplinary investigation followed, much of which is summarized in the first edition of *Human Walking* (14). This effort inspired many other scientists and clinicians to further investigate and expand our basic knowledge of the kinematics of normal human walking.

Human walking is a relatively unique form of ambulation in that it is bipedal. While there are animal examples of bipedal locomotion (bears, primates, marsupials), the bipedal gait in man is uniquely efficient and functional. Some researchers feel that it is the evolution of the foot, allowing a stable platform for bipedal walking, which allowed development of man's hands as tool users. Human bipedal walking has been described by many authors using simple analogies to make a complex phenomenon more understandable. The pattern of leg motions has been likened to bicycling (2), to pendulum action, and to a controlled fall. Lettre and Contini (21) have described human and animal locomotion in three distinct stages:

1) *development* stage (from rest to some velocity),
2) *rhythmic* stage (some constant average velocity), and
3) *decay* stage (coming back to rest) (Fig. 3-1).

Most research has concentrated on the rhythmic stage of *free speed walking*. Many observations have confirmed that the rhythmic stage of human walking is very consistent and is directly related to the optimal efficiency for an individual. The patterns of movements of the body during free speed-walking are remarkably consistent between individuals and form the basis of the data to be presented in this chapter.

An important concept to understand is that smooth passage of the common center of mass is essential for efficient walking (13,27). Elevation of the center of mass begins in early single limb support during the phase of forward deceleration. When the center of mass reaches its greatest height (approximately 30% of gait cycle), potential energy is maximal and kinetic energy is minimal. This reciprocal relationship between potential and kinetic energy is retained, but the order is reversed during double limb support, in which kinetic energy is maximal and potential energy is at its lowest level. Muscle action is required, and oxygen must be consumed both to initiate and sustain walking. For the movements of the common center of mass to be smooth, the movements of the lower extremities, and to a lesser extent the movements of the upper extremities, must follow normal or near normal pathways. While our task in this chapter is to describe kinematics, not kinetics, the two are intertwined. However, accurate measurement of kinematics provides a foundation on which to build kinetic analysis, which will be described in the next chapter. In this chapter, we will provide a fundamental background of the engineering principles used to quantify human motion, describe the basic events of the gait cycle, explain how these events subdivide the phases and periods of the cycle, and give an in-depth description of the normal average dynamic joint angle measurement of the pelvis and lower extremity body segments/joint in the three standard frames of reference (sagittal, coronal, and transverse planes).

PRINCIPLES OF MOTION MEASUREMENT

Motion analysis is the set of methods and techniques aimed at quantitative analysis of human movement. The scientific foundation of gait analysis is based on rigid body mechanics. Bioengineers have contributed the most in this area. Nonetheless, it is important for all to have some basic

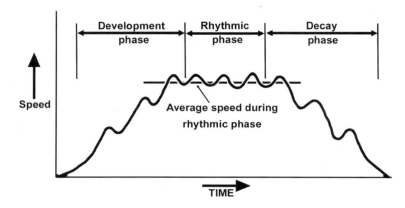

FIGURE 3-1. Three phases of walking. (Adapted from Lettre, Contini, 1967.)

understanding of the concepts that are shaping the discipline of gait analysis. Confusion sometimes arises regarding the use of terms in the literature that describe the study of motion. The study and analysis of humans in motion and the forces acting upon humans in motion is known as biomechanics. The prefix "bio" is from the Greek, and it means "life." The suffix "mechanics" is an area of Newtonian physics designed to study the effect of forces on bodies and motion. Understanding the biomechanics of human movement has both basic and applied value. There are a number of fundamental concepts and definitions that are required as a foundation for the understanding of human movement.

There are two types of physical quantities: scalars and vectors. Scalars are those fundamental quantities that require only a single number to specify them. Examples include volume, mass, density, electric charge, and speed. Vectors require specification of both magnitude and direction to completely characterize them. Examples include displacement, velocity, and acceleration.

Kinematics is the subdivision of mechanics that deals with the description of motion without regard to the forces causing this motion. Kinematics describes motion in terms of displacement, velocity, and acceleration in space. Kinematic analysis relates further to the study of relative motion between rigid bodies and finds application in analysis of gait and other body movements where each limb segment is considered a rigid body. The body segments are usually defined as the HAT (head, arms, and trunk), pelvis, thigh, shank, and foot.

External markers are used to define orthogonal coordinate systems affixed to each body segment, whose axes define the position of these body segments. With a camera-based system, either passively reflective or actively illuminated markers are used (Fig. 3-2a). These markers are commonly attached to the subjects as either discrete points or rigid clusters with multiple markers on each cluster. Placement of these external markers on the surface of the body segments are aligned with particular bony landmarks. As the patient walks along a marked walkway, the cameras track and record the marker trajectories.

Using stereophotogrammetric principles, the planar projections of markers viewed by each camera are used to reconstruct the 3-dimensional instantaneous position of the markers relative to an inertially fixed laboratory coordinate system. If the position of at least three noncolinear points fixed to the body segment can be obtained (and the body segment is assumed to be rigid) then the six degrees-of-freedom associated with the position and orientation of each segment can be obtained. Initially, a body-fixed coordinate system is computed for each body segment (Figure 3-2b). For instance, consider the markers on the shank at an instant in time. A vector, S_{TZ}, can be formed from the lateral malleolus to the lateral knee marker. Another vector can be formed from the lateral malleolus to the marker on the shank wand. The vector cross-product of these two vectors is a vector S_{TX}, which is perpendicular to the plane containing all three markers. The unit vector, S_{TY}, may be determined as the vector cross-product of S_{TZ} and S_{TX}. Thus, the vectors S_{TX}, S_{TY}, and S_{TZ} form an orthogonal body fixed coordinate system, called a technical coordinate system. In a similar manner, the marker based, or technical, coordinate system may be calculated for the thigh, i.e., T_{TX}, T_{TY}, and T_{TZ}. These segments are linked and thus lack independence of movement. Hence their points of attachment, i.e., the joints, are the points of principal kinematic significance. Once the position of adjacent limb segments has been determined, it is possible to determine the relative angle between adjacent limb segments in three dimensions. This assumes that the technical coordinate systems reasonably approximate the anatomic axes of the body segments, e.g., T_{TZ} approximates along the axis of the thigh and S_{TZ} approximates the long axis of the shank. Alternatively, additional data can be collected that connects the technical coordinate system to the underlying anatomic coordinate system. This more rigorous approach adapts a subject calibration procedure to relate the technical coordinate systems with pertinent anatomic landmarks (5). The subject calibration is performed as a static trial with the subject standing. Additional markers are typically added to the medial femoral condyles and the medial malleoli during the static

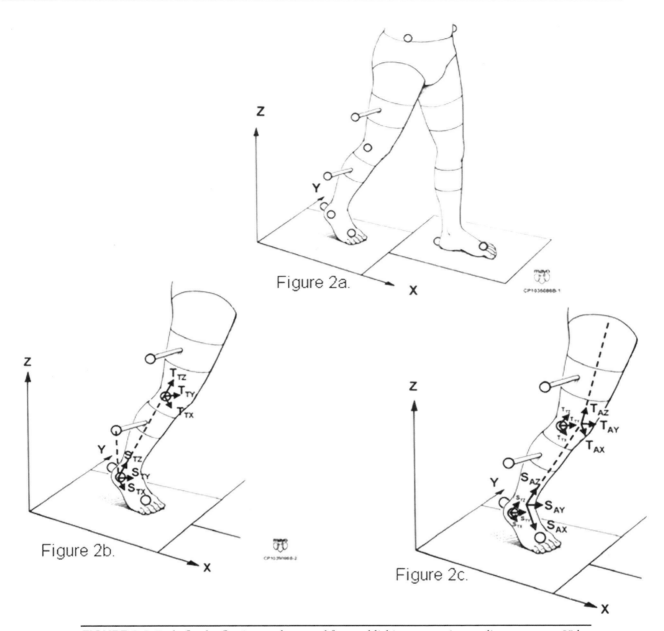

Figure 2a.

Figure 2b.

Figure 2c.

FIGURE 3-2. Body-fixed reflective markers used for establishing anatomic coordinate systems. Video camera motion measurement systems calculate the location of external markers placed on the body segments and aligned with specific bony landmarks (Fig. 3-2a). A body-fixed external coordinate system is computed from three or more markers on each body segment (Fig. 3-2b). Subsequently, a subject calibration relates the external coordinate system with an anatomic coordinate system through the identification of anatomic landmarks, e.g. the medial and lateral femoral condyles and medial and lateral malleoli (Fig. 3-2c).

calibration trial. These markers serve as anatomic references for the knee axis and ankle axis. The hip center location is estimated from markers placed on the pelvis (31). The technical coordinate system is then transformed into alignment with the anatomic coordinate system for each limb segment, e.g. S_{AX}, S_{AY}, S_{AZ} (Figure 3-2c). The marker system is coupled to a biomechanical model (15). Once the position of adjacent limb segments has been determined

(and each body segment is assumed to be rigid), it is possible to determine the relative angles between adjacent limb segments in three dimensions.

These measurements are made in three dimensions with reference to standard anatomic planes: sagittal, coronal, and transverse, utilizing embedded coordinate systems (7). Presently, there is a lack of uniformity in the human locomotion literature on the specification of the local and global coordinate systems. This lack of uniformity leads to ambiguities in the description of locomotion performance. For example, one author may describe a certain motion or joint moment positive while a second author may term the same quantity negative. Standardization is needed. Currently, the International Society of Biomechanics is attempting to address this issue.

Degrees-of-freedom is a term in mechanics that describes the ability of an object to move in space. The number of degrees-of-freedom of a system is the number of independent coordinates that must be specified to define the location and orientation of the object. A rigid body in space without any constraint has six degrees-of-freedom. This means that three coordinates of a reference point on the body are needed to specify its location, and three angles with respect to a set of reference axes are needed to specify its orientation. In reality, all anatomic joints have six degrees-of-freedom that consist of three rotations and three translations about the coordinate axes. However, if the motion of the joint is limited by anatomic constraints, the number of degrees-of-freedom is reduced. Depending on the anticipated application, various degrees of simplification have been considered for kinematic modeling of joints. The interphalangeal joints of the foot have been assumed to have one degree-of-freedom (flexion/extension). The ankle, able to rotate about two axes, can be assumed to have two degrees-of-freedom (plantar/dorsiflexion, in/eversion). The hip, able to rotate about three axes, has three degrees-of-freedom (flexion/extension, abduction/adduction, internal/external rotation).

Displacement is a change of position in space and may be either linear or angular. Displacement represents the motion that is measured. Displacements are vector quantities requiring a definition of magnitude as well as direction. Generally, three-dimensional motion of a rigid body is defined by six independent quantities, usually three translational and three rotational degrees-of-freedom. Translation, or linear displacement, is a special term that describes motion during which all points on a body or line describe parallel lines as being either straight or curved. The term, therefore, can apply to either linear or angular motions where there is no tendency for rotation. Rotation, or angular displacement, refers to an angular change in position of a line in space (or a line drawn on a body) in relation to some reference in which all points on a body or line describe circular arcs about a fixed axis or point. All limb segments undergo angular displacement during human movement. Points on the limb may also undergo linear displacement.

Given the wide range of possible types of motion, care must be taken when describing or interpreting the biomechanics of human movement. The type of movement (linear or angular), the reference frame, as well as the dimensions of the movement (degrees-of-freedom), must be defined. The motion of a rigid body may be grouped into three general categories (1) which will be described in the next section.

ANALYTICAL DESCRIPTION OF JOINT MOVEMENT

Planar Motion

A hinge joint is the simplest but most common model used to represent an anatomic joint in planar motion about a single axis embedded in a fixed segment (i.e., a single degree-of-freedom). In this case, points on the limb describe a circular path around a fixed center of rotation. The limb undergoes simple angular motion. The center of rotation is the point that has zero velocity relative to all points on the body that are rotating around it. Assume that from a motion study, the velocity (time and displacement) is known for the two points A and B on the shank (Fig. 3-3), which is behaving as a rigid body. Points A and B undergo angular displacement in space as shown by the two velocity vectors. At any instant there will be a center of rotation for the knee. Surprisingly, it is easy to find the location of the center of rotation, which need not be on the body in question. Lines are drawn perpendicular to each of the two velocity vectors. A velocity vector has no component perpendicular to itself and therefore velocity is zero along these lines. The point where the two zero velocity components intersect is the instant center of rotation. By

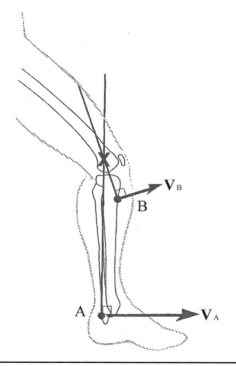

FIGURE 3-3. Determination of the instant center of rotation of the knee using the velocities of points A and B. The perpendiculars to the velocity vectors of points A and B intersect at the instant center of rotation.

definition, it has zero velocity relative to the points rotating around it.

In general planar motion, the moving limb segment can have both translation and rotation about the fixed segment. Because of the translational component of motion, the center of rotation or axis of rotation for the moving segment will change through the course of motion. At any point in time, an approximate center of rotation can be determined, which is defined as the instantaneous center of rotation (ICR). As shown in the previous example, the velocity of a point on a rigid body experiencing rotation must be perpendicular to a line joining the point and the center of rotation. This specific property can be used to determine the ICR graphically. In experimental measurements, however, it is difficult to determine the velocity of different points on a body in motion. An alternate method for approximating the ICR was described by Franz Reuleaux in 1876 (26). In this method, the instantaneous location of two points on the moving segment are identified from two consecutive positions within a short period of time, and the intersection of the bisectors of the line joining the same points at the two positions defines the ICR (Fig. 3-4). For a true hinged motion, the ICR will be a fixed point throughout

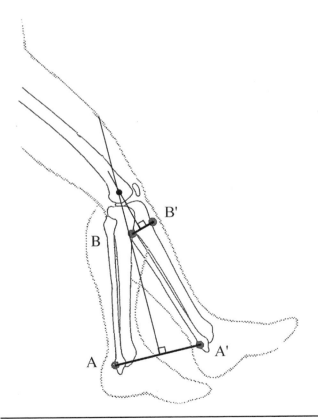

FIGURE 3-4. Determination of the instant center of rotation using Reuleaux's method. The points A and B are displaced to A′ and B′, respectively, during the rotation of the moving segment. Straight, connecting lines are drawn between A and A′, and between B and B′. Perpendicular bisectors of these displacement lines intersect at the instant center of rotation.

the movement. Otherwise, loci of the ICR or centrodes will result. In practice, determination of the ICR by the above described method is highly sensitive to error in locating the points used to define the individual ICRs. The errors increase exponentially as the individual displacements are made smaller. Conversely, increasing the displacement increments decreases the error in determining the ICR (24). However, with larger intervals, the true kinematics are not accurately reproduced.

Rotational Three-Dimensional Motion

Very commonly, when describing or modeling an anatomic joint, only the rotational motions are considered. A spherical joint is commonly used to represent a joint that allows three degrees-of-freedom in rotation. Three angles are required in order to specify the relative position between the moving and fixed segments. For finite spatial rotation, the sequence of rotation is extremely important and must be specified for a unique description of joint motion (10). For the same amount of rotation, different final orientations will result from different sequences of rotation (Fig. 3-5). However, with proper selection and definition of the axes of rotation between two bony segments, it is possible to make the finite rotation sequence independent or commutative (6,11).

The concept of Eulerian angles has been adopted in the field of orthopedic biomechanics to unify the definition of finite spatial rotation (6,11). In the selection of reference axes, one axis is fixed to the stationary segment and another axis is fixed to the moving segment (Fig. 3-6). In the knee joint, for example, the flexion-extension angle φ occurs about a mediolaterally directed axis defined by a line connecting the medial and lateral femoral condyles. The axial rotation angle ψ is measured about an axis defined by the line along the shaft of the tibia. The third axis (also defined as the floating axis) is orthogonal to the other two axes and defines abduction/adduction θ. These rotations match the Eulerian angle description and are thought to be performed in such a way as to bring the moving segment from the reference orientation into the current orientation. If a unit vector triad ($\vec{I}$, $\vec{J}$, $\vec{K}$) is attached to a fixed segment along the X, Y, Z axis and another triad ($\vec{i}$, $\vec{j}$, $\vec{k}$) is fixed to the moving segment along the x, y, z, axes, the relationship between them after any arbitrary finite rotation can be expressed by a rotational matrix in terms of the Eulerian angles ϕ, ψ, θ.

$$\begin{bmatrix} i \\ j \\ k \end{bmatrix} = \begin{bmatrix} c\psi \cdot c\phi + s\psi \cdot s\theta \cdot s\phi & s\psi \cdot c\theta & -c\psi \cdot s\phi + s\psi \cdot s\theta \cdot c\phi \\ -s\psi \cdot c\phi + c\psi \cdot s\theta \cdot s\phi & c\psi \cdot c\theta & s\psi \cdot s\phi + c\psi \cdot s\theta \cdot c\phi \\ c\theta \cdot s\phi & -s\theta & c\theta \cdot c\phi \end{bmatrix} \begin{bmatrix} I \\ J \\ K \end{bmatrix}$$

Where s and c stand for sine and cosine, respectively. The Eulerian angles can be calculated based on the known orientation of these unit vector triads attached to the proximal and distal body segments.

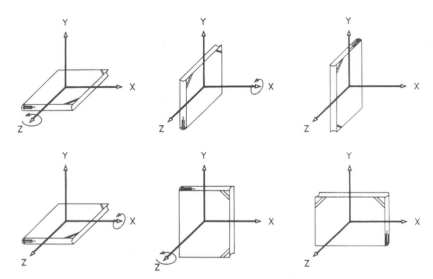

FIGURE 3-5. The sequence of rigid body rotation is extremely important. For the same amount of rotation different final orientations will result from different sequences of rotation.

The advantage of using this system for description of the spatial rotation of anatomic joints is that the angular rotations do not have to be referred back to the neutral position of the joint because the rotation sequence can be independent, and the measurement can be easily related to anatomic structures (6,11). However, it is important to recognize that two of the rotational axes in the system are nonorthogonal when the joint departs from its neutral position. Consequently, the system is difficult to use in kinetic analysis. Angular velocity and acceleration have to be transformed into a set of inertial axes in terms of the Eulerian angles defined (17). Another disadvantage is the "gimbal lock" situation (6) when the first and third (embedded) rotation axes are parallel. In this situation, if the angles are inexact because of noisy measurements, strong nonorthogonality will result in highly correlated, large errors in the rotational angles of the embedded axes (37). This problem can be resolved by selecting the proper axis of rotation or by using special mathematical manipulation (23).

Generalized Six Degree-of-Freedom Joint Motion

For a more general unconstrained movement in 3-D space, three translations and three rotations are required to describe the joint motion. The displacement of a rigid body may take place along any one of an infinite number of paths. It is convenient to describe the displacement in terms of the simplest motion that can produce it. The most commonly used analytical method for the description of six degree-of-freedom displacement of a rigid body is the screw displacement axis (SDA) (19,20,28,36). This is Chaslés' Theorem (8). The motion of the moving segment from one position to another can be defined in terms of a

$$\bar{r}_1 = [T]\,\bar{\rho} + \bar{r}_0$$

where

$$[T] = [T_\psi]\,[T_\theta]\,[T_\phi]$$

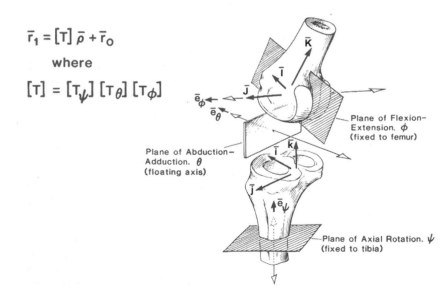

FIGURE 3-6. Description of knee joint motion using the Eulerian angle system. The axis fixed to the distal femur defines the flexion/extension motion, φ. The axis fixed to the proximal tibia along its anatomic axis defines internal-external rotation, ψ. The floating axis is orthogonal to the other two axes and is used to measure abduction-adduction, θ.

$$\bar{r}_{p_2} = [\mathrm{T}]\,\bar{r}_{p_1} + \bar{d}$$

also

$$\bar{r}_{p_2} = \bar{r}_{p_1} + t\bar{\rho} + \Delta\bar{r}$$

where

$$\Delta\bar{r} = (1 - \cos\Phi)(\bar{\rho} \times (\bar{\rho} \times \bar{r})) + \sin\Phi\,(\bar{\rho} \times \bar{r})$$

$$\bar{r} = \bar{r}_{p_1} - \bar{s}$$

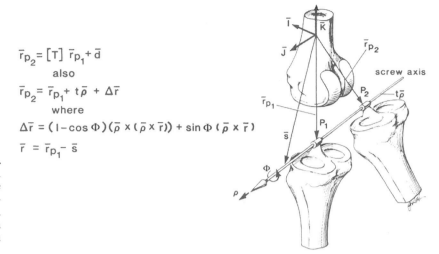

FIGURE 3-7. The screw displacement axis can be used to describe general spatial motion. The tibia moves from position 1 to position 2 by rotation about the screw axis by an amount ϕ and by translating along the screw axis, ρ, by an amount τ. (Reproduced with permission from Mayo Clinic.)

simultaneous rotation Φ around and a translation t along a unique axis, called a screw displacement axis, which is located in the fixed segment (Fig. 3-7). Four additional parameters are required to completely describe the displacement of the moving body. These additional parameters are the inclination and location of the SDA. The screw displacement axis is a true vector quantity. Its magnitude can be decomposed along any coordinate axes used for the analysis. However, the amount of the finite screw rotation is not a vector quantity and the decomposition of it must be carefully interpreted because of the noncommutative nature of finite rotation. Woltring (16) recommended that the component rotations (flexion/extension, abduction/adduction, endo-/exorotation) can be defined as components of the product $\Phi = \Phi\,\rho$, where ρ is the screw axis unit direction vector.

The orientation of the SDA and screw rotation is based on a rotational matrix used to define the location of reference points with respect to a coordinate system after finite rotation. This rotational matrix can be expressed in terms of directional cosines between the coordinate axes before and after rotation or in terms of Eulerian angles. For the SDA, if the direction angles for the SDA are u_x, u_y, u_z letting Φ be the screw rotation, the rotation matrix [R] can also be derived (18).

$$R = \begin{bmatrix} (u_x^2\,\text{vers}\,\Phi + \cos\Phi) & (u_x u_y\,\text{vers}\,\Phi - u_z\sin\Phi) & (u_x u_z\,\text{vers}\,\Phi + u_y\sin\Phi) \\ (u_x u_y\,\text{vers}\,\Phi + u_z\sin\Phi) & (u_y^2\,\text{vers}\,\Phi + \cos\Phi) & (u_y u_z\,\text{vers}\,\Phi + u_x\sin\Phi) \\ (u_z u_x\,\text{vers}\,\Phi - u_y\sin\Phi) & (u_y u_z\,\text{vers}\,\Phi + u_x\sin\Phi) & (u_z^2\,\text{vers}\,\Phi + \cos\Phi) \end{bmatrix}$$

Where vers $\Phi = 1 - \cos\Phi$. The screw rotation Φ may be found from the trace of the matrix $[R]$

$$\Phi = \cos^{-1}\{(\text{tr}[R] - 1)/2\}$$

With Φ known, the components for the orientation of the screw axis can be calculated. From the translation vector, which can be obtained by comparing the position vectors of the reference points on the moving body, the amount

of translation along the SDA and the position vector of a point on the SDA can be calculated.

There are several advantages of using the screw displacement axis. First, the orientation of the screw axis remains invariant, regardless of the reference coordinate axis used. Second, the gimbal lock situation can be avoided when using the SDA approach (30). Third, the SDA can be decomposed into orthogonal axes, which may be better suited for decomposing other vectorial entities such as force and moment vectors (37). Unfortunately, just like determination of the center of rotation for planar motion, determination of the screw displacement axis is highly sensitive to measurement error as well. The ratio of error increases exponentially with decreasing displacement (20). In practice, use of more than three reference points on the moving segment helps to minimize experimental error. Implementation of these procedures for defining a screw displacement axis description of human body movement has been explored in the literature (28).

GAIT EVENTS

A gait cycle is defined in terms of an interval of *time* during which one sequence of regularly recurring succession of *events* is completed. During free speed (self selected), walking a cycle of repeated events has been consistently observed. These events are simply 1) foot strike and 2) foot-off (30). Since there are two extremities, there are four events: *foot strike (FS)*, *opposite foot-off (OFO)*, *opposite foot strike (OFS)*, and *foot-off (FO)*. Typically, initial foot contact is at the heel, but in pathologic gait other areas of the foot may strike first (i.e., toe walkers). Hence the term foot strike is used instead of heel strike. Similar reasoning applies to using the term foot-off rather than toe-off. The entire cycle repeats itself with the second foot strike (Fig. 3-8). The two phases (stance and swing) and most of the periods of the

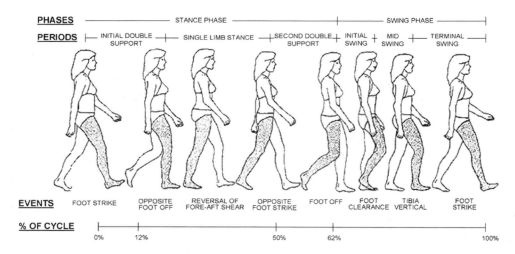

FIGURE 3-8. Normal walk cycle illustrating the events of gait.

basic gait cycle can be described in reference to these basic repeated events (30,34). Today, the commonly accepted convention is to describe the cycle in terms of percentage, rather than the time elapsed, as we have observed that the events occur in a remarkably similar sequence and are independent of time, thus allowing normalization of the data for multiple subjects. Therefore, initial foot strike is designated as 0% and the second ipsilateral foot strike as 100% (0%–100%). Furthermore, in normal subjects, the opposite limb repeats the same sequence of events, but is 180 degrees out of phase so that opposite foot strike = 50% and the second opposite foot strike = 150% of the gait cycle.

The phases of the basic walking cycle are simple: the *stance phase* is defined by the percentage of the cycle when the foot is in contact with the ground and the *swing phase* by the time when the foot is in the air. The four basic events of gait define these phases (30). Stance phase comprises the period between foot strike (0%) and ipsilateral foot-

off (62%). Swing phase starts a foot off (62%) and ends at second ipsilateral foot strike (100%) (see Fig. 3-8).

The major subdivisions of the cycle/phases (Table 3-1) describe the transitions that have to occur while the body's center of mass passes over the oscillating limbs. Stance phase is commonly divided into three periods: 1) *initial double limb support* (foot strike to opposite foot-off), 2) *single limb support* (opposite foot-off to opposite foot strike), and 3) *second double limb support* (opposite foot strike to foot-off). These periods are again defined by their respective events of gait. Swing phase can also be subdivided into three periods: 1) *initial swing* (foot-off to foot clearance), 2) *mid swing* (foot clearance to tibia vertical), and 3) *terminal swing* (tibia vertical to foot strike). It is important to recognize that, from the standpoint of function, second double support (preswing) prepares the limb for swing. The average cycle consists of 62% stance phase and 38% swing phase. Swing time is identical with the time of contralateral single limb stance.

▶ **TABLE 3-1 Gait Cycle: Events, Periods, and Phases**

Event	% Gait Cycle	Period	Phase
Footstrike	0		
		Initial double limb support	
Opposite foot-off	12		Stance, 62% of cycle
		Single limb support	
Opposite foot strike	50		
		Second double limb support	
Foot-off	62		
		Initial swing	
Foot clearance	75		
		Mid swing	Swing, 38% of cycle
Tibia vertical	85		
		Terminal swing	
Second foot strike	100		

▶ TABLE 3-2 Gait Cycle: Periods and Functions

Period	% Cycle	Function	Contralateral Limb
1. Initial double limb support	0–12%	Loading, weight transfer	Unloading and preparing for swing (preswing)
2. Single limb support	12–50	Support of entire body weight; center of mass moving forward	Swing
3. Second double limb support	50–62	Unloading and preparing for swing (preswing)	Loading, weight transfer
4. Initial swing	62–75	Foot clearance	Single limb support
5. Mid swing	75–85	Limb advances in front of body	Single limb support
6. Terminal swing	85–100	Limb deceleration, preparation for weight transfer	Single limb support

Initial double limb support (Table 3-2) is characterized by a very rapid loading onto the forward limb with shock absorption and slowing of the body's forward momentum. The foot usually progresses to foot flat, and the knee acts as a shock absorber (see specific sagittal motion curves for more discussion). After opposite foot-off, the opposite leg is in swing, and the weight-bearing limb is in single limb stance. As the body passes over the fixed foot, the center of mass rises to its peak while both forward and vertical velocity decrease. Forward shear then reverses to aft shear, the center of mass falls, and forward and vertical velocity increase. This transition from fore to aft shear occurs around 30% of the cycle (mid stance in normal subjects). It is very difficult to determine this transition point precisely in the walking cycle without a laboratory environment, while the other events are clearly observable. Once this peak in elevation of the center of mass is achieved, the center of mass falls until the end of single limb stance at opposite foot strike (50% of the cycle). Second double limb support (opposite foot strike to foot-off) is also defined as preswing. As

weight is transferred rapidly to the forward limb, the trailing limb is ending its extension movement in preparation to swing forward in front of the body. The preparation for swing limb acceleration actually occurs during the period of second double limb support. At this time, the leg must be flexed at the knee and hip and plantar flexed at the ankle to prepare for "toe off".

The subdivision of swing phase can best be understood by comparing the leg to a compound pendulum. Such a pendulum is able to change its period through the action of muscles and hence the cadence of walking (9,22). The duration of swing is determined by the mass moment of inertia of the parts (body segments) and their configuration in space (12). The critical event of foot clearance occurs around 75% of the cycle when the swinging limb passes the standing limb. The time when the tibia becomes perpendicular to the floor heralds the beginning of limb deceleration.

Terminology has developed to describe the linear measurement parameters of the gait cycle (Fig. 3-9) (34).

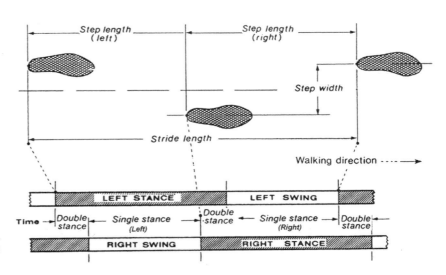

FIGURE 3-9. Linear distance measurements of the gait cycle.

▶ **TABLE 3-3 Age-Related Temporal-Distance Factors**

Age (yr)	Velocity (cm/sec)	Cadence (steps/min)	Opposite Toe-Off (% of cycle)	Duration of Stance (%)	Duration of Swing (%)	Stride Length (cm)
1	64	176	17.5	67.3	33.4	43.0
1.5	71	171	17.5	67.6	33.4	4935
2	72	156	16.7	66.8	34.2	54.9
2.5	81	156	153.5	65.7	35.3	61.8
3	86	154	15.5	65.5	35.5	66.8
4	100	152	14.2	63.7	37.3	77.9
5	108	154	13.4	63.5	37.5	84.3
6	109	146	13.4	63.6	37.4	89.3
7	114	143	12.4	62.4	38.6	96.5
20–25	153	115	9.0	60.0	41.0	158.8
30–35	145	111	11.0	61.0	39.0	156.9
40–45	159	122	11.0	61.0	39.0	155.9
50–55	155	118	10.0	60.0	40.0	157.9
60–65	147	115	11.0	61.0	39.0	153.0

Cadence is defined as the number of steps in a standard time frame (steps/minute). *Step length* is defined by the distance (in centimeters) between the same point on each foot (usually the heel), during double limb support. Right step length refers to the distance from the right heel to the left heel. The converse is true for left step length. *Stride length* is defined by the distance (in centimeters) traveled between two successive foot strikes of the same foot. Therefore, each stride is composed of one right and one left step length (measured in centimeters). *Walking speed* is the average speed attained after approximately three steps (rhythmic stage) expressed in distance covered per unit of time (cm/sec or m/minute).

It should be emphasized that these parameters of the human gait cycle are comparable only when limited to free speed walking on level ground. The temporal distance parameters vary with age (Table 3-3). Therefore, age-matched normal controls are required when comparing with children or older adults. Introducing other variables such as fixed slow/fast walking velocities, ramps, stairs, or even neurologic immaturity can change these relationships markedly and make comparison with normal data difficult or impossible.

maturation. Initial heel strike, reciprocal arm/leg swing, and initial knee flexion wave were present in the majority of normal 2-year-old children. Maturation of the dynamic joint angles was well-established between 3 and 4 years of age (4). Five important determinates of mature gait were: 1) duration of single limb stance, 2) walking speed, 3) cadence, 4) step length, and 5) the ratio of pelvic spread to ankle spread. The ability to walk seemed to depend primarily on motor control system maturation. Myelination is an important element of this process (32). In children aged 1 to 7 years there was a linear relationship between step length and leg length (Fig. 3-10). There was also a linear relationship between age and walking speed; however, the slope changed around 4 years of age due to a change in the rate of growth (Fig. 3-11). Even though the pattern of mature walking was well-established between 3 and 4 years of age, growth changes continue throughout puberty. The body's increase in stature continues to influence the temporal/distance factors of step length, walking speed (increases) and cadence (decreases). The temporal/distance parameters stabilize by age 20 and remain largely unchanged throughout most of adult life (see Table 3-3 and Chapter 8 for more details).

GAIT MATURATION

An extensive study of gait maturation has been performed (31,32) and is reviewed in Chapter 7. The joint angle rotations of 415 children aged 1 to 7 years were measured in the sagittal, coronal, and transverse planes. When the joint angles were grouped by age, they were remarkably similar during free speed walking, although they showed evidence of age-related gait

MOTION CURVES

The gait kinematics described here are associated with a group of twenty adult subjects (9 males and 11 females) evaluated at Mayo Clinic. Subjects range in age from 20 to 42 years and had a mean age of 30 years (± 8). Their mean weight was 75 kg (± 17) and their mean height was 173 cm (± 11). These individuals had normal strength, full range of motion of the lower extremities, no neurologic deficits,

STEP LENGTH vs. LEG LENGTH

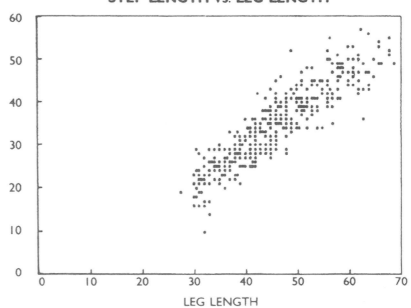

FIGURE 3-10. Scatter plot showing linear relationship between step length and leg length of subjects aged 1–7 years. (From Sutherland DH, Olshen RA, Biden EN, Wyatt MP. *The development of mature walking.* London: MacKeith Press; 1988:57.)

no arthritis, and no previous major lower extremity joint surgery. The subjects walked at a self-selected speed (117 ± 14 cm/sec). The user is referred to Kaufman et al. (16) for a description of the methods used in the data collection. Description of the lower extremity motion is typically reported using Eulerian angles. The 3-D motion of the pelvis, hip, knee, and angle is commonly available using current technology. In order to remember these curves, we have found it useful to break down each curve into separate recognizable segments and emphasize certain *key points* when teaching this material to other colleagues.

SAGITTAL PLANE (SIDE VIEW)

The sagittal plane measurements are probably the most commonly studied, best understood, and most accurately reproduced.

Anterior Pelvic Tilt

The sagittal movements of the pelvis are controlled by gravity, inertia, and the action of the hip flexor and extensor muscles (Fig. 3-12). The role of the thoracopelvic muscles has produced speculation, but objective data

WALKING VELOCITY (CM/SEC.)

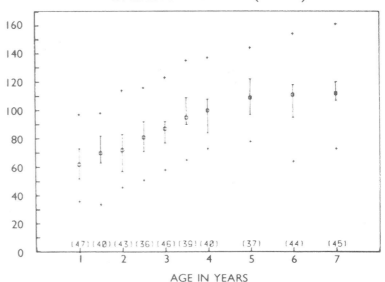

FIGURE 3-11. The lines in the center connect the 25th, 50th, and 75th percentiles. The dots represent minimal and maximal values. (From Sutherland DH, Olshen RA, Biden EN, Wyatt MP. *The development of mature walking.* London: MacKeith Press; 1988:57.)

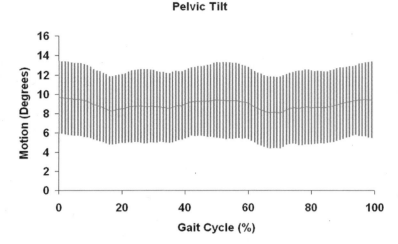

FIGURE 3-12. Sagittal movements of the pelvis (anterior pelvic tilt represented by all values above the zero axis).

relative to their contribution are not available. The center of gravity is within the pelvis when the body is in the anatomic (upright) position; however, dynamic postural changes can alter the location of the center of mass. It is therefore necessary, under dynamic conditions, to calculate the position of the center of mass rather than ascribe it to an anatomic location. The pelvis is inclined forward (anterior) or flexed and moves in a sinusoidal manner with two peaks and two valleys. The pelvis is most horizontal (least amount of tilt) at foot-off and opposite foot-off, with maximum flexion occurring in mid- to late stance and terminal swing. The curve is very similar to the sagittal curve of the body center of mass (Figure 3-13) but lags behind it. Forward pelvic tilt decreases during the period of loading (first and second double limb support) and the increases while the body's center of mass passes over the fixed foot (mid-stance and terminal swing). The tilt begins to flatten once again as the body center of mass is decelerated during late single limb stance (following heel rise).

KEY POINTS

✔ Pelvic tilt oscillates like body center of mass
✔ Flattest (least tilt at end of double limb support)

Hip Flexion/Extension

The sagittal plane motion is very simple and can be seen to be a single, sinusoidal curve (Fig. 3-14). One leg progresses forward in order to advance the body while the other remains behind to support the body. The hip is flexed at initial contact and extends until opposite foot contact. As soon as the opposite foot strikes the ground, weight is transferred to the forward limb, and the trailing leg begins to flex at the knee and hip, while pivoting on the forefoot.

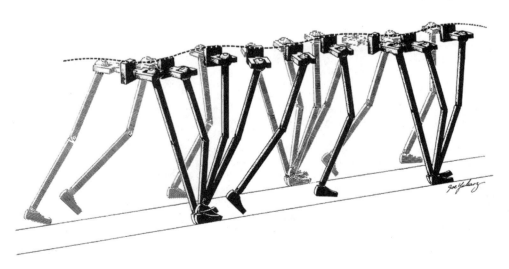

FIGURE 3-13. Sagittal curve of the body center of mass. (From Saunders JB, Enmanm VT, Eberhart HD. The major determinants in normal and pathological gait. *J Bone Joint Surg* 1953; 35A:544–553.)

Hip Flexion

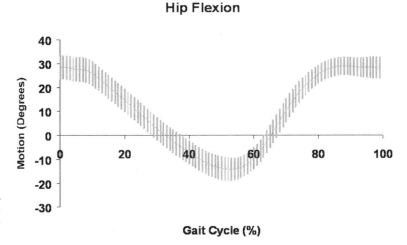

FIGURE 3-14. Normal hip flexion-extension. A positive value indicates hip flexion and a negative value indicates hip extension.

Preswing is synonymous with second double limb support and describes this period. It is followed by slight extension just before foot strike. The hip extensor muscles decelerate the thigh and diminish the hip flexion in preparation for weight acceptance.

Knee Flexion/Extension

The sagittal motion of the knee is known as the knee flexion and extension curve (Fig. 3-15). This motion curve can be described as two flexion waves, each starting in relative extension, progressing into flexion, then returning again to the starting point in extension. The first flexion wave, or stance phase knee flexion, acts as a shock absorber to aid in weight acceptance. This curve peaks in early stance at opposite foot-off. The mechanical source for this shock absorber is the eccentrically contracting quadriceps muscles, which are active until the ground reaction force line pro-

gresses anterior to the knee, creating an extension force and bringing the knee joint back into extension by mid stance. It should be noted that this passive extension cannot occur without the strong eccentric contraction of the plantar flexors restraining the shank from progressive forward rotation (29,33). The second flexion wave is necessary in order to clear the foot in early swing phase. Flexion at the knee actually precedes the onset of hip flexion at opposite foot strike. The knee is rapidly flexed beginning just after heel rise to a maximum in swing phase just as the swinging foot passes the opposite limb. This flexion effectively shortens the limb allowing for foot clearance of the swinging limb to prevent foot dragging. The knee joint is then rapidly extended by a combination of inertial force of the compound inverted pendulum (thigh and shank), and the activity of the gluteus maximus, hamstrings, and quadriceps muscles. Nearly full extension is achieved just prior to foot strike.

Knee Flexion

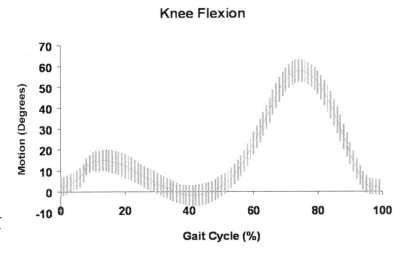

FIGURE 3-15. Normal knee flexion-extension. A positive value indicates knee flexion.

KEY POINTS

✔ *First flexion wave: shock absorber*

✔ *Second flexion wave: foot clearance*

Ankle Plantar Flexion/Dorsiflexion

This is the most complex of the sagittal curves and can be broken down into four separate functional segments (Fig. 3-16).

This first segment occurs between foot strike and opposite foot-off. The ankle is positioned at approximately neutral when foot strike occurs (normally heel first), and the position of the ground reaction force posterior to the ankle center causes plantar flexion until foot flat is achieved, prior to opposite foot-off. This portion of the ankle motion curve is also known as the first rocker (25).

The second segment occurs during single limb stance (between the events of opposite foot-off and opposite foot strike). It is typically convex superiorly and reflects the body passing over the fixed flat foot (second rocker) (25). Toward the end of the single limb stance, at approximately 40% of the cycle, the heel begins to rise as the plantar flexors increase their force of contraction and act concentrically (29,33). This is also known as the third rocker. At opposite foot strike the ankle has lost some dorsiflexion but has not returned to neutral.

The third segment continues with opposite foot strike and ends with foot-off. Rapid plantar flexion occurs to a maximum of 20 to 25 degrees just as the foot is lifted off the ground. Some individuals confuse this period with the period of acceleration of the ankle (actually heel rise) due to the concentric action of the plantar flexors. This association would require simultaneous muscle activity and plantar flexion movement, but electromyography has consistently shown that the plantar flexors are silent after opposite foot strike (29,33). The transfer of weight to the

opposite limb occurs very rapidly, and the plantar flexion movement occurring after opposite foot strike is passive. This movement may be entirely due to gravity and inertia or there may be passive tension in the plantar flexors after cessation of the electromyographic signal.

The fourth segment is rapid ankle dorsiflexion. The timing of this swing phase movement is found to coincide with the maximum foot clearance effort and also with the second knee flexion wave. Hence this segment is functionally connected to foot clearance. The ankle is maintained in this neutral position by isometric contraction of the anterior compartment muscles until foot strike when these same muscles are again needed to eccentrically restrain the plantar flexion that repeats the first segment of the cycle.

KEY POINTS

✔ Foot flat occurs in initial double support

✔ Single limb stance contains, in sequence, progressive dorsiflexion, and reversal of movement towards plantar flexion (due to eccentric then concentric action of the plantar flexors muscles)

✔ Second double support (preswing), ends in foot-off and is passive with respect to the plantar flexor muscles

✔ Limb shortening to clear the foot begins at foot-off and peaks during swing when the swinging ankle passes the supporting ankle

CORONAL PLANE (FRONT VIEW)

Pelvic Obliquity

Pelvic obliquity can be viewed with respect to each lower extremity or with both together (Fig. 3-17). Although the same motion curve is associated with the movements of both lower extremities, it is necessary to correlate pelvic

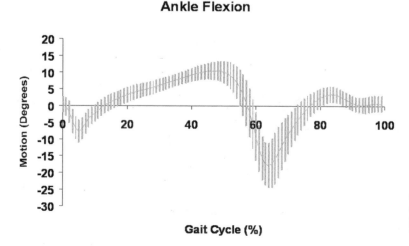

Ankle Flexion

FIGURE 3-16. Normal ankle plantar-dorsiflexion. A positive value indicates dorsiflexion and a negative value indicates plantarflexion.

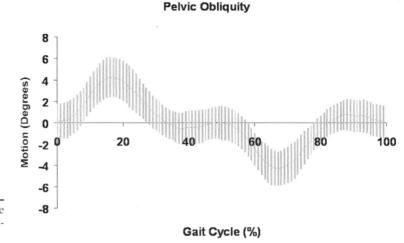

FIGURE 3-17. Normal pelvic obliquity. A positive value indicates that the pelvis is higher on the ipsilateral side than on the contralateral side.

obliquity functionally with the movement of both sides of the pelvis. We find it easier to understand the motion curve when we study the events and motion measurements of one side at a time rather than with both together. The key functional correlation is to remember that the motion classically described by Trendelenburg (35) is normal. The *contralateral* pelvis normally drops in early stance phase, and a rise or positive curve is produced ipsilaterally, where the measurement is referenced. In Trendelenburg gait the contralateral pelvic drop is excessive. In normal subjects, the pelvic obliquity peak occurs just after opposite foot-off, corresponding with early single limb stance. There is a small secondary rise during the acceleration period of single stance phase and then the pattern inversely duplicates itself, beginning at opposite foot strike as the opposite leg repeats the same functional tasks. The rise in the ipsilateral pelvis functionally shortens the limb and acts like a shock absorber for the body center of mass, decreasing the required vertical translation needed to pass over the fixed foot.

KEY POINTS

✔ Some drop of the contralateral pelvis during stance is normal (in Trendelenburg gait the drop is excessive)

✔ Pelvic obliquity serves as a shock absorber and limb length adjustment

HIP ABDUCTION/ADDUCTION

In normal subjects, the hip abduction/adduction curve (Fig. 3-18) is remarkably similar to the pelvic obliquity curve (Fig. 3-17). This makes perfect sense. Since the foot is basically fixed to the floor, there is very little coronal plane motion at the ankle or knee, and the pelvis is acting as a shock absorber. The hip abduction/adduction wave gives the coronal plane dynamic alignment of the thigh with respect to the pelvis. The hip, which is neutral at foot strike, rapidly adducts during first double support and rapidly abducts during second double support. In swing phase, the hip adducts from near maximum

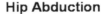

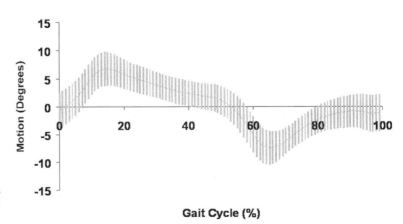

FIGURE 3-18. Normal hip abduction (AB)/adduction. A positive value indicates hip adduction.

Pelvic Rotation

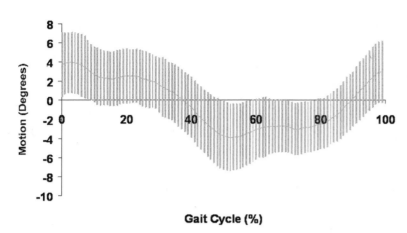

FIGURE 3-19. Normal pelvic rotation. A positive value indicates internal pelvic rotation.

abduction at toe off to a neutral or perpendicular position relative to the pelvis just before foot strike. There is no abduction motion during swing phase, which implies that there is no circumduction occurring in normal subjects.

KEY POINTS

✔ Similar to pelvic obliquity in normal subject
✔ Adduction peaks at opposite foot-off
✔ Maximum abduction at toe-off
✔ Relative adduction in swing phase

TRANSVERSE PLANE (AXIAL VIEW)

Pelvic Rotation

This curve reports movement of the pelvis with respect to the laboratory coordinates (Fig. 3-19). The motion is a single sinusoidal curve with the peak at foot strike and a minimum at opposite foot strike (50%). Initially, the pelvis is internally rotated and it externally rotates until opposite foot strike when it begins to internally rotate again. Functionally, this curve is closely related to the sagittal plane hip flexion and extension curve. Both pelvic rotation and hip flexion serve to effectively lengthen the limb and increase stride length.

KEY POINTS

✔ Single sinusoidal curve similar to hip flexion/extension
✔ Maximum internal rotation at foot strike
✔ Maximal external rotation at opposite foot strike

Hip Rotation

Hip rotation describes the motion of the femur with respect to the pelvis (Fig. 3-20). Internal rotation of the hip begins in late swing phase and continues through stance

Hip Rotation

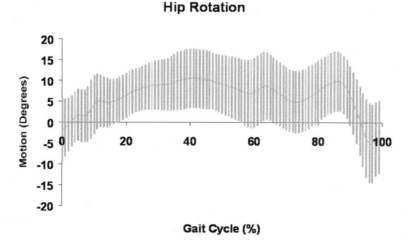

FIGURE 3-20. Normal hip rotation. A positive value indicates internal hip rotation.

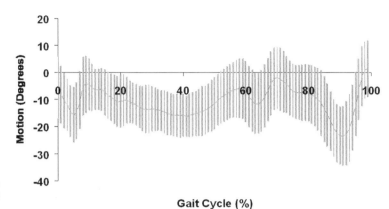

FIGURE 3-21. Normal knee rotation. A positive value indicates internal knee rotation.

to opposite foot strike. The hip then externally rotates until late swing, completing one sinusoidal motion curve. Hip rotation changes direction from internal to external in late stance phase.

KEY POINTS

✔ Sinusoidal curve
✔ Peak internal rotation coincides with opposite foot strike
✔ External rotation in swing

Knee Rotation

The shank is closely coupled to the fixed foot and the obliquely oriented mitre-hinge apparatus of the subtalar joint (Fig. 3-21) (14). Pronation of the hind foot produces obligatory internal rotation of the shank while supination causes external rotation (14). At foot strike the tibia is in neutral rotation in relation to the laboratory coordinates, and the foot (heel) is in supination. As loading occurs

(first rocker) and the foot transitions to foot flat, the hind foot and mid foot must pronate to accommodate the walking surface, producing a coupled internal torsion of the shank, reaching a maximum at opposite toe-off. The shank begins to externally rotate slowly in early single limb support and increases as the plantar flexors increase their effort, thereby causing heel rise. The hind foot then moves into supination and stiffens the ankle joint, while the knee internally rotates until foot-off.

KEY POINTS

✔ Internal rotation during pronation
✔ External rotation during supination

Foot Progression Angle

This measurement is made with respect to the laboratory coordinate frame (Fig. 3-22). It describes the position of the foot with respect to the line of walking progression.

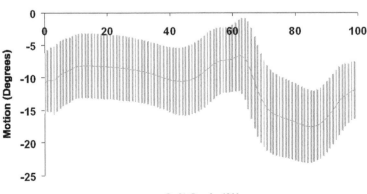

FIGURE 3-22. Normal foot progression. The negative values indicate that the long axis of the foot is externally rotated with respect to the line of progression.

This measurement is closely related to clinical observations and is of great clinical importance. The first segment of the curve shows a relatively constant amount of external rotation. During single limb support the foot externally rotates further as the opposite limb advances during swing. Between the event of opposite foot strike and foot-off (the period of second double support), there is an internal rotation movement. Beginning at foot-off, the foot is rotated externally as it simultaneously dorsiflexes to clear the foot during swing phase. In late swing the foot internally rotates as it prepares for foot contact.

KEY POINTS

✔ Foot rotation remains in external rotation throughout entire gait cycle

✔ Further external rotation during single limb support as opposite limb is advanced in swing

✔ Small internal rotation during second double support (third rocker)

✔ External rotation in initial swing

✔ Internal rotation in terminal swing

The motion curves that we have described are in clinical use in gait laboratories, and provide an important basis for clinical assessment. They do not replace dynamic electromyographic or force studies. It is necessary to use all three types of measurements to arrive at a robust knowledge of the causal factors in abnormal gait.

SUMMARY

The study of movements in human walking has produced rich information that lays the cornerstone for kinetic analysis. Most of the early clinically oriented gait literature emphasized sagittal motion; however, coronal plane and transverse plane movements are now being used with equal importance as better analytic methods and improved technology have evolved. Clinicians who provide treatment to patients with gait disorders expect high quality biomechanical analyses to result from gait laboratory referrals. If this expectation is to be met, accurate and meaningful movement measurements must form the foundation for clinical analysis and treatment plans. All clinicians who treat patients with disorders of walking should become familiar with at least the rudiments of the scientific basis of gait analysis. This is essential if they are to use appropriate biomechanical principles in treatment planning and post-treatment evaluation. Gait laboratory physicians have a particular responsibility for meeting this challenge because of their prominent role in the treatment of patients with musculoskeletal disorders.

ACKNOWLEDGMENT

We gratefully acknowledge Barbara Iverson-Literski for her careful preparation of this manuscript.

REFERENCES

1. An KN, Chao EY. Kinematic analysis of human movement. *Ann Biomed Eng* 1984;12:585–597.
2. Basmajian JV. The human bicycle: an ultimate biological convenience. *Orthop Clin North Am*, 1976;7:1027–1029.
3. Bell AL, Pederson DR, Brand RA, Prediction of hip joint center location from external landmarks. *Hum Move Sci* 1989;8:3–16.
4. Biafore S, Cottrell G, Focht LM, et al. Neural network analysis of gait dynamics. In: *Transactions of the Orthopaedic Research Society;* 1991.
5. Cappozzo A, Catani F, Croce UD, et al., Position and orientation in space of bones during movement: Anatomic frame definition and determination. *Clin Biomech* 1995;10:171–178.
6. Chao EYS. Justification of triaxial goniometer for the measurement of joint rotation. *J Biomech* 1980;13:989–1006.
7. Chao E. Justification of triaxial electrogoniometer for the measurement of joint rotation. *J Biomech* 1980;13:987–1006.
8. Chasles M. Bulletin de la Universite des Sciences (Ferussac). 1830;XIV:321.
9. Gage JR. An overview of normal walking. *Instructional Course Lectures* 1990;39:291–303.
10. Goldstein H. *Classical Mechanics*. Reading, MA: Addison-Wesley; 1959.
11. Grood E, Suntay W. A joint coordinate system for the clinical description of three-dimensional motions: Applications to the knee. *J Biomech Eng* 1983;105:136–143.
12. Hicks R, Tashman S, Cary JM, et al. Swing phase control with knee friction in juvenile amputees. *J Orthop Res* 1985;3:198–201.
13. Inman VT. *The Joints of the Ankle*. Baltimore: Williams and Wilkins, 1976.
14. Inman VT. Ralston HJ, Todd F. *Human Walking*. Baltimore, Williams & Wilkins; 1981.
15. Kadaba MP, Ramakrishnan HK, Wootten ME. Measurement of lower extremity kinematics during level walking. *J Orthop Res* 1990;8:383–392.
16. Kaufman K, Hughes C, Morrey B, et al. Gait characteristics of patients with knee osteoarthritis. *J Biomech* 2001;34:907–915.
17. Kaufman KR, An KN, Chao EY. A comparison of intersegmental joint dynamics to isokinetic dynamometer measurements. *J Biomech* 1995;28:1243–1256.
18. Kinzel GL, Hall AS, Jr, Hillberry BM. Measurement of the total motion between two body segments. I. Analytical development. *J Biomech* 1972;5:93–105.
19. Kinzel GL, Hillberry BM, Hall AS, Jr, et al. Measurement of the total motion between two body segments. II. Description of application. *J Biomech* 1972;5:283–293.
20. Kinzel GL. On the design of instrumented linkages for the measurement of relative motion between two rigid bodies, in *Ph.D. Thesis*. West Lafayette, IN: Purdue University, 1973.
21. Lettre C, Contini R. *Accelerographic analysis of pathological gait*. New York University School of Engineering and Science Technical Report 1368-01. New York, 1967.
22. Mena D, Mansour JM, Simon SR. Analysis and synthesis of human swing leg motion during gait and its clinical applications. *J Biomech* 1981;14:823–832.
23. Mital NK. Computation of rigid body rotation in three-dimensional space from body-fixed acceleration measurements, in *Ph.D. Thesis*. Detroit: Wayne State University, 1978.
24. Panjabi MM. Centers and angles of rotation of body joints: a study of errors and optimization. *J Biomech* 1979;12:911–920.
25. Perry J. *Gait Analysis: Normal and Pathological Function*. Thorofare, NJ: Slack; 1992.

26. Reuleaux F. *The kinematics of machinery: Outline of a theory of machines.* London; 1876.
27. Saunders JB, Inman VT, Eberhart HD. The major determinants in normal and pathological gait. *J Bone Joint Surg Am* 1953:35A: 543.
28. Spoor C, Veldpaus F. Rigid body motion calculated from spatial coordinates of markers. *J Biomech* 1980;13:391–393.
29. Sutherland DH, Cooper L, Daniel D. The role of the ankle plantar flexors in normal walking. *J Bone Joint Surg Am,* 1980;62:354–363.
30. Sutherland DH, Cooper L. The events of gait. *Bulletin of Prosthetic Research* 1981;10–35:281–282.
31. Sutherland DH, Olshen R, Cooper L, et al. The development of mature gait. *J Bone Joint Surg Am* 1980;62:336–353.
32. Sutherland DH, Olshen RA, Biden EN, et al. *The Development of Mature Walking.* Oxford, England: Mac Keith Press; 1988.
33. Sutherland DH. An electromyographic study of the plantar flexors of the ankle in normal walking on the level. *J Bone Joint Surg Am* 1966;48:66–71.
34. Sutherland DH. *Gait Disorders in Childhood and Adolescence.* Baltimore: Williams & Wilkins; 1984.
35. Trendelenburg FV. *Deutsche mechanische Wochenschrift.* 1924;2: 21–24.
36. Woltring HJ, Huiskes R, Lange DA, et al. Finite centroid and helical axis estimation from noisy landmark measurements in the study of human joint kinematics. *J Biomech* 1985;18:379–389.
37. Woltring HJ. Analytical body-segment photogrammetry. In: *Models, Connection with Experimental Apparatus and Relevant DSP Techniques for Functional Movement Analysis.* Dipartimento di Elettronica ed Automatica: Universita di Ancona, 1990.
38. Woltring HJ. Representation and calculation of 3-D joint movement. In: Leo T, Fioretti S, eds. Workshop on Assessment of Clinical Protocols. Internal Report Dipartimento di Elettronica ed Automatica: Universita degli Studi do Ancona, 1989.

Kinetics of Normal Walking

Roy B. Davis and Kenton R. Kaufman

A number of clinical centers routinely use information derived from quantitative gait analysis in the decision-making process for the treatment of gait-related abnormalities (22,47,51,67,71). Kinematic data augmented by electromyographic (EMG) tracings compliment clinical examination and observational gait findings (15). Increasingly, the results of joint kinetic analyses, specifically intersegmental moments and powers, are also used in the evaluation and assessment of normal (21,29,46,65,76) and pathologic gait (18,22,34,48,59,73,74). For example, the evaluation of the relationship of intersegmental power generation in persons with hemiplegia suggests that the noninvolved limb shows greater than normal power generation to compensate for the weaker involved limb (41,42). In clinical gait analysis, an appreciation of compensatory mechanisms and secondary abnormalities is often as valuable as an understanding of primary gait deviations. Other clinical investigators have used joint kinetic parameters to examine the biomechanical performance of orthoses in children with cerebral palsy and myelomeningocele (26,44,68).

An understanding of knee joint loading is important in subjects with angular deformities. In many studies, the methods for determining joint loads have been based on static analysis when an individual stands on one limb. This posture is easily obtained from a standing radiograph. It is implied that this represents single limb support during gait. However, in reality, this is not the case. Several studies have clearly demonstrated that there is no correlation between the angular deformity of the knee measured on radiographs and the dynamic force distribution in the joint during gait (24,28,70). Further, it has been shown that dynamic loading during gait is more closely correlated with clinical outcome than static measurements (54,69).

Gait kinematics can be observed, to a degree, directly. Consequently, quantitative measurements can be compared with observed motions to develop an understanding of the quantitative results. This does not suggest that understanding the relationship between observed patterns and quantitative measurements is without challenge, particularly as it relates to pathologic gait with its often complex three-dimensional (3-D) motion. Gait kinetic results, however, are inherently more difficult to understand because they cannot be directly observed. Moreover, while the focus of gait kinematics may be concentrated on variables familiar to many readers, such as joint angles, gait kinetic results involve perhaps less well-understood concepts such as intersegmental moments, work, mechanical energy, and power. The objectives of this chapter are therefore to introduce and define kinetic concepts that are relevant to human locomotion and to present and describe the underlying kinetics of the gait of normal ambulators (i.e., without locomotor impairment).

GROUND REACTIONS

Standing quietly, a person's weight (force of gravity) tends to pull the person down toward the ground (Figure 4-1). That person does not move downward because the ground is pushing upward with a total force equal in magnitude to the individual's weight (Newton's third law). If that individual's body is relatively symmetric and the person is standing without "leaning to one side," then their weight is evenly shared by each lower extremity (Figure 4-1A). The loads under each foot can be represented by one resultant ground reaction force (GRF) that combines the two loads, i.e., the resultant GRF magnitude equals body weight. Analogously, a bathroom scale combines the load under each foot when it reports body weight. With one half of body weight supported by each foot/leg, the point of application of the resultant GRF passes approximately midway between the subject's two feet (Figure 4-1B). In this case, there is no motion because the external forces applied to the person, i.e., body weight and the GRF, are balanced, that is, they are equal and opposite in magnitude. When the person leans to one side (Figure 4-1C), the point of application of the GRF shifts in that direction. Clearly, overall body posture can affect the GRF. Additional trunk lean would leave that person unstable, i.e., the downward weight vector (or weight line) would fall outside of the base of support. To remain in static equilibrium, the subject requires

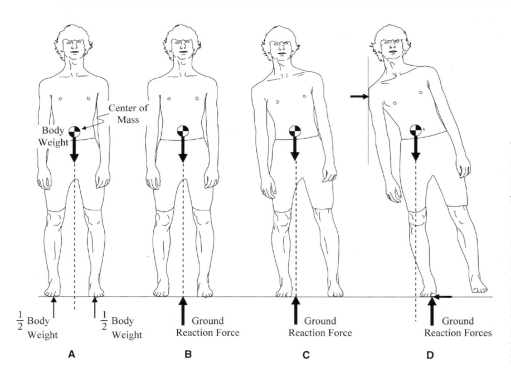

FIGURE 4-1. (**A**) Standing quietly with body weight evenly distributed under each foot, the subject is in "static equilibrium." (**B**) The loads under each foot are combined into a single ground reaction force equal to the sum of the forces under the two feet and located approximately midway between the feet. (**C**) As body weight is shifted laterally, the point of application of the ground reaction force shifts as well. (**D**) When the body weight vector is shifted beyond the base of support, additional lateral forces are required to maintain equilibrium.

additional support (Figure 4-1D). The horizontal force applied to the upper body by the wall is balanced with an equal and opposite horizontal GRF component. Note also that the two equal and opposite vertical forces are no longer aligned (i.e., colinear). They form a "force couple" that would tend to rotate the body in a counterclockwise direction. A second, clockwise force couple formed by the two equal and opposite horizontal forces balances the counterclockwise force couple. Consequently, the subject is in both translational and rotational static equilibrium.

A change in motion occurs when a net imbalance of external forces acts on a rigid body or a system of rigid bodies. Consider a ball that is resting on an icy surface without motion, as shown in Figure 4-2A. Again, there is no motion because the upward ground reaction force, $\mathbf{F_{GRF}}$, balances the downward weight (force) of the ball, $\mathbf{W}$. If the ball is kicked as shown in Figure 4-2B, with a hori-

zontal force passing through the center of the ball, then the ball accelerates horizontally due to the applied horizontal force. Newton's second law,

$$\mathbf{F} = m\mathbf{a}$$

where $\mathbf{F}$ represents the imbalanced force vector, m is the mass of the object, and $\mathbf{a}$ is the translational (or linear) acceleration of the object (in the same direction as $\mathbf{F}$), allows a prediction of the motion that results from the force application. Consequently, if the horizontal forces due to air resistance and the friction between the ball and the icy ground are assumed to be small, then the kicking force will produce a horizontal acceleration of the ball that is proportional to the mass of the ball, or

$$\mathbf{F_{kick}} = m_{ball}\,\mathbf{a_{ball}}$$

where $\mathbf{F_{kick}}$ represents the kick force, m_{ball} is the mass of the ball, and $\mathbf{a_{ball}}$ is the acceleration of the ball. If the kick is stronger (i.e., the magnitude of the force increased), then the acceleration of the ball will be greater. Note also that if the ball is sodden with water (i.e., its mass is increased), then a greater kicking force would be required to produce the same acceleration realized with a dry ball.

In mechanics, mass represents resistance to a change in translational motion or a measure of the inertia of the object. It is also the property of the object that gives rise to its gravitational attraction. Taken together, the product of the mass and acceleration of the object represent an inertial force. This inertial force and its associated acceleration are in opposite directions. For example, when a player kicks

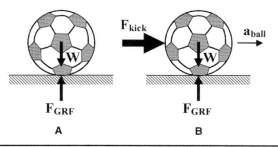

FIGURE 4-2. Acceleration of a ball due to the force applied during a kick.

the ball (Figure 4-2) by applying $\mathbf{F_{kick}}$ to the right, the ball accelerates to the right. The ball simultaneously pushes back (to the left) on the kicker's foot with an inertial force equal in magnitude to $m_{ball}\,\mathbf{a_{ball}}$ (and to $\mathbf{F_{kick}}$). Newton's third law states this explicitly, i.e., the forces between interacting bodies (e.g., the player's foot and the ball) are equal in magnitude, opposite in direction, and lie along the same line of action.

The "center of mass" of an object is that point where all of the mass of the object could be concentrated and still have the same mechanical effect. In a uniform gravitational field, the center of mass (COM) and the center of gravity of an object are located at the same point. In a multi-segmented object such as the human body, the location of the center of mass of the object is affected by the location of the center of mass of each of the segments. When the subject in Figure 4-1C leaned his upper body to his right, it shifted the trunk COM, the head COM, and the right and left arm COM to his right. As a result, his body COM shifted to his right as well.

Note that the application of force causes an immediate acceleration of the object. Since acceleration is the rate of change in velocity

$$a = \frac{\Delta v}{\Delta t}$$

or

$$\Delta v = a\Delta t$$

a change in velocity is not immediately produced. That is, it takes a change in time to result in a change in velocity. Moreover, since velocity is the rate of change in displacement

$$v = \frac{\Delta s}{\Delta t}$$

or

$$\Delta s = v\Delta t$$

a change in displacement is not immediately produced either. Again, it takes time to result in a change in displacement.

In this same way, external forces that are applied to the human body can also produce motion. For example, immediately before a vertical jump, the magnitude of the vertical ground reaction force equals the subject's weight (Figure 4-3A and Figure 4-3D, Point A). As the individual begins his downward motion to prepare to jump, i.e., accelerating downward, the vertical GRF drops in magnitude to less than body weight (Figure 4-3B and Figure 4-3D, Point B). With the generation of additional muscle force, the downward motion is halted and the hips and knees begin to extend and ankles begin to plantar flex (Figure 4-3C). The subject actively pushes down on the ground and the ground pushes up on the subject with a GRF that is

greater than body weight (Figure 4-3D, Point C). This vertical force imbalance (i.e., vertical GRF minus body weight) accelerates the center of mass of the subject upward. Note that the GRF is not directly applied to the body COM like the kicking force was applied to the ball. The external force imbalance is transmitted from the ground upward through the joints and ultimately applied to the trunk through the hip joints. The muscle forces cause the legs to push down on the ground and up on the trunk, simultaneously. Humans walk using this same action–reaction relationship, that is, muscle forces continually modify the magnitude and direction of the ground reaction loads to produce and control ambulation.

During walking, the body COM is accelerated upward and downward over the gait cycle (Figure 4-4). One might anticipate that the GRF would vary over the gait cycle because of this upward and downward acceleration, as was seen in the previous jumping example. An examination of the ground reaction loads during walking presented in Figure 4-5 demonstrates this relationship.

The magnitude of the vertical GRF under each foot depends on whether the limb of interest is in double support, single support, or swing phase. Consider a limb that is transitioning from swing phase to stance phase. During double support, when both feet are in contact with the ground, the vertical GRF rapidly increases in magnitude as the external load is transferred from one lower extremity to the other (Figure 4-5, Point A). One might anticipate that the magnitude of the vertical GRF be equal to the subject's weight during single support, with a constant value from approximately 12% to 50% of the gait cycle. In reality, however, the magnitude of the vertical GRF oscillates above and below the value of the subject's weight due to the upward and downward acceleration of the body COM. That is, during the first part of single support, the body COM translates from its lowest to its highest elevation in the gait cycle (Figure 4-4). Consequently, this upward acceleration coincides with a vertical GRF that is greater than body weight (Figure 4-5, Point B). Before reaching its highest elevation at about 30% of the gait cycle (Figure 4-5, Point C), the upward velocity of the body COM begins to decrease. This vertical deceleration upward (or acceleration downward) coincides with a vertical GRF that is less than body weight. From this highest elevation, the body COM falls vertically, resulting in an increasing downward acceleration that coincides with a vertical GRF that continues to drop in magnitude. After reaching a relative minimum, the vertical GRF increases in magnitude, reflecting a downward acceleration that is now decreasing (Figure 4-5, Point D). The second rise in the vertical GRF above body weight, later in single support (Figure 4-5, Point E), coincides with a second upward acceleration that slows and controls the downward movement of the body COM. Finally, during second double support body weight is

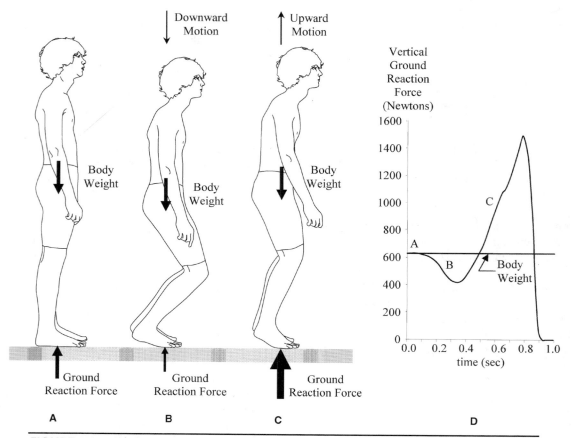

FIGURE 4-3. Vertical GRF changes during a vertical jump: (**A**) subject standing, (**B**) downward motion, (**C**) jumping motion, and (**D**) trace of the vertical ground reaction force during this movement sequence. The points A, B, and C in plot (*D*) correspond to illustrations (*A*), (*B*) and (*C*).

transferred from one limb to the other and the GRF drops to zero (Figure 4-5, Point F).

In addition to the vertical GRF, friction between the foot and the ground produces anterior and posterior shear ground reaction forces (i.e., forces that are parallel to the ground). These anterior and posterior shear ground

reaction forces reflect forward and backward accelerations of the body. During the first double support interval, the ground pushes backward on the lower extremity, producing a backward acceleration that decelerates and controls the forward movement. This posterior (Figure 4-5, Point G) shear force reaches a maximum at the end of the first

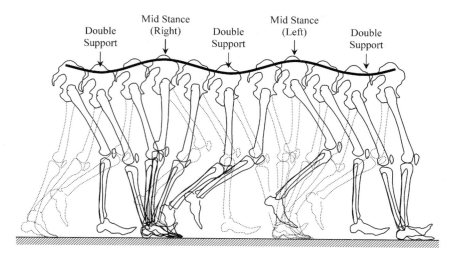

FIGURE 4-4. Vertical displacement of the body center of mass during ambulation. The highest elevation occurs at midstance and the lowest elevation occurs during double support.

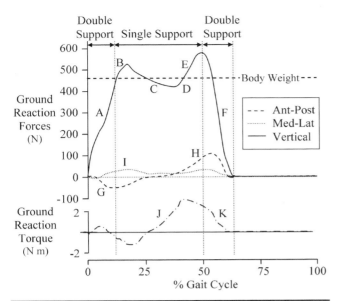

FIGURE 4-5. Ground reaction loads (forces and vertical torque) for one adult female walking at 71 m/min. Letters A through K are identified in the text.

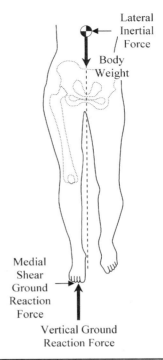

FIGURE 4-6. Schematic of a person in single support. The body weight and vertical GRF force couple tend to rotate the body toward the swing limb (clockwise). The medial shear GRF and the corresponding lateral inertial force balance this effect (i.e., produce a counterclockwise force couple) in order to achieve dynamic equilibrium.

double support interval after which it deceases in magnitude. The relatively small shear force values in midstance reflect relatively low backward or forward acceleration of the body during this brief time interval, i.e., the body COM moves forward at approximately a constant speed. Later in single support, muscle forces accelerate the body COM forward as reflected in an anterior (Figure 4-5, Point H) shear force. During second double support, muscle forces accelerate the stance limb forward into swing. These relationships between the external shear ground reaction forces and the associated accelerations of the body COM hold true for single support. During first double support, however, a posterior shear force is applied to the leading limb while an anterior shear force is applied to the trailing limb. Consequently, depending on the relative magnitudes of these two shear forces, the net imbalance in shear force might be quite small, reflecting little horizontal (forward or backward) acceleration of the body COM during double support.

A third GRF component, a medial shear force (Figure 4-5, Point I) applied to the stance limb, increases during double support to a relatively constant value for all of single support. This relatively small medial GRF force produces a medial acceleration of the body COM (along with a corresponding lateral inertial force). This mechanism allows humans to walk with a step width. Since the vertical GRF component generally passes lateral to the body COM during gait (Figure 4-6), the vertical GRF and the subject's weight create a force couple that tends to rotate the body (i.e., the body COM would fall toward the swing limb). The medial shear force and the lateral inertial force, as a force couple, tend to rotate the body in the opposite direc-

tion, thereby dynamically balancing the weight/GRF force couple.

In addition to the ground reaction forces, a vertical ground reaction torque is also applied to the foot during gait. There is a tendency for the foot to twist about a vertical axis while on the ground during normal locomotion. This tendency is resisted or constrained by the friction between the foot and the ground. During the second half of single support, for example, the advancing swing limb and other upper body motions tend to rotate externally the stance limb foot. The vertical ground reaction torque prevents this motion with a resistance that tends to rotate the foot internally (Figure 4-5, Point J). As the magnitude of the vertical ground reaction torque falls off during the second double support (Figure 4-5, Point K), the foot is less constrained by the torque and externally rotates with respect to the direction of progression.

During normal ambulation, the foot lands on its heel and lifts off from its toes. Consequently, the point of application of the ground reaction load, referred to as the center of pressure (COP), moves from the heel forward to the toes, as illustrated in Figure 4-7. The COP progresses rapidly forward so that by midstance, the ground reaction load is concentrated under the metatarsals. With the COP positioned under the forefoot, the GRF can more

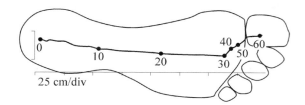

FIGURE 4-7. Center of pressure for one adult female walking at 71 m/min. Times during the gait cycle (i.e., 0%, 10%, 20%, etc.) are indicated on the plantar surface of the foot.

effectively stabilize the stance limb, as will be described later.

INTERSEGMENTAL FORCES AND MOMENTS

Muscle forces produce and control joint motion. As was seen in the jumping example, muscle forces controlled the lower extremity joints as the subject moved downward and then provided additional force to extend those joints in his jump upward. Those muscle forces were also channeled through the joints to allow the subject to "push down" on the ground and produce an upward acceleration of the body COM. Muscles are able to both influence joint motion and channel force through the joints because muscles cross those joints at some distance away from their centers of rotation. These mechanisms are illustrated in the following simple example.

Assume that a foot is loaded with an external vertical GRF, $\mathbf{F_{GRF}}$, as shown in Figure 4-8A. Other external loads such as the weight of the foot are neglected in this example. Further assume that the foot is held in this static

position by the plantar flexor muscles (gastrocnemius and soleus) in opposition to external force $\mathbf{F_{GRF}}$. That is, assume that force $\mathbf{F_{GRF}}$ is sufficiently strong to dorsiflex the ankle. Consequently, the plantar flexor muscles must produce an internal muscle force that is sufficiently strong to prevent that dorsiflexion. To explore this relationship between this external force $\mathbf{F_{GRF}}$ and the internal muscle force, a "free-body-diagram" of the foot is created in which the foot is separated from the leg to reveal the internal muscle force, $\mathbf{F_{muscle}}$ (Figure 4-8B). Note that the internal force at the ankle joint, $\mathbf{F_{joint}}$, is added to the diagram to represent the internal force that the tibia and fibula would apply to the foot to keep external force $\mathbf{F_{GRF}}$ and internal muscle force $\mathbf{F_{muscle}}$ from translating the foot upward. For the joint force $\mathbf{F_{joint}}$ to effectively counter this influence by the external force $\mathbf{F_{GRF}}$ and the muscle force $\mathbf{F_{muscle}}$, the magnitude of $\mathbf{F_{joint}}$ must be equivalent to the combined magnitudes of $\mathbf{F_{GRF}}$ and $\mathbf{F_{muscle}}$, expressed mathematically as

$$\mathbf{F_{joint}} = \mathbf{F_{GRF}} + \mathbf{F_{muscle}}$$

The diagram is simplified further by representing the foot as a rigid lever with a fulcrum at the ankle (Figure 4-8C). In this way, one can appreciate that the distances between GRF $\mathbf{F_{GRF}}$ and muscle force $\mathbf{F_{muscle}}$ and the fulcrum, d_1 and d_2, respectively, are important. Levers work because these distances, called "lever arms," increase the mechanical effectiveness or advantage of an applied force. The use of common tools illustrates this point. To tighten a nut on a bolt, a turning force is more effectively applied at the end of the wrench away from the nut. To pull a nail, force is more effectively applied at the end of the hammer handle away from the head of the hammer. The forces applied to a lever produce moments about the fulcrum that reflect both

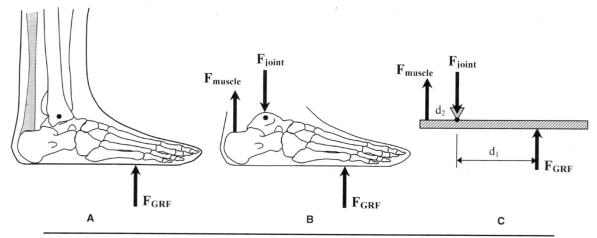

FIGURE 4-8. Static equilibrium of the lower leg. (**A**) An external force F_{GRF} is resisted by plantar flexor muscle force (*shaded area*). (**B**) The "free-body-diagram" of the foot illustrates the internal muscle and joint forces, F_{muscle} and F_{joint}, respectively, which counterbalance the external force F_{GRF}. The weight of the foot is neglected. (**C**) The equivalent loading of the foot is illustrated as a lever with a fulcrum at the ankle.

the magnitude of the force and the distance between the force and fulcrum. Returning to the example (Figure 4-8C), the external moment produced by the external force $\mathbf{F_{GRF}}$ about the fulcrum is the product of the magnitude of $\mathbf{F_{GRF}}$ and d_1. Similarly, the internal moment produced by the muscle force $\mathbf{F_{muscle}}$ is the product of the magnitude of $\mathbf{F_{muscle}}$ and d_2. Note that $\mathbf{F_{joint}}$ does not produce a moment about the fulcrum because it passes through the fulcrum, i.e., it has no lever arm (also referred to as "moment arm"). Observe that $\mathbf{F_{GRF}}$ tends to rotate the foot in a counterclockwise direction while $\mathbf{F_{muscle}}$ tends to rotate the foot in a clockwise direction. Consequently, for the foot to remain in this position, the counterclockwise moment associated with $\mathbf{F_{GRF}}$ is balanced by the clockwise moment associated with $\mathbf{F_{muscle}}$, or expressed mathematically,

$$d_1 \times F_{GRF} = d_2 \times F_{muscle}$$

It can be observed from this relationship that if the external force $\mathbf{F_{GRF}}$ increases, then the muscle force $\mathbf{F_{muscle}}$ must increase as well (keeping d_1 and d_2 constant). Observe that if both the external force $\mathbf{F_{GRF}}$ and the internal muscle force $\mathbf{F_{muscle}}$ increase, then the internal joint force $\mathbf{F_{joint}}$ must increase as well. The converse is also true. That is, if the muscle force $\mathbf{F_{muscle}}$ changes, then both the external force $\mathbf{F_{GRF}}$ and the joint force $\mathbf{F_{joint}}$ change in response. In this way, the muscle force influences both the position of the joint and the force applied to the joint. Note also that this relationship is directly related to the magnitudes of the moment arms. For example, if the magnitude of the external force $\mathbf{F_{GRF}}$ and the muscle moment arm d_2 are held constant, then the muscle force $\mathbf{F_{muscle}}$ must increase (or decrease) if d_1 is increased (or decreased). One can anticipate from the previous discussion pertaining to ground reactions during gait that muscle force magnitudes will vary to produce changes in the GRF magnitude and COP location as well as in response to that external loading. The muscle moment arm values also vary with joint position

during gait, thereby changing the mechanical advantage of the internal muscle forces (63).

Muscle forces are generally not produced in isolation. For walking, Figure 4-9A depicts a more realistic scenario where multiple tendons carry internal muscle forces across the ankle joint. Also shown are external loads that are applied to the foot, including the weight of the foot and a distributed force (or pressure) on the plantar surface of the foot. Figure 4-9A also depicts a distributed force loading on the ankle articular surface that reflects the joint contact force (also referred to as a bone-on-bone force) that is transmitted from the tibia and fibula to the dome of the talus. Not shown is the distributed shear force under the foot. Ideally, a mechanical analysis would provide values for the several "unknown" muscle forces and the "unknown" ankle joint loading if the kinematics of the foot and ground reaction loads are measured and the inertial properties, e.g., mass, mass moment of inertia, of the foot are estimated. This is a very challenging analytical problem, however. Fundamentally, there are more unknowns in this scenario than there are equations to solve for the unknowns. A good deal of work has been done in this area, employing optimization strategies to predict values for the unknown muscle forces (10,12,31). While these techniques may provide some insight in normal locomotion, assumptions required in these approaches limit their applicability in pathological gait analysis.

More commonly in clinical gait analysis, several muscle forces and the distributed load on the ankle are expressed as a single concentrated intersegmental force vector, $\mathbf{F_A}$, and moments produced by the muscle forces (and any other structures that cross the joint) are represented as a single net intersegmental moment vector, $\mathbf{M_A}$ (Figure 4-9B). The distributed loads on the plantar surface of the foot are presented as a resultant ground reaction force, $\mathbf{F_{GRF}}$, and torque, $\mathbf{T_{GR}}$, both applied at the COP. The kinematics of the foot and ground reaction loads are measured and the inertial properties, e.g., mass and mass moment of inertia,

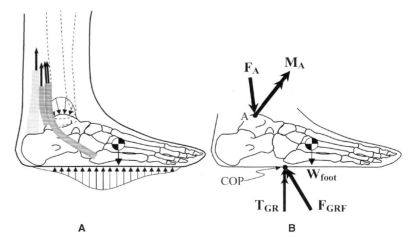

FIGURE 4-9. Schematic of the lower leg during gait. (**A**) Some of the forces (concentrated and distributed) that would be applied to the foot during the stance phase of gait are illustrated. (**B**) A "free-body-diagram" of the foot showing the ankle intersegmental force and moment, weight of the foot, and ground reactions associated with a three-dimensional inverse dynamics analysis.

A

B

of the foot are estimated. Newton's translational equation of motion,

$$\Sigma \mathbf{F} = m\ \mathbf{a}$$

where $\Sigma \mathbf{F}$ represents the sum of the forces applied to the body segment, m is the mass of the body segment, and $\mathbf{a}$ is the linear acceleration vector of the body segment COM, allows for the solution of unknown $\mathbf{F_A}$. Newton's rotational equation of motion,

$$\Sigma \mathbf{M_g} = I_g \alpha$$

where $\Sigma \mathbf{M_g}$ represents the sum of the moments of force acting about the body segment COM, I_g is the centroidal mass moment of inertia of the body segment, and α is the angular acceleration of the body segment, is employed to solve for the unknown ankle moment, $\mathbf{M_A}$.

This kinetic analysis begins with the foot to solve for the intersegmental reactions at the ankle and then moves up from the ground to the hip. For the foot, the translational equation of motion becomes

$$\Sigma \mathbf{F} = \mathbf{F_A} + \mathbf{F_{GRF}} + \mathbf{W_{foot}} = m_{foot}\ \mathbf{a_g}$$

where m_{foot} is the mass of the foot and $\mathbf{a_g}$ is the linear acceleration of the foot COM. Consequently, the unknown ankle intersegmental force can be expressed as

$$\mathbf{F_A} = m_{foot}\ \mathbf{a_g} - \mathbf{F_{GRF}} - m_{foot}\ \mathbf{g}$$

where the weight of the foot, $\mathbf{W_{foot}}$, is represented by the product of the mass of the foot and the gravitational constant $\mathbf{g}$. The expanded rotational equation of motion becomes

$$\Sigma \mathbf{M_g} = \mathbf{M_A} + \mathbf{r_1} \times \mathbf{F_A} + \mathbf{r_2} \times \mathbf{F_{GRF}} + \mathbf{T_{GR}} = I_{foot}\ \alpha_{foot}$$

where $\mathbf{r_1}$ and $\mathbf{r_2}$ are position vectors (not shown in Figure 4-9B) that describe the location of the ankle joint center and the COP relative to the foot COM, respectively, $\mathbf{T_{GR}}$ is the vertical ground reaction torque, I_{foot} is the centroidal mass moment of inertia of the foot, and α_{foot} is the angular acceleration of the foot. The moment that force $\mathbf{F_A}$ produces about the foot COM is the vector cross product of $\mathbf{r_1}$ and $\mathbf{F_A}$. Similarly, the moment that force $\mathbf{F_{GRF}}$ produces about the foot COM is the vector cross product of $\mathbf{r_2}$ and $\mathbf{F_{GRF}}$. The unknown ankle reaction moment can be expressed as

$$\mathbf{M_A} = I_{foot}\ \alpha_{foot} - \mathbf{r_1} \times \mathbf{F_A} - \mathbf{r_2} \times \mathbf{F_{GRF}} - \mathbf{T_{GR}}$$

Mass moment of inertia was referenced in Newton's rotational equation of motion. Just as the mass of an object represents the resistance to a change in translational motion, the mass moment of inertia represents the resistance to a change in rotational motion. Similarly, as mass is a measure of the translational inertia of a segment, mass moment of inertia is associated with the rotational inertia of a segment. The product of the mass moment of inertia and the angular acceleration may be thought of as an inertial moment. The mass moment of inertia combines

two inertial properties of the object: the mass of the object and the distribution of mass within the object. Commonly found objects illustrate this relationship. For example, a hammer offers a different resistance to rotation depending on whether it is held and rotated about its handle or its head. The mass of the hammer does not change in the two scenarios, but the distribution of that mass about the two reference axes does change. Consequently, with respect to mass moment of inertia, the choice of reference axes is important.

Inertial properties of body segments are often estimated from regression models based on human cadaveric studies (8,11,19). For example, the locations of the COM of the thigh, shank, and foot might be expressed as a function of segment length, e.g., the shank COM is distal to the knee center by approximately 43% of the shank length (19). Alternatively, other investigators (27,72) map the surface geometry of the limb segment and then divide the segment into elliptical slices of constant density. The inertial properties of the entire segment are then determined by combining the contributions of the individual elements. Still other investigators approximate entire segments as simple geometric solids, e.g., ellipsoids, cylinders, of constant density, such as the Hanavan (23) 15-segment model. The time required to quantify the surface geometry of individual segments from photographic images or numerous anatomic measurements, e.g., over 200 in the Hatze (25) detailed model, limits the feasibility of some of these latter approaches in the clinical setting. Cappozzo and Berme (6) conclude that when extreme accuracy is desired, the Hatze model appears to offer the best current approach. These authors advise that if a statistical model is used, then the test subject should be consistent with the body composition and gender of the study population employed to develop the regression relationships. For example, the work of Dempster (19) is based on eight male subjects ranging in age from 52 to 83 years. Note that these techniques provide estimates of the "principal" mass moments of inertia about principal axes passing through the segment COM. A principal axis is based on the symmetric distribution of the mass of the segment about that axis. The principal axes of the thigh, for example, might be approximated by a longitudinal axis from the knee to hip center and two transverse axes that are perpendicular to each other and the longitudinal axis. Generally, the anatomically aligned coordinate systems constructed to compute the kinematics of the segment approximate the principal axes of the segment as well.

For greater accuracy, a technique, known variously as stereophotometrics, biostereometrics or stereophotogrammetry, has also been used as a means of mathematical segmentation to obtain mass distribution properties of body segments in a living subject. This technique involves three-dimensional photography of the subject by cameras placed at strategic locations. The coordinates of a number of points on the body serve as input to a digital computer that can then recreate the geometric subtlety of the body segments. This technique is used to determine the mass distribution properties of the body segments, which can be calculated from anthropometric dimensions using regression equations (36). Detailed analysis has shown that the principal axes are not aligned with the anatomic axes. Nonetheless, a cosine matrix of the principal axes with respect to the anatomic axes is available (36).

To summarize, the unknown intersegmental force and moment at the ankle, $\mathbf{F_A}$ and $\mathbf{M_A}$, respectively, can be solved through the application of Newton's translational and rotational equations of motion. A number of measurements are required for this computational process, including:

- The ground reactions, $\mathbf{F_{GRF}}$ and $\mathbf{T_{GR}}$, and COP location, measured using instrumented force platforms, and
- The location of the ankle joint center (and other anatomic reference points on the foot), measured with laboratory-based motion measurement technology, e.g., motion data capture cameras (14,15).

A number of intermediate computational estimates and results are provided as well, including:

- The relative and absolute angular position of the foot, either computed from the motion capture data or measured directly, e.g., electromagnetic sensors,
- The location of the foot COM, the mass of the foot, m_{foot}, and the mass moment of inertia of the foot, I_{foot}, typically estimated based on the anthropometric characteristics of the subject, and
- The linear acceleration of the foot COM, $\mathbf{a_g}$, and the angular acceleration of the foot, $\mathbf{\alpha_{foot}}$, calculated through numerical differentiation of the location of the COM and the foot attitude, respectively (80–82).

The intersegmental forces and moments are determined from the measurement of the external ground reaction loads and estimates of segment weight and inertia.

Once the reactions at the ankle, $\mathbf{F_A}$ and $\mathbf{M_A}$, have been determined, then the process can be repeated for an analysis of the shank, or lower leg, to determine the knee intersegmental force and moment. In this step of the process, the ankle intersegmental force, $\mathbf{F_A}$ and intersegmental moment, $\mathbf{M_A}$, are treated as the known external loads to the distal shank in order to determine the unknown knee intersegmental force and moment, $\mathbf{F_K}$ and $\mathbf{M_K}$, respectively. Again, a number of measured values are required, e.g., the locations of the ankle and knee joint centers, attitude of the shank. Estimated values are required, e.g., the location of the shank COM, the mass of the shank, and the mass moment of inertia of the shank. Intermediate computed values are required as well, e.g., the linear acceleration of the shank COM and the angular acceleration of the

shank. The same process is then repeated to solve for the hip intersegmental force and moment.

The mechanical power associated with joint kinematics and intersegmental moments can be computed from the combination of the intersegmental moment and the joint angular velocity, i.e.,

$$P_J = \mathbf{M_J} \cdot \omega_J$$

where P_J is the intersegmental power, $\mathbf{M_J}$ is the net intersegmental moment, and ω_J is the joint angular velocity at joint J. Intersegmental power represents the rate at which work is done by or on the intersegmental moment in producing or controlling joint rotational displacement. Intersegmental power "generation" (positive intersegmental power) may be related to concentric muscle contraction and intersegmental power "absorption" (negative intersegmental power) may be related to eccentric muscle contraction. However, these relationships are not always valid. Intersegmental power absorption may also be associated with the passive elongation of muscles and other soft tissue structures that cross the joint.

Intersegmental power is a scalar quantity that reflects the sum of the products of the vector components of the intersegmental moment and joint angular velocity. As such, power does not have directionality. In the interpretation of clinical data, however, it is often advantageous to display each of the planar contributions to intersegmental power separately in order to better appreciate the mechanical effect of an intersegmental moment about a particular anatomical axis. Consequently, in the normative data presented later in the chapter, sagittal and coronal intersegmental power will be described separately.

Other investigators (5) have examined both rotational and translational intersegmental power through the use of a six degree-of-freedom gait model (i.e., three degrees of rotation and three degrees of translation at each joint), expressed as

$$P_J = \mathbf{M_J} \cdot \omega_J + \mathbf{F_J} \cdot \mathbf{v_J}$$

where $\mathbf{F_J}$ is the net intersegmental force and $\mathbf{v_J}$ is the translational velocity of one segment relative to the other at joint J. Translational ankle intersegmental power values were found to be small relative to the associated rotational intersegmental power contributions during normal gait, approximately an order of magnitude smaller. While these translational power contributions were statistically significant, their clinical significance and relevance is not known.

The computational process outlined above is referred to as "inverse dynamics," where movement kinematics and external loads are measured and internal reactions are computed (9). This process contrasts with a "forward dynamics" analysis or a "forward simulation" model, where internal forces, e.g., muscle forces, are numerically applied and the resulting kinematics and ground reactions are predicted (83,85). The validity of each of these techniques is predicated on the quality of the measured data and the appropriateness of the assumptions associated with the specific biomechanical model.

The primary assumption in the inverse dynamics approach is that soft tissue movement relative to underlying bony structures is small. The body segments are assumed to be "rigid" and not to deform when loaded. Moreover, joint center locations are assumed to be well estimated and to remain fixed relative to the associated segment coordinate system. An appreciation of the implications of these assumptions is particularly important in the assessment of clinical results (35). For example, excessive soft tissue movement of a patient with obesity can reduce the quality of estimates of the joint center locations as well as distort kinematic quantities such as angular velocities and accelerations.

Two fundamental limitations associated with inverse dynamics should be reiterated as well. The *net* intersegmental moment combines moments due to individual muscle forces and other soft tissue structures that cross the joint. Moreover, the intersegmental force underestimates the joint contact force produced between articulating surfaces of the joint (77). Paul (50) reports peak hip force magnitudes of 3.9 times body weight compared to peak intersegmental force magnitudes of approximately 1.1 times body weight (4).

A reconsideration of the previous example illustrates this dilemma. Shown in Figure 4-10A, the static foot is again loaded with a known external GRF F_{GRF} at known distance d_1 anterior to the ankle. Other external loads such as the weight of the foot are again neglected. Unknown internal muscle (F_{pfm}) and joint (F_{J1}) forces are also shown. From the previous discussion, it was appreciated that the joint contact force was the sum of the external

force F_{GRF} and the internal force F_{muscle}, or

$$F_{J1} = F_{GRF} + F_{pfm}$$

and the moment associated with the muscle force was expressed as

$$d_2 \times F_{pfm} = d_1 \times F_{GRF}$$

For an inverse dynamics analysis (Figure 4-10B), the muscle force has been incorporated into the intersegmental force F_A and the moment due to muscle force has been incorporated into the intersegmental moment M_A. Inverse dynamics again predicts an intersegmental moment M_A based on the external force and distance d_1, is

$$M_A = d_1 \times F_{GRF}$$

Inverse dynamics, however, predicts an intersegmental force F_A that is equal in magnitude to the external force F_{GRF},

$$F_A = F_{GRF}$$

and underestimates the joint contact force by an amount equal to F_{muscle}.

If agonist and antagonist muscle forces are introduced, the dilemma becomes more challenging. From Figure 4-10C, it can be seen that the joint contact force counters both a plantar flexor muscle force F_{pfm}, a dorsiflexor muscle force F_{dfm} as well as the external force F_{GRF}, or

$$F_{J2} = F_{GRF} + F_{pfm} + F_{dfm}$$

The same free-body-diagram (Figure 4-10B) applies in this scenario. That is, both agonist and antagonist muscle forces have been incorporated into the intersegmental force F_A and the moments due to both muscle forces have been incorporated into the intersegmental moment M_A. Inverse dynamics continues to predict an intersegmental

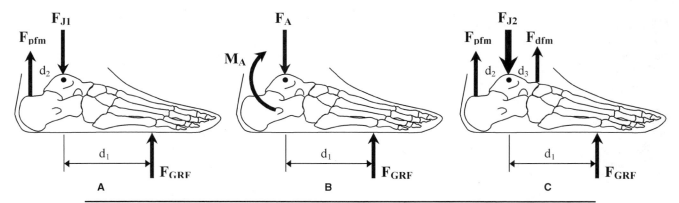

FIGURE 4-10. Static equilibrium of the lower leg. (**A**) An external force F_{GRF} and internal plantar flexor muscle and joint forces, F_{pfm} and F_{J1}, respectively, are shown. The weight of the foot is neglected. (**B**) The two-dimensional "free-body-diagram" of the foot associated with the loading shown in (*A*) and (*C*). (**C**) The same schematic of the foot/ankle (*A*) with the addition of co-contraction, an internal dorsiflexor muscle force F_{dfm} is depicted. Note that co-contraction does not change the value of the net intersegmental moment M_A and that the joint contact forces F_{J1} and F_{J2} are not equal, nor are they equal to the intersegmental force F_A.

force $\mathbf{F_A}$ equal in magnitude to only the external force $\mathbf{F_{GRF}}$ and consequently, underestimates the joint contact force by an amount equal to $\mathbf{F_{pfm}} + \mathbf{F_{dfm}}$. In Figure 4-10C, the plantar flexor muscle moment must now balance the internal dorsiflexor muscle moment as well as the external moment due to the force $\mathbf{F_{GRF}}$, or

$$d_2 \times F_{pfm} = d_1 \times F_{GRF} + d_3 \times F_{dfm}$$

Alternatively, it can be seen that the combination of plantar flexor and dorsiflexor moments balance the moment due to the external force $\mathbf{F_{GRF}}$, or

$$d_2 \times F_{pfm} - d_3 \times F_{dfm} = d_1 \times F_{GRF}$$

Intersegmental moment $\mathbf{M_A}$ predicted by inverse dynamics remains unchanged, or

$$M_A = d_1 \times F_{GRF}$$

and has analytically combined the moment due to the plantar flexor muscle force with the moment due to the dorsiflexor muscle force. Inverse dynamics underestimates the joint contact force and cannot distinguish internal moments produced by separate (and perhaps antagonistic) muscles.

For additional details associated specifically with the calculation of intersegmental moments and powers, readers are referred to Winter (77), Davis et al. (17), Kaufman et al. (30), Õunpuu et al. (45), and Palladino and Davis (49). Readers are also encouraged to consider the classical contributions of Braune and Fischer (republished 3), Elftman (20), Bresler and Frankel (4), and Paul (50).

INTERSEGMENTAL MOMENTS AND POWERS DURING WALKING

The intersegmental moments and powers described here are associated with a group of 27 pediatric subjects (17 females, 10 males, mean age: 9.9 ± 3 years, mean mass: 33 ± 12 kg, mean height: 137 ± 17 cm) evaluated at Newington Children's Hospital (Newington, Connecticut) in 1988 and 1989. All of the pediatric subjects were without neuromuscular and orthopaedic impairment and walked at a self-selected speed (119 ± 14 cm/sec) and cadence (130 ± 13 steps/min). Readers are referred to Õunpuu et al. (46) for a description of the protocols and methods used in the data collection and analysis.

All of the moments presented in this section are the "internal" intersegmental moments that are produced by the body to either modify or control the effects of "external" loads. Perry (52) describes this as an internal response to an external demand. As illustrated in Figure 4-11, a GRF that passes anterior to the hip by distance d creates an *external* hip flexor moment. The external hip flexor moment is balanced with an equal and opposite *internal* hip extensor moment. Presentations of both external and internal

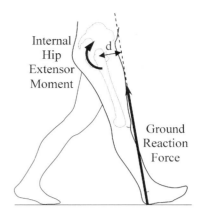

FIGURE 4-11. Schematic of a person just after right foot contact. The external ground reaction force produces an *external* hip flexor moment that is resisted by an opposite and equal *internal* hip extensor moment.

moments are found in the literature, i.e., the display convention varies between journals. Also, the intersegmental moment and power results are normalized with respect to body mass in this chapter. The literature is inconsistent with respect to this display convention as well.

The intersegmental moments described in this section reflect the net moment applied across the joint, consistent with the discussion presented above. A net intersegmental moment reflects the moments of both agonist and antagonist muscles as well any other soft tissue structures that cross the joint. Consequently, for example, a net "extensor moment" reflects a dominance of internal extensor forces over flexor forces. It does not imply the presence of only extensor muscle forces or the absence of flexor muscle forces.

Ankle – Sagittal Plane of the Talocrural Joint

At and immediately following foot contact, the ground reaction force is applied to the heel and its line of action passes posterior to the ankle center. Consequently, it produces an external moment that tends to plantar flex the ankle. This external plantar flex moment is countered by an internal ankle dorsiflexor moment (Figure 4-12, Point A). This dorsiflexor moment (associated with eccentric activity of the ankle dorsiflexors) controls the lowering of the mid- and forefoot to the ground. The magnitude of this dorsiflexor moment is small, because the GRF passes relatively near the ankle center and the magnitude of the GRF is still small (relative to its peak value at the end of this double support interval); refer to Point A in Figure 4-5. Note that the mass of the foot is small relative to the other segments of the body and consequently the contribution of segment weight and segment inertia to the ankle intersegmental moment can be considered negligible in stance.

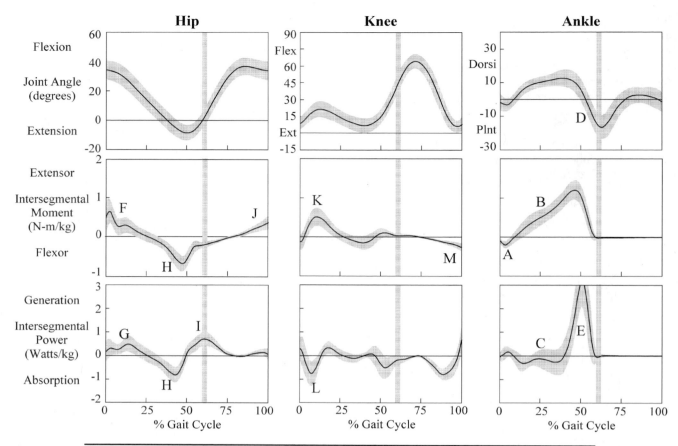

FIGURE 4-12. Sagittal plane joint angles, moments and powers for the hip, knee and ankle associated with a group of 27 pediatric subjects evaluated at Newington Children's Hospital (Newington, Connecticut) in 1988 and 1989, as described in (46). Shown are average values (*solid line*), one standard deviation in average value (*gray band*), and average foot off (*vertical gray line*).

Once the foot is flat, the COP moves quickly forward under the plantigrade foot and the line of action of the GRF passes anterior to the ankle center. Consequently, the GRF produces an external dorsiflexor moment that increases rapidly in magnitude. This external dorsiflexor moment is balanced by an internal plantar flexor moment (Figure 4-12, Point B). This internal plantar flexor moment (associated with eccentric activity of the ankle plantar flexors) controls the forward advancement of the shank over the plantigrade foot and is commonly referred to as the "plantar flexion-knee extension couple."

Note that ankle power magnitudes remain small during this interval (Figure 4-12, Point C), despite the rapid increase in internal plantar flexor moment. Recall that intersegmental power is the product of intersegmental moment and joint angular velocity. The magnitude of joint angular velocity is reflected by the slope (or steepness) of the joint angle plot. During this interval, the ankle is dorsiflexing, but at a slower and slower rate (as reflected in a decreasing slope). Consequently, although the internal plantar flexor moment is increasing, the ankle angular velocity is diminishing and the intersegmental power remains small. Intersegmental power is being absorbed because the plantar flexor moment is associated with a dorsiflexing motion.

The ankle begins to plantar flex after reaching a peak dorsiflexion angle at about 40% of the gait cycle. The velocity of this plantar flexing motion increases as reflected by the increasing slope of the ankle angle plot (Figure 4-12, Point D). Consequently, the internal plantar flexor moment is combined with a significant plantar flexing angular velocity to produce a significant ankle power generation burst (Figure 4-12, Point E). This ankle power generation lifts the heel off the ground and accelerates the ankle center upward and forward. This power generation is attributed to concentric activity of the ankle plantar flexors and has been termed "push-off" (75). However, the electrical (EMG) activity of the primary plantar flexor muscles (gastrocnemius and soleus) begins to subside in the middle of this power generation burst (at about 50% of the gait cycle) (52). Perry (52) suggests that the plantar flexors stiffen the ankle allowing the leg to rotate over a forefoot fulcrum, referring to this as "roll-off." Results from induced acceleration analysis (33) and forward simulation

(39), however, demonstrate a significant contribution to forward progression of the body by this plantar flexor "push-off" mechanism.

Hip – Sagittal Plane of the Joint

In the first part of stance, the body COM is pulled forward and upward with a hip extensor moment (associated with concentric contraction of the hip extensors) (Figure 4-12, Point F). Hip power generation (Figure 4-12, Point G) aids in elevating the body COM to its highest elevation in mid-stance while contributing to forward momentum. Later in single support, the body COM continues to translate forward and also falls downward under the influence of gravity. The resulting hip flexor moment and power absorption is associated with the passive elongation of the hip flexor musculature (Figure 4-12, Point H).

The hip reaches full extension and begins to flex at 50% of the gait cycle. The hip flexor moment produces the hip flexing motion as realized in the hip power generation burst (Figure 4-12, Point I) that continues to increase in magnitude until foot off. This hip power burst (attributed to concentric contraction of the hip flexors) helps propel the lower extremity into swing. Note that the timing of the onset of this power generation (50% of the gait cycle) is closely aligned with peak ankle power generation. This provides evidence that the ankle initially propels the stance limb toward swing in terminal stance and then the hip assumes that role in double support and into swing phase. This observation is further supported by a principle component analysis of the hip and ankle moments (60).

The hip extensor moment in the second half of swing (Figure 4-12, Point J) decelerates the lower extremity in preparation for foot contact. It is observed that both the hip flexor moment/acceleration in late stance and early swing and the hip extensor moment/deceleration mechanisms affect knee motion, as will be described in the next section.

Knee – Sagittal Plane of the Joint

A net internal knee extensor moment in early stance (Figure 4-12, Point K) supports and controls knee flexion during the first double support interval, also referred to as loading response or weight acceptance. The corresponding initial knee power absorption wave (Figure 4-12, Point L) is consistent with a knee extensor moment and a simultaneously flexing knee. This is followed by a smaller knee power generation wave that is also consistent with the knee extensor moment and an extending knee motion. This power absorption and generation may be associated with eccentric followed by concentric contraction of the knee extensors. Aside from the early extensor moment, knee moments during stance are remarkably small given the 5 to 10 degrees of knee flexion found during single support. Moreover, the mechanism that produces the sig-

nificant motion of the knee in swing is not apparent from the knee moment and power.

During single support, the knee is stabilized by the plantar flexion–knee extension couple described earlier. The increasing internal ankle plantar flexor moment seen at this time controls forward advancement of the shank and thus helps stabilize knee position. The hip extensor moment in stance also aids in stabilizing the knee by controlling the motion of the thigh. Sadeghi et al. (60) substantiates this high degree of coordination between the ankle and hip in providing support during stance.

Peak knee extension in stance occurs at approximately 40% of the gait cycle, at which point the swing phase knee flexion wave begins. Recall that at this same point in the gait cycle, the ankle is maximally dorsiflexed and ankle power generation begins to produce ankle plantar flexion, thereby displacing the ankle center upward and forward. This action may also accelerate the knee center upward and forward as well, thereby initiating the swing phase knee flexion wave. A second source of power for the production of knee flexion in swing is the late stance hip flexor moment with its associated hip power generation that begins at approximately 50% of the gait cycle (51,53,84). A hip flexor moment accelerates the thigh and the knee joint center forward. The proximal end of the shank translates forward as well, but segment inertia limits the simultaneous rotation of the shank. This combination of thigh rotation and shank translation results in knee flexion.

A knee flexor moment (Figure 4-12, Point M) is produced in the second half of swing phase at the same time that the knee is rapidly extending. One might have more readily anticipated that this rapid knee extension would have required a net knee extensor moment. This apparent contradiction can be explained by again examining the simultaneous hip kinetics. Recall, that a hip extensor moment is seen in the second half of swing. This hip extensor moment decelerates the thigh and the knee joint center. Consequently, the proximal end of the shank decelerates, but the center of mass and distal end of the shank are carried forward by momentum, causing the shank to rotate forward. The forward rotation of the thigh is slowed while the forward rotation of the shank is facilitated, thus the knee is extended. The knee flexor moment controls the rate of knee extension to avoid injury to posterior ligamentous structures. The hamstrings, in crossing both the hip and the knee, may aid in simultaneously producing a hip extensor moment that promotes knee extension and a knee flexor moment that controls that motion.

Hip – Coronal Plane of the Joint

During ambulation, the line of action of the body weight vector typically passes medial to the hip center (Figure 4-13). Consequently, during single support, gravity pulls the body COM downward. An internal hip abductor

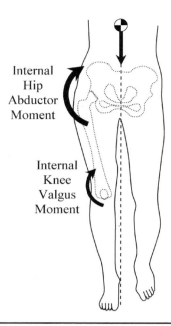

FIGURE 4-13. Schematic of a person in single support. The weight of the head, arms, and trunk would tend to cause hip adduction and knee varus. The internal hip and knee moments counter this tendency.

moment (Figure 4-14A, Point A) counters this effect and supports the pelvis and upper body during single support (commonly associated with eccentric contraction of the hip abductors). The magnitude of the coronal plane hip moment during each double support interval is small, consistent with the loading and unloading of the ground reactions during this interval (assuming that the contributions to the moment by segment weight and segment inertia are also small). Early in stance, hip power absorption (Figure 4-14A, Point B) results from the combination of the hip abductor moment and hip adduction (caused by the drop of the contralateral pelvis). Later in stance, power generation (Figure 4-14A, Point C) is realized as the hip abductor moment aids in elevating the depressed contralateral pelvis.

Knee – Coronal Plane of the Joint

With respect to the knee, the line of action of the weight vector also typically passes medial to the knee center (Figure 4-13). The distance between the force line of action and the knee center is less than at the hip. Consequently, the pattern of the internal valgus knee moment (Figure 4-14B) is similar but reduced in magnitude.

For additional detail pertaining to intersegmental moments and powers during normal gait, readers are referred to Davis and Õunpuu (16).

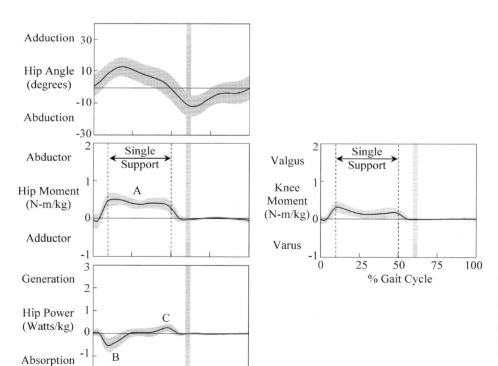

FIGURE 4-14. (A) Coronal plane hip angle, moment and power, and (B) coronal plane knee moment associated with a group of 27 pediatric subjects evaluated at Newington Children's Hospital (Newington, Connecticut) in 1988 and 1989, as described in (46). Shown are average values (*solid line*), one standard deviation in average value (*gray band*), and average foot off (*vertical gray line*).

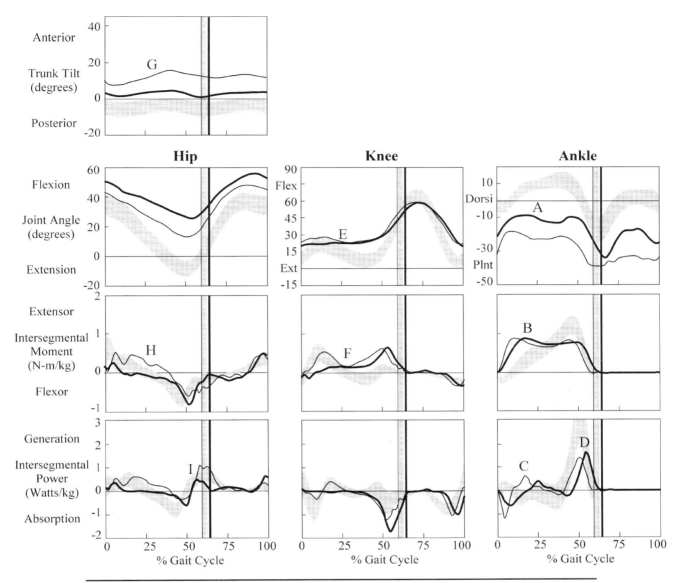

FIGURE 4-15. Sagittal plane joint angles, moments and powers for the hip, knee and ankle for two ten-year-old subjects, one with hemiplegic type cerebral palsy (*thin line*) and one with congenital proximal myopathy (*thick line*). Shown also are one standard deviation in average value (*gray band*) and average foot off (*vertical gray line*) associated with the normative data presented in Figure 4-12.

Example—Kinetics in Pathological Gait

With respect to clinical application, intersegmental moment and power data should not be examined in isolation. A comprehensive interpretation of a patient's walking pattern for clinical decision-making should include their medical history, observational gait findings documented by a video record, clinical examination results (e.g., lower extremity joint ranges of motion, muscle strength and tone, evidence of muscle spasticity and contracture, bony deformity) as well as quantitative gait data: stride and temporal measurements, segment and joint kinematics (i.e., angular displacement), EMG tracings, and joint kinetics (15,18).

A systematic review of this information by a multidisciplinary clinical team affords an opportunity to distinguish primary deviations from compensatory mechanisms. Subtle abnormalities seen in the joint kinematics may be highlighted by the intersegmental moment and power results.

To illustrate these points, the data for two ten-year-old females, one with right hemiplegic type cerebral palsy (CP) and the other with congenital proximal myopathy, are presented in Figure 4-15. While their diagnoses are quite different, with one exhibiting primarily muscle spasticity and hypertonicity (that overlays muscle weakness) and motor control deficits and the other presenting with proximal muscle weakness, their sagittal kinematic patterns are quite similar.

Both girls are toe walkers with excessive ankle plantar flexion throughout the gait cycle (Figure 4-15, Point A) resulting from plantar flexor tightness and over-activity. This results in an elevated plantar flexor moment in early stance (Figure 4-15, Point B). Moreover, the peak plantar flexor moment later in stance is reduced because the equinus (excessive plantar flexion) ankle position reduces the moment arm between the GRF and the ankle center. Premature ankle power generation is seen with both subjects (Figure 4-15, Point C) but for different reasons. For the girl with CP, a spastic stretch reflex ends an ankle dorsiflexing motion in early stance and produces a slight plantar flexing motion. The girl with proximal myopathy produces the slight plantar flexing motion in midstance as a "vault" compensation to aid in clearance for the contralateral swing limb. The magnitude of ankle power generation in late stance (Figure 4-15, Point D) is reduced for both girls. For both girls, the excessively plantar flexed position of their ankles throughout stance predisposes them to poor plantar flexion velocity in late stance. That is, the already-shortened plantar flexor muscles may be poorly positioned to produce additional contractile force. Producing significantly more plantar flexion in late stance is also counterproductive with respect to foot attitude, that is, a more vertically-oriented foot in early swing presents a greater challenge with respect to clearance later in swing.

For both girls, their knees are excessively flexed at foot contact and throughout stance (Figure 4-15, Point E). The knee intersegmental moment in stance is reasonably well "compensated" in both cases (Figure 4-15, Point F). That is, one might anticipate greater knee extensor moment magnitudes with 20 to 30 degrees of knee flexion in single support. The excessive ankle plantar flexion-knee extension couple restrains the forward motion of the shank and supports the knee during single support. For the girl with CP, an anterior trunk lean (Figure 4-15, Point G) shifts her body COM forward and moves the GRF vector closer to the knee center. This also elevates her hip extensor moment in stance (Figure 4-15, Point H). The elevated hip extensor moment controls forward motion of the thigh, also supporting the knee during single support. Her adequate hip extensor strength (documented in the clinical examination) facilitates this compensation. With hip extensor weakness associated with proximal myopathy, the other girl is more limited with respect to using her trunk posture to control the GRF. Alternatively, she walks with a shorter step length (73% relative to an age-matched normal). In this way, the moments at both the hip and knee are reduced as the excursion of the GRF will be reduced and the elevated plantar flexor moment is sufficient to control the knee. It is observed that her precise control of the GRF significantly reduces her need to produce an internal hip extensor moment.

A comprehensive surgical package was recommended for the girl with CP, including right femoral derotational rotational osteotomy, right medial hamstring lengthening, and right rectus femoris transfer. These recommendations were based on her clinical examination, kinematics, and EMG. The excessive plantar flexor moment and premature ankle power generation in early stance, along with the excessive plantar flexion throughout stance and tightness on clinical examination, supported a recommendation for right gastrocnemius recession.

The referring physician for the girl with proximal myopathy was considering bilateral gastrocnemius recession given her equinus gait pattern. Based on this girl's limited hip power production (Figure 4-15, Point I) and her finely tuned control of the GRF to minimize hip extensor moment requirements, the gait analysis team recommended only continued clinical follow-up with no surgery. For additional information related to the interpretation of pathological gait patterns, readers are referred to Sutherland and Davids (66) and Õunpuu (43).

WORK AND ENERGY

Work is done when a force is displaced linearly some distance along its line of action or a moment is displaced rotationally through some angular displacement. When a book is put up on a shelf, work is done on the book (i.e., its weight is displaced upward). When a wrench tightens a bolt, work is done by the wrench (i.e., the applied moment is displaced in the direction of its application) and work is done on the bolt (i.e., the resisting moment offered by the bolt is displaced opposite to its direction of resistance). The rate at which work is done is defined as power. More power is required to tighten the bolt quickly than slowly. In mechanics, work and energy are intimately related. When work is done on a "system," the energy level of the system increases. Conversely, when work is done by a system, the energy level of the system decreases. System definition depends on the scope of the analysis. In placing the book on the shelf, the system might be defined to include only the book or it might be expanded to include the book and the person performing the task as well.

The muscles that produce internal intersegmental moments during a sit-to-stand task do work. That is, the downward weight (force) of the head, arms, and trunk (HAT) is displaced vertically upward. Consequently, the lower extremity muscles have done work on the HAT segment. Alternatively, this work may be characterized as a change in the gravitational potential energy of the segment (defined as the product of the weight of the segment and its height above some reference level or datum), expressed mathematically as

$$E_P = mgh$$

where mg is the segment weight (the product of mass and gravitational constant) and h is the height of the segment COM above some datum. In this case, the gravitational potential energy of the HAT segment is increased as the HAT COM is displaced upward. In this same way, the gravitational potential energy of the HAT segment increases and decreases over the gait cycle (as described below).

Another type of potential energy is elastic potential energy. The elastic potential energy of a mechanical spring is increased when it is compressed (or stretched). Observe that, again, this elastic potential energy is related to the linear displacement of the spring force, i.e., the work done on the spring. In this same way, the elastic potential energies of the muscles and tendons of the lower extremity change during activities such as walking. Elastic potential energy cannot be directly assessed during gait, however, as this would require measures of muscle force and displacement as well as tendon force and displacement. This represents the most significant limitation of this technique because elastic potential energy stored in and returned from soft tissue structures may be significant in gait during intervals with coactivity of agonists and antagonists muscles, e.g., transitions from swing to stance.

Kinetic energy, the "energy of motion," can, however, be computed. Translational kinetic energy, E_{KT}, is a function of the mass, m, and linear velocity, v, of the segment of interest, expressed as

$$E_{KT} = \frac{1}{2}mv^2$$

Similarly, rotational kinetic energy, E_{KR}, is expressed as

$$E_{KR} = \frac{1}{2}I\omega^2$$

where I is the centroidal mass moment of inertia about an axis that coincides with the angular velocity, or a vector component of the angular velocity, ω. For example, if the motion of walking is assumed to lie in one plane, i.e., a sagittal plane, then the axis associated with segmental angular velocity and the centroidal mass moment of inertia would be perpendicular to that plane. In 3D analyses, the relationship is easily expanded to include the three components of the angular velocity vector along with the associated principal mass moment of inertia, i.e.,

$$E_{KR} = \frac{1}{2}I_{xx}\,\omega_x{}^2 + \frac{1}{2}\,I_{yy}\,\omega_y{}^2 + \frac{1}{2}\,I_{zz}\omega_z{}^2$$

The interplay between potential and kinetic energy is quite interesting. Consider the simple pendulum comprised of a small ball (concentrated mass) and a lightweight string shown in Figure 4-16. As this pendulum swings back and forth, kinetic and potential energy are exchanged. Immediately after the pendulum is released from its highest elevation (Figure 4-16, Point A), its potential energy is maximum and its kinetic energy is zero (the pendulum is released from a stationary position). As the pendulum swings down and the ball loses elevation and gains speed (Figure 4-16, Point B), the potential energy decreases while the kinetic energy increases. When the pendulum reaches its lowest point and the ball is moving at its fastest velocity (Figure 4-16, Point C), the potential energy is minimized while the kinetic energy is maximized. Note that in this example, if gravitational potential energy is referenced to the lowest elevation of the pendulum path, then the gravitational potential energy would be equal to zero at this point. As the pendulum swings away from vertical and the ball gains elevation and loses speed, the potential energy increases while the kinetic energy decreases (Figure 4-16, Point D). At its highest point when the ball stops momentarily (Figure 4-16, Point E), all of the available kinetic energy has been transformed into potential energy, which is maximized at this point. In this idealized example, energy losses to air resistance (friction) and strain in the string have been neglected and the transfer between kinetic and potential energy is complete. Its total mechanical energy (the sum of kinetic and potential energy) remains constant and illustrates the law of conservation of energy. This idealized pendulum would continue to swing in perpetuity.

In an extension of this example, agonist and antagonist muscles are added to the simple pendulum (Figure 4-17). Immediately after the pendulum is released, both muscles are inactive and the total energy level of the system (which now includes both muscles as well as the pendulum)

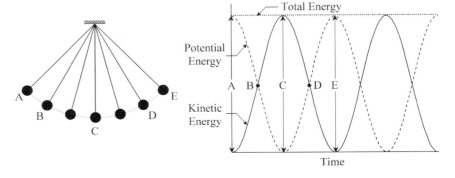

FIGURE 4-16. Energy changes due to motion of a simple pendulum. If air resistance and strain in the string are neglected, there is a complete transfer between potential and kinetic energy during motion. Consequently, the total energy of the pendulum remains constant.

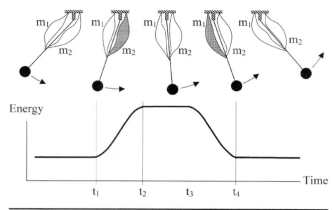

FIGURE 4-17. Agonist and antagonist muscles are added to a simple pendulum. Concentric muscle contraction (m_2 from t_1 to t_2) increases the energy level of the pendulum, and eccentric muscle contraction (m_1 from t_3 to t_4) decreases the energy level of the pendulum.

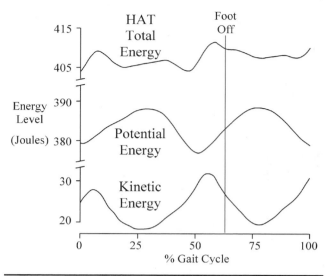

FIGURE 4-18. Potential energy, kinetic energy, and total energy of the HAT for an adult female walking at 71 m/min.

is constant. It is assumed in this illustration that the energy change associated with the passive elongation of the muscles is negligible. Muscle m_2 concentrically contracts from time t_1 to t_2. The muscle does work as its contractile force results in muscle shortening (i.e., force and displacement are in the same direction). Consequently, energy is added to the system. From t_2 to t_3 both muscles are again inactive and the system energy level remains constant. Eccentric contraction of muscle m_1 from t_3 to t_4 removes energy from the system. Work is done on the muscle since its contractile force results in muscle lengthening (i.e., force and displacement are in opposite directions).

This transfer between kinetic and potential energy can be seen in gait (7), as illustrated by the representative data presented in Figure 4-18 for the HAT. The gravitational potential energy reaches a minimum twice in the gait cycle during each period of double support, when the COM of the HAT is at its lowest point vertically. The kinetic energy (the sum of translational and rotational kinetic energies) is greatest at these same points, coincident with the maximum velocities of the HAT. The gravitational potential energy peaks at midstance, at about 30% and 80% of the gait cycle in the data shown in Figure 4-18, when the COM of the HAT has been lifted to its highest elevation. Note that 80% in the gait cycle for the ipsilateral limb is coincident with midstance for the contralateral limb. The velocity of the COM of the HAT has also slowed at midstance; consequently, kinetic energy is minimal at this point. The change in total HAT energy over the gait cycle (8 Joules) is less than either the change in gravitational potential energy (11 Joules) or kinetic energy (14 Joules). The exchange between kinetic and potential energy, although incomplete, reduces the lower extremity muscular effort (and metabolic energy) required for walking (7).

The energy requirements of a lower extremity segment and each associated leg segment depicted in Figure 4-19 are consistent with other investigators (7). The change in the total energy for the leg segments over the gait cycle is due principally to the change in translational kinetic energy in swing. However, for this subject, rotational kinetic energy did contribute up to 7% of the total energy of the shank in swing (78). With each leg segment, the total energy is minimal in midstance when segment velocities and kinetic energies are minimal as well. For gravitational potential energy, the vertical displacement of each segment is measured relative to the ground. Energy is added to each leg segment in late stance and taken away from each leg segment in late swing.

The change in energy requirements for both legs is less than the energy change for one leg during gait, 12 Joules compared with 18 Joules for the individual's data presented in Figure 4-19. That is, the minimal energy of one (stance) leg combines with maximal energy of the other (swing) limb to result in a biphasic pattern for both legs. A similar biphasic pattern is seen for the total energy requirement of the entire body during gait, with change in energy seen in late single support and during the second double support interval for each side. An asymmetry in the energy requirements between the two lower extremities can be appreciated for this individual with the peak body total energy level in swing greater than the peak body total energy level in stance (coinciding with swing for the contralateral limb), i.e., 516 Joules as compared to 511 Joules.

The rate of change of these energy values reflects the power requirements of the body during gait, i.e., power is the rate that energy is supplied or taken away. For the subject whose data are depicted in Figure 4-20, the whole body in early and late stance requires power. During both

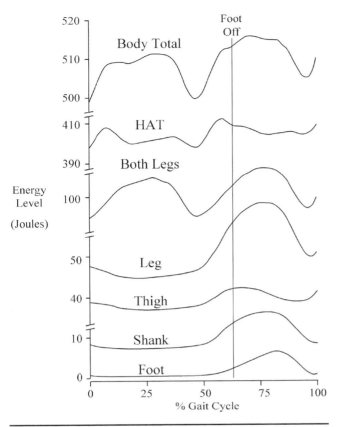

FIGURE 4-19. Energy levels for the whole body, HAT, both lower extremities, right lower extremity, thigh, shank, and foot for one adult female walking at 71 m/min.

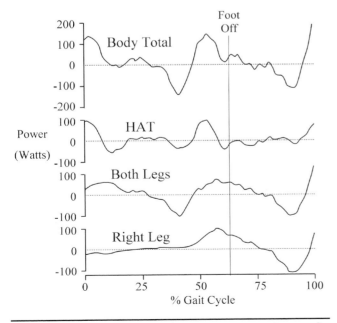

FIGURE 4-20. Rate of energy change or power requirement for the whole body, HAT, both legs, and the right leg for one adult female walking at 71 m/min.

of these intervals, power is required to lift the body COM from first double support to midstance and to propel the stance limb into swing. Sources of energy include muscles acting on the body segments, e.g., the lower extremities, or the release of stored elastic energy. Power is also taken away (energy is released or lost) from the whole body during the second half of single support and in late swing. During both of these intervals, the body COM falls from its highest elevation at midstance and a swing leg is decelerated in preparation for foot contact. Work is done on structures capable of absorbing energy, e.g., the passive elongation of muscles shortened by contraction, such as the hip flexors in single support and the hamstrings in late swing.

These power "requirements" were derived mathematically from the segmental mechanical energy profiles. An alternative power flow analysis during gait employs the rate of displacement (i.e., linear and angular velocity) of the intersegmental forces and moments (58). For example, the power flow within the shank can be computed through a consideration of the ankle and knee moments rotating with the shank and the ankle and knee forces translating with the ankle and knee centers, respectively. Robertson and Winter (58) found good agreement between the rate of energy change and power flow in the lower extremity. Siegel et al. (61) improved this correlation for the foot through a full 3D analysis that also included the power contributions of the ground reactions. The results of a power flow analysis for one adult subject are presented in Figure 4-21 along with her rate of mechanical energy change data for comparison. The correlation between the rate of energy change and power flow over the gait cycle ranged from 0.796 for the thigh to 0.997 for the foot, again, comparable to values reported previously (58,61).

To appreciate the mechanisms associated with segmental power flow data depicted in Figure 4-21, the different contributors, e.g., joint force and moment, are presented in Figure 4-22. For the foot in stance, ankle moment power generation is largely offset by ankle force power absorption. Ankle force power generation in the first half of swing increases the translational kinetic energy of the foot (as was seen in Figure 4-19). Conversely, ankle force power absorption in the second half of swing decreases the translational kinetic energy of the foot. For the shank, a dominant ankle force power generation (moderated by ankle moment, knee moment, and knee force power absorption) provides initial shank power generation in late stance. Knee force power generation is the primary contributor to shank power generation just before toe-off and into early swing. This phasing of power generation is consistent with an early contribution by the plantar flexor muscles followed by a later contribution by the hip flexors. In late swing, ankle force power generation is offset by knee force power absorption. Consequently, shank power absorption in the second half of swing is primarily due to knee

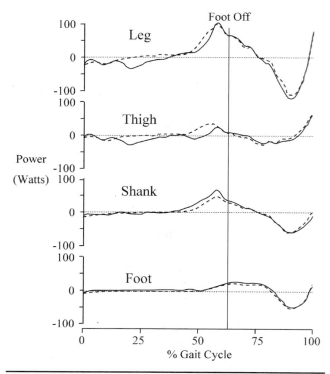

FIGURE 4-21. Power flow of each right leg segment and the entire leg (*solid line*) shown with the associated mechanical power requirements for the same segments (*dashed line*) for one adult female walking at 71 m/min.

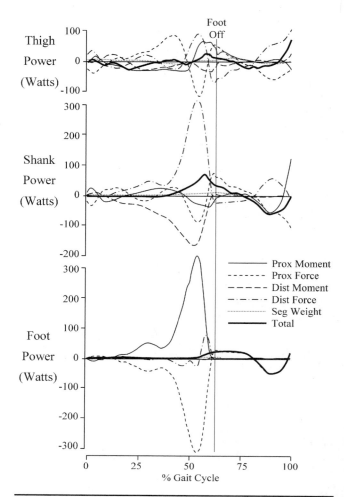

FIGURE 4-22. Contributions to power flow of each right leg segment for one adult female walking at 71 m/min.

moment power absorption, consistent with hamstring power absorption. The sharp rise in knee moment power generation at the end of the gait cycle for this particular individual is associated with an aberrant flexing of the knee in preparation for foot contact (a slight correction for knee hyperextension during terminal swing). A coincident increase in knee force power absorption is seen as well at this time. For the thigh, excessive hip moment power absorption in stance for this individual results in overall thigh power absorption in stance. Hip moment power generation at foot off (moderated by the other contributors) results in thigh power generation, increasing the mechanical (translational kinetic) energy of the thigh. Hip and knee forces contribute to thigh power absorption during midswing. Knee force power generation is balanced by hip force power absorption in late swing. The sharp rise in thigh power generation in late stance is attributed to knee force power generation and results in a small increase (2 Joules) in the energy level for the thigh (Figure 4-19). Readers are referred to the work of Robertson and Winter (58,79) for additional details pertaining to these energy transfer processes.

A power flow analysis provides a measure of the power into and out of individual lower extremity segments. By tracking the power flow between the segments in the leg and assuming that segmental energy increases only with intersegmental power generation, Meinders et al. (37) used this technique to estimate the role of the plantar flexors on HAT energy. More recently, other investigators have used forward dynamics techniques in conjunction with power flow analysis to examine more directly the effect of intersegmental moments on trunk propulsion (57) and the effect of intersegmental moments in one leg on the dynamics of the contralateral leg as well as the trunk (62). These latter approaches indicate that *both* positive and negative intersegmental power can contribute to the increase in the energy level of other segments. Inferences can be made from power flow analysis based on intersegmental moments computed through inverse dynamics, but this technique cannot directly identify those muscles that are responsible for propulsion and support during locomotion.

SUMMARY

Human locomotion is fundamentally related to the production of muscle force that either creates or controls that motion. Muscle forces act at some distance away from the joints that they span. These moment arms provide the muscles with the leverage to generate intersegmental moments that produce and control the rotations of those joints. It also allows the muscle forces to be transmitted to the joints so that these joint forces can accelerate and move the HAT, referred to as the passenger unit by Perry (52). The ground reaction loads are an external reflection of these internal forces. Muscles provide "local" control over the joints that they span, but as described by Zajak and his colleagues (40,85), the primary function of muscles can be the redistribution of power and energy among the body segments.

Inverse dynamics approaches provide some insight into the mechanisms that move and control the lower extremity joints. This information can be useful in assessing treatment options or evaluating treatment approaches clinically. Inverse dynamics is limited with respect to the prediction of muscle forces during walking. Net internal intersegmental moments combine contributions of both agonist and antagonist muscles. Intersegmental forces are underestimated, i.e., do not reflect joint contact force magnitudes. Optimization techniques to allow the prediction of muscle force from computed intersegmental forces and moments are improving (64), but are still limited with respect to clinical application. The direct measurement of muscle force with miniature intramuscular pressure transducers may ultimately resolve this empirical quandary (13,32).

Forward dynamics approaches show good promise in elucidating the relationships between muscle force production and gait kinematics as these techniques can provide estimates of muscle force. Sophisticated whole-body forward simulations afford an excellent platform from which to investigate the role of different muscles and muscle groups in locomotion (1,2). The sensitivity of the conclusions of these simulations to uncertainty in the underlying model and the model parameters needs to be further clarified (85). Current efforts to build models that incorporate subject-specific parameters related to muscle characteristics and bone geometry are expected to provide assistance in clinical decision-making (55,56). Significant challenges lie ahead, however. For example, forward simulations require optimization criteria to direct the computational process. It is not clear that the optimization strategy that is appropriate in the investigation of able-body gait will apply in pathological gait analysis.

REFERENCES

1. Anderson FC, Goldberg SR, Pandy MG, Delp SL. Contributions of muscle forces and toe-off kinematics to peak knee flexion during the swing phase of normal gait: an induced position analysis. *J Biomech* 2004;37:731–737.
2. Anderson FC, Pandy MG. Dynamic optimization of human walking. *J Biomech Eng* 2001;123:381–390.
3. Braune W, Fischer O. *The Human Gait* (translation). Berlin: Springer, 1987.
4. Bresler B, Frankel JP. The forces and moments in the leg during level walking. *Trans ASME* 1950;72:27–36.
5. Buczek FL, Kepple TM, Siegel KL, Stanhope SJ. Translational and rotational joint power terms in a six degree-of-freedom model of the normal ankle complex. *J Biomech* 1994;27:1447–1457.
6. Cappozzo A, Berme N. Body segment inertial parameter determination. In: Berme N, Cappozzo A, eds. *Biomechanics of Human Movement: Applications in Rehabilitation, Sports and Ergonomics.* Worthington, Ohio: Bertec Corporation; 1990;179–185.
7. Cappozzo A, Figura F, Marchetti M. The interplay of muscular and external forces in human ambulation. *J Biomech* 1976;9:35–43.
8. Chandler RF, Clauser CE, McConville JT, Reynolds HM, Young JW. Investigation of inertial properties of the human body. AMRL-TR-74-137, AD-A016-485. DOT-HS-801-430. Aerospace Medical Research Laboratories, Wright-Patterson Air Force Base, Ohio; 1975.
9. Chao EYS. Determination of applied forces in linkage systems with known displacements: with special application to biomechanics. PhD Dissertation, University of Iowa, Iowa City; IA, 1971.
10. Chao EY, Rim K. Application of optimization principles in determining the applied moments in human leg joints during gait. *J Biomech* 1973;6:497–510.
11. Clauser CE, McConville JT, Young JW. Weight, volume and center of mass of segments of the human body. AMRL-TR-69-70. Aerospace Medical Research Laboratory, Wright-Patterson Air Force Base, Ohio; 1969.
12. Crowninshield RD. Use of optimization techniques to predict muscle forces. *J Biomech Eng* 1978;100:88–92.
13. Davis J, Kaufman KR, Lieber RL. Correlation between active and passive isometric stress and intramuscular pressure in the isolated rabbit tibialis anterior muscle. *J Biomech* 2003;36:505–512.
14. Davis RB. The motion analysis laboratory. In: Gage JR, ed. *The Treatment of Gait Problems in Cerebral Palsy.* London: MacKeith Press; 2004;90–98.
15. Davis RB, DeLuca PA, Õunpuu S. Analysis of gait. In: Schneck DJ, Bronzino JD, eds. *Biomechanics: Principles and Applications* Boca Raton: CRC Press; 2002;8:1–9.
16. Davis RB, Õunpuu S. Kinetics of normal gait. In: Gage JR, ed. *The Treatment of Gait Problems in Cerebral Palsy.* London: MacKeith Press; 2004;120–134.
17. Davis RB, Õunpuu S, Tyburski DJ, Gage JR. A gait analysis data collection and reduction technique. *Hum Mov Sci* 1991;10:575–587.
18. DeLuca, PA. Gait analysis in the treatment of the ambulatory child with cerebral palsy. *Clin Orthop Rel Res* 1991;264:5–75.
19. Dempster WT. Space requirements of the seated operator: Geometrical, kinematic, and mechanical aspects of the body with special reference to the limbs. WADC-55-159, AD-087-892. Wright Air Development Center. Wright-Patterson Air Force Base, Ohio; 1955.
20. Elftman H. Forces and energy changes in the leg during walking. *Am J Physiol* 1939;125:339–356.
21. Eng JJ, Winter DA. Kinetic analysis of the lower limbs during walking: What information can be gained from a three-dimensional model? *J Biomech* 1995;28:753–758.
22. Gage JR, Perry J, Hicks RR, Koop S, Werntz JR. Rectus femoris transfer to improve knee function of children with cerebral palsy. *Dev Med Child Neurol* 1987;29:159–166.
23. Hanavan EP A mathematical model of the human body. AMRL-TR-64-102, AD-608-463. Aerospace Medical Research Laboratories, Wright-Patterson Air Force Base, Ohio; 1964.
24. Harrington IJ. Static and dynamic loading patterns in knee joints with deformities. *J Bone Joint Surg* 1983;65-A(2):247–259.
25. Hatze HA. A mathematical model for the human body. *J Biomech* 1980;13:833–843.
26. Hullin MG, Robb JE, Loudon IR. Ankle-foot orthosis function in low-level myelomeningocele. *J Pediatric Orthop* 1992;12:518–521.
27. Jenson RK. Body segment mass, radius and radius of gyration proportions of children. *J Biomech* 1986;19:359–368.
28. Johnson F, Leitl S, Waugh W. The distribution of load across the knee: a comparison of static and dynamic measurements. *J Bone Joint Surg* 1980;62-B:346–349.

29. Judge J, Davis RB, Õunpuu S. Step length reductions in advanced age: the role of ankle and hip kinetics. *J Gerontology: Med Sci* 1996;51A:M303–M312.

30. Kaufman KR, An KN, Chao EYS. A comparison of intersegmental joint dynamics to isokinetic dynamometer measurements. *J Biomech* 1995;28:1243–1256.

31. Kaufman KR, An KN, Litchy WJ, Chao EYS. Physiological prediction of muscle forces: Part I - Theoretical formulation. *Neurosci* 1991;40:781–792.

32. Kaufman KR, Wavering T, Morrow D, Davis J, Lieber RL. Performance characteristics of a pressure microsensor. *J Biomech* 2003;36:283–287.

33. Kepple TM, Siegel KL, Stanhope SJ. Relative contributions of the lower extremity joint moments to forward progression and support during gait. *Gait Posture* 1997;6:1–8.

34. Lai KA, Kuo KN, Andriacchi TP. Relationship between dynamic deformities and joint moments in children with cerebral palsy. *J Pediatric Orthop* 1988;8:690–695.

35. Manal K, McClay I, Richards J, Galinat B, Stanhope S. Knee moment profiles during walking: errors due to soft tissue movement of the shank and the influence of the reference coordinate system. *Gait Posture* 2002;15:10–17.

36. McConville JT, Churchill TD, Kaleps I, Clauser CE, Cuzzi J. Anthropometric relationships of body and body segment moments of inertia. Technical report AFAMRL-TR-80-119, Air Force Aerospace Medical Research Laboratory, Aerospace Medical Division, Air Force Systems Command, Wright-Patterson Air Force Base, Ohio; Yr.

37. Meinders M, Gitter A, Czerniecki JM. The role of plantar flexor work muscle work during walking. *Scan J Rehab Med* 1998;30:39–46.

38. Meriam JL, Kraige LG. *Engineering Mechanics—Dynamics*. New York: John Wiley & Sons; 1997.

39. Neptune RR, Kautz SA, Zajac FE. Contributions of the individual ankle plantar flexors to support, forward progression and swing initiation. *J Biomech* 2001;34:1387–1398.

40. Neptune RR, Zajac FE, Kautz SA. Muscle force redistributes segmental power for body progression during walking. *Gait Posture* 2004;19:194–205.

41. Olney SJ, Costigan PA, Hedden DM. Mechanical energy patterns in gait of cerebral palsied children with hemiplegia. *Phys Ther* 1987;67:1348–1354.

42. Olney SJ, MacPhail HA, Hedden DM, Boyce WF. Work and power in hemiplegic cerebral palsy gait. *Phys Ther* 1990;70:431–438.

43. Õunpuu S. Patterns of gait pathology. In: Gage JR, ed. *The Treatment of Gait Problems in Cerebral Palsy*. London: MacKeith Press; 2004;217–237.

44. Õunpuu S, Bell KJ, Davis RB, DeLuca PA. An evaluation of the posterior leaf spring orthosis using joint kinematics and kinetics. *J Pediatric Orthop* 1996;16:378–384.

45. Õunpuu S, Davis RB, DeLuca PA. Joint kinetics: methods, interpretation and treatment decision-making in children with cerebral palsy and myelomeningocele. *Gait & Posture* 1996;4:62–78.

46. Õunpuu S, Gage JR, Davis RB. Three-dimensional lower extremity joint kinetics in normal pediatric gait. *J Pediatric Orthop* 1991;11:341–349.

47. Õunpuu S, Muik E, Davis RB, Gage JR, DeLuca PA. Part I: the effect of the rectus femoris transfer location on knee motion in children with cerebral palsy. *J Pediatric Orthop* 1993;13:325–330.

48. Õunpuu S, Thompson JD, Davis RB, DeLuca PA. An examination of knee function during gait in children with myelomeningocele. *J Pediatric Orthop* 2000;20:629–635.

49. Palladino J, Davis RB. Biomechanics. In: Enderle J, Blanchard S, Bronzino J, eds. *Introduction to Biomedical Engineering*. Amslerdam: Elsevier Academic Press; 2005;127–210.

50. Paul JP. Forces transmitted by the joints in the human body. *Proc Inst Mech Eng* 1967;181:8–15.

51. Perry J. Distal rectus femoris transfer. *Dev Med Child Neurol* 1987;29:153–158.

52. Perry J. *Gait Analysis: Normal and Pathological Function*. Thorofare, NJ: Slack; 1992.

53. Piazza SJ, Delp SL. The influence of muscles on knee flexion during the swing phase of gait. *J Biomech* 1996;29:723–733.

54. Prodromos CC, Andriacchi TP, Galante JO. A relationship between gait and clinical changes following high tibial osteotomy. *J Bone Joint Surg* 1985;67–A:1188–1194.

55. Riemer RF. Validated, subject-specific model for predicting tibiofemoral knee force distribution from intersegmental forces. MS Thesis, Department of Mechanical Engineering, Houghton, Michigan: Michigan Technological University; 2003.

56. Riemer RF, Haut Donahue T, Kaufman KR. Tibiofemoral load distribution during gait of normal subjects. *Proceedings of American Society of Biomechanics*, 2004.

57. Riley PO, Dela Croce U, Kerrigan DC. Effect of age on lower extremity joint moment contributions to gait speed. *Gait Posture* 2001;14:264–270.

58. Robertson DGE, Winter DA. Mechanical energy generation, absorption and transfer amongst segments during walking. *J Biomech* 1980;13:845–854.

59. Rose SA, DeLuca PA, Davis RB, Õunpuu S, Gage JR. Kinematic and kinetic evaluation of the ankle following lengthening of the gastrocnemius fascia in children with cerebral palsy. *J Pediatric Orthop* 1993;13:727–732.

60. Sadeghi H, Somaye S, Prince F, Allard P, Labelle H, Vaughan CL. Functional roles of the ankle and hip sagittal muscle moments in able-bodied gait. *Clin Biomech* 2001;16:688–695.

61. Siegel KL, Kepple TM, Caldwell GE. Improved agreement of foot segmental power and rate of energy change during gait: Inclusion of distal power terms and use of three-dimensional models. *J Biomech* 1996;6:823–827.

62. Siegel KL, Kepple TM, Stanhope SJ. Joint moment control of mechanical energy flow during normal gait. *Gait Posture* 2004;19:69–75.

63. Spoor CW, van Leeuwen JL, Meskers CGM, Titulaer AF, Huson A. Estimation of instantaneous moment arms of lower-leg muscles. *J Biomech* 1990;23:1247–1259.

64. Stansfield BW, Nicol AC, Paul JP, Kelly IG, Graichen F, Bergmann G. Direct comparison of calculated hip joint contact forces with those measured using instrumented implants. An evaluation of a three-dimensional mathematical model of the lower limb. *J Biomech* 2003;36:929–936.

65. Sutherland DH, Cooper L, Daniel D. The role of the ankle plantar flexors in normal walking. *J Bone Joint Surg* 1980;62-A:354–363.

66. Sutherland DH, Davids JR. Common gait abnormalities of the knee in cerebral palsy. *Clin Orthop* 1993;288:139–147.

67. Sutherland DH, Santi M, Abel MF. Treatment of stiff-knee gait in cerebral palsy: a comparison by gait analysis of distal rectus femoris transfer versus proximal rectus release. *J Pediatric Orthop* 1990;10:433–441.

68. Thomson JD, Õunpuu S, Davis RB, DeLuca PA. The effects of the ankle foot orthoses on knee and ankle motion in persons with myelomeningocele: an evaluation using three-dimensional gait analysis. *J Pediatric Orthop* 1999;19:27–33.

69. Wang J-W, Kuo KN, Andriacchi TP, Galante JO. The influence of walking mechanics and time on the results of proximal tibial osteotomy. *J Bone Joint Surg* 1990;72-A:905–909.

70. Wang H, Olney SJ. Relationships between alignment, kinematic and kinetic measures of the knee of normal elderly subjects in level walking. *Clin Biomech* 1994;9:245–252.

71. Waters RL, Garland DE, Perry J, Habig T, Slabaugh P. Stiff-legged gait in hemiplegia: surgical correction. *J Bone Joint Surg* 1976;927–933.

72. Weinbach A. Contour maps, center of gravity, moments of inertia and surface area of the human body. *Hum Bio* 1938;10:356–371.

73. Winter DA. Overall principle of lower limb support during stance phase of gait. *J Biomech* 1980;13:923–927.

74. Winter DA. Use of kinetic analyses in the diagnostics of pathological gait. *Physiotherapy Canada* 1981;33:209–214.

75. Winter DA. Energy generation and absorption at the ankle and knee during fast, natural, and slow cadences. *Clin Orthop Rel Res* 1983;175:147–154.

76. Winter DA. Kinematic and kinetic patterns in human gait: variability and compensating effects. *Hum Mov Sci* 1984;3:51–76.

77. Winter DA. *Biomechanics and Motor Control of Human Movement*. New York: John Wiley and Sons; 2005;86–117.

78. Winter DA, Quanbury AO, Reimer GD. Analysis of instantaneous energy of normal gait. *J Biomech* 1976;9:253–257.
79. Winter DA, Robertson DGE. Joint torque and energy patterns in normal gait. *Biol Cybernet* 1978;29:137–142.
80. Winter DA, Sidwell HG, Hobson DA. Measurement and reduction of noise in kinematics of locomotion. *J Biomech* 1974;7:157–159.
81. Woltring HJ. On smoothing and derivative estimation from noisy displacement data in biomechanics. *Hum Mov Sci* 1985;4:229–245.
82. Wood GA. Data smoothing and differentiation procedures in biomechanics. *Exerc Sport Sci Rev* 1982;10:308–362.
83. Yamaguchi GT. *Dynamic Modeling of Musculoskeletal Motion.* Boston: Kluwer Academic Publishers; 2001;3–21.
84. Yamaguchi GT, Zajac FE. Restoring unassisted natural gait to paraplegics via functional neuromuscular stimulation: a computer simulation study. *IEEE Trans Biomed Eng* 1991;37:886–902.
85. Zajac FE, Neptune RR, Kaytz SA. Biomechanics and muscular coordination of human walking: Part I: Introduction to concepts, power transfer, dynamics and simulations. *Gait Posture* 2002;16:215–232.

APPENDIX

Glossary of Gait Kinetics Terminology*

Acceleration – The rate of change of velocity with respect to time; a vector quantity with characteristics of magnitude and direction.

Angular acceleration – Acceleration associated with rotational displacement. Unit of measure: radians per second squared (rad/s^2).

Linear acceleration – Acceleration associated with translational displacement. Unit of measure: meters per second squared (m/s^2).

Body – In mechanics, a generic term that refers to the object under analysis (e.g., the entire human body or just a particular body segment such as the foot); in biomechanics, it generally refers to the entire human body.

Rigid body – An object whose deformation under the application of a set of forces may be considered negligible, i.e., the distance between any two points in the object is assumed to remain constant.

Center of gravity – The point through which the concentrated gravitational force (weight) of the body or a body segment passes. In a uniform gravitational field, the center of gravity and the center of mass are located at the same point.

Center of mass – The point where all of the mass of the body or a body segment could be concentrated and still have the same mechanical effect. In a uniform gravitational field, the center of mass and the center of gravity are located at the same point.

Center of pressure – The point of application of the ground reaction force.

Force – The action of one object on another that tends to change the state of rest or state of motion of the object to which it is applied; a vector quantity with characteristics of magnitude, direction, and point of application (or line of action). Unit of measure: Newtons (N).

Concentrated force – The effect of a distributed force acting at a point of application.

Distributed force – Forces acting between two bodies that are dispersed over the contact area shared by the two bodies, e.g., pressure under the foot during gait. Unit of measure: Newtons per meter squared (N/m^2) or Newtons per centimeter squared (N/cm^2). See also pressure.

External force – A force that is applied between the body and its environment. Examples include ground reaction force, body (or body segment) weight, and inertial force.

Ground reaction force – A concentrated force that represents the summation of the distributed forces (e.g., pressure) applied to the plantar surface of the foot at the center of pressure during activities such as gait.

Inertial force – A force that is associated with the acceleration of an object. This force resists a change in motion and consequently, it is directed opposite to the acceleration of the object.

Internal force – A force that is produced within the body. Examples include muscle force, ligamentous force, and joint contact force.

Intersegmental force – A force acting across the joint that dynamically balances the body segment under investigation. The magnitude of the intersegmental force underestimates the joint contact force, i.e., it does not reflect the entire compressive load applied to the joint.

Joint contact force – The compressive force applied to the joint, including all forces produced by muscles crossing the joint and those caused by gravity and any movement inertia.

Normal force – A force applied perpendicular to a surface, e.g., the vertical component of the ground reaction force.

Shear force – A force applied parallel to a surface, e.g., the anterior-posterior component of the ground reaction force.

Force couple – The torque produced by two equal and opposite forces that are noncollinear (not lying along the same line of action).

Forward dynamics – A process by which movement kinematics are predicted through the application of governing equations of motion that incorporate assumed (or derived) muscle activation patterns and estimated (e.g., segment inertial properties, muscle properties, musculoskeletal geometry) quantities.

*Readers are also referred to the engineering mechanics text by Meriam and Kraige (38).

Inertia – A resistance to a change in motion, i.e., velocity. See also mass and mass moment of inertia.

Inverse dynamics – A process by which intersegmental forces and moments are calculated through the application of governing equations (e.g., Newton's equations of motion) that incorporate measured (e.g., kinematics, ground reactions) and estimated (e.g., segment inertial properties) quantities.

Kinematics – The study of motion without reference to the forces that cause that motion. See also kinetics.

Kinetics – The study of motion that relates the action of forces to motion. See also kinematics.

Lever arm – Synonymous with moment arm.

Mass – A measure of the resistance of an object to a change in translational motion, i.e., its translational inertia. Unit of measure: kilogram (kg).

Mass moment of inertia – A measure of the resistance of an object to a change in rotational motion, i.e., its rotational inertia. The mass of the object and the distribution of that mass about particular axes passing through the object determine the magnitude of the mass moment of inertia. Unit of measure: kilogram-meters squared ($kg \cdot m^2$).

Mechanical energy – The capacity of an object or a system to do work; the sum of kinetic and potential energy.

  Kinetic energy – The energy associated with motion. Kinetic energy combines either the mass of the object and its translational velocity or the mass moment of inertia of the object and its rotational velocity. Unit of measure: Joule (J).

  Potential energy (gravitational) – The energy associated with work done against or by gravity. Gravitational potential energy combines the weight of the object and the height of its center of mass above some reference height or datum. Unit of measure: Joule (J).

  Potential energy (elastic) – The energy associated with work done against or by the force of elastic elements within the object, e.g., passive muscle tissue, ligaments. Elastic potential energy combines the force of the elastic structure and the distance that the force is displaced along its line of action. Unit of measure: Joule (J).

Moment – The tendency of a force to rotate an object about an axis; a vector quantity with characteristics of magnitude and direction. A moment is the vector cross product of the position vector from any point on the axis to any point on the line of action of the force and the force vector.

In two dimensional analyses, a moment is the product of the magnitude of the force and the moment arm. Unit of measure: Newton-meter (N·m).

  External moment – The moment produced by an external force.

  Internal Intersegmental moment – The moment acting about the joint that dynamically balances the body segment under investigation; sometimes referred to as "joint moment" or "muscle moment."

Moment arm – The shortest (perpendicular) distance between the line of action of a force and an axis of rotation. Synonymous with lever arm.

Momentum – The resistance of a moving object to acceleration; defined mechanically as the product of the mass of an object and its linear velocity or the mass moment of inertia of an object and its angular velocity. See also inertia.

Pressure – Distributed normal forces. Unit of measure: Newtons per meter squared (N/m^2) or Newtons per centimeter squared (N/cm^2).

Power – The rate at which work is done on or by a system; the rate of change in mechanical energy in a system per unit time. Unit of measure: Watt (W).

  Intersegmental power – The rate at which work is done on or by an intersegmental moment.

Torque – The moment produced by a force couple. Note that a torque or force couple can only produce rotation of an object. Unit of measure: Newton-meter (N·m).

  Ground reaction torque – The vertical torque produced by friction between the foot and ground.

Velocity – The rate of change of displacement with respect to time; a vector quantity with characteristics of magnitude and direction.

  Angular velocity – Velocity associated with rotational displacement. Unit of measure: radians per second (rad/s).

  Linear velocity – Velocity associated with translational displacement. Unit of measure: meters per second (m/s).

Weight – The force on an object due to gravity represented as a concentrated force passing through the center of gravity of the object. Weight is the product of the mass of an object and the acceleration due to gravity (approximately $9.81 \, m/s^2$ on the surface of the Earth). Unit of measure: Newton (N).

Work – The change in energy associated with the linear displacement of a force (along its line of action) or the rotational displacement of a moment. Unit of measure: Joule (J).

Chapter 5

Energetics of Walking

Jessica Rose, Don W. Morgan, and James G. Gamble

People naturally walk in a manner that conserves energy. To accomplish this, limb and trunk motions are integrated to smooth the forward progression of the body and decrease the displacement of the center of gravity. Walking speeds are selected which minimize the energy expended per distance walked. Deviation from the normal walking pattern increases energy expenditure and limits ambulation. Thus, for a person with a disability, energy expenditure is a primary consideration in decisions regarding therapeutic treatment.

METABOLIC ENERGY

The human body utilizes metabolic energy in the form of ATP to support physiologic processes, such as muscle contraction and relaxation, and for cellular reactions such as active transport systems, hormone receptor signaling, and protein synthesis. The fuel for the body's energy requirements comes from ingested nutrients or from stored glycogen and fat.

Energy Transductions in the Body

Cells convert energy stored in the chemical bonds of food sources to free energy that can be used for the molecular reactions of cellular metabolism. These physiologic processes involve several forms of energy transduction, from chemical energy of molecular bonds to thermal energy of heat or to mechanical work of organ movements such as that which occurs in the heart and lungs. Mechanical energy is used at a cellular level as well. For instance, a single microtubule transport system within the cell generates 2.6×10^{-7} dynes (3). All metabolic energy transductions obey the first law of thermodynamics, which states that energy is conserved as it is interconverted. This means that at rest, the chemical energy from blood glucose can be released as heat (thermal energy) or converted to the chemical and mechanical energy of resting metabolism that is ultimately released as heat (15). Only about 1% of the resting energy is converted directly to pressure-volume work on the atmosphere, such as exhalation. Thus, at rest, the

vast majority of chemical energy from food is released as heat (Fig. 5-1). Measuring the heat production of the body closely approximates the total amount of energy utilized in that state.

During exercise, skeletal muscle uses the chemical energy from the hydrolysis of ATP to produce mechanical and chemical work. In the process of this irreversible transduction, movement occurs and energy is dissipated in the form of heat. Part of this heat arises from friction of the mechanochemical coupling that produces physical work (Fig. 5-1) (15,93). When performing physical work, human energy efficiency approaches 30%; 70% of the energy utilized is ultimately released as heat (15). Humans are ~24% efficient while walking at a comfortable speed. At a slow walking speed, efficiency decreases to 14%. This is comparable with the internal combustion engine of an automobile, which is only 10% to 20% efficient at converting the chemical energy of gasoline to heat and transducing heat into the mechanical energy of torque at the drive shaft (90).

Metabolic Energy Storage and Utilization

Cellular reactions, including skeletal muscle contraction, utilize chemical energy derived from ingested carbohydrates (glucose) and fat (lipids). Carbohydrates provide 4.2 kcal/g and lipids 9.5 kcal/g of energy. Heat of combustion is the same whether it occurs inside or outside the body except for protein, which provides 26% more kilocalories when combusted outside the body (owing to the mechanism of amino acid metabolism). While protein is not generally considered a primary energy source, protein use can increase during extreme conditions such as starvation and during hard and protracted exercise (48). Ingested protein provides essential amino acids that are required to synthesize enzymes and other cellular proteins.

The chemical energy of carbohydrates and fats is not used directly for metabolic work, but is first transferred to the high-energy phosphate bond of ATP. Energy in the terminal phosphate bond is available for molecular synthesis, active transport, muscle contraction, and other cellular

77

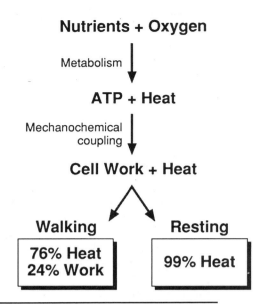

FIGURE 5-1. Energy transductions in the body.

reactions. The terminal phosphate bond of ATP has a high free energy of hydrolysis, designated as a "high-energy" phosphate bond. Current estimates of the free energy of hydrolysis per phosphate bond for physiologic conditions (such as those occurring in contracting muscle) are as high as 12–14 kcal/mole (112).

Muscle utilizes phosphate bond energy to slide the actin and myosin protein filaments relative to each other, leading to shortening and increased tension of the muscle (20). In the presence of intracellular Ca^{2+}, one phosphate bond is cleaved by myosin ATPase per actin-myosin protein interaction. Additional ATP is required to pump Ca^{2+} back into the sarcoplasmic reticulum, disengaging the proteins and allowing muscular relaxation. An average person at rest requires 72 kcal per hour, utilizing six mol ATP every hour. Level walking at 80 m per minute requires 240 kcal per hour or 18 mol ATP.

Oxidative and Glycolytic Metabolism

Under normal conditions, ATP is produced by glycolytic and oxidative reactions in the cytosol and mitochondria of the cell. Carbohydrates are metabolized to pyruvate in the cytosol by a series of glycolytic reactions. Glycolysis is the source of anaerobic energy, yielding 2 mol ATP/mol glucose. Fats are metabolized in the cytosol to free fatty acids. Acetyl coenzyme A, derived mostly from pyruvate and free fatty acids, is the initial substrate for the Krebs Cycle. In the mitochondria, electrons and hydrogen ions released from metabolic substrates are transferred to nicotinamide and flavin adenine dinucleotide, which act as hydrogen acceptors and electron carriers, delivering the reducing equivalents to the electron transport chain. The electron transport chain creates an electrochemical gradient across the inner mitochondrial membrane and this gradient is used

to drive the synthesis of ATP from ADP and inorganic phosphate (39).

For each pair of electrons transferred to oxygen in the electron transport chain, sufficient free energy is released to form approximately three ATP molecules. The complete oxidation of a glucose molecule to carbon dioxide and water yields a net total of 36 or 38 ATP molecules, depending on the location of ATP synthesis (48). This compares quite favorably with the net gain of two ATP molecules per glucose molecule resulting from anaerobic metabolism. Oxidative (aerobic) ATP production provides most of the body's energy needs at rest and at submaximal workloads. Energy for muscular contraction predominantly comes from aerobic metabolism that involves the continuous oxidation of metabolites in the mitochondria. Only a small amount of the total energy is provided by phosphagen and glycolytic metabolism. In the absence of oxygen, ATP production occurs exclusively in the cytosol of the cell. These anaerobic sources of energy are primarily available for short-term, high-intensity work. At submaximal workloads, such as walking on a level surface, the ATP produced in the cytosol represents a very small amount of the total ATP produced (15).

In the absence of oxygen, pyruvate from glucose metabolism is reduced to lactic acid. At high work rates, lactic acid is produced faster than it can be utilized, and lactate accumulation causes intracellular and extracellular acid-base imbalance with unfavorable consequences such as muscle fatigue and hyperventilation. At higher work rates, both aerobic and anaerobic ATP production share in energy generation. Anaerobic metabolism provides an increasing proportion of the energy requirements at higher work rates (15).

MEASUREMENT AND UNITS

Historically, the measurement of heat production and the changes in gas content of respired air were used to investigate metabolism. In the 1780s, Lavoisier studied the central role of oxygen in metabolism (43). He compared the combustion of food inside and outside the body and recognized that the same amount of heat was released during the two processes. Lavoisier named the element that took up approximately one-fifth of the volume of air "oxygen," which means "acid former" because carbonic acid, sulfuric acid, or phosphoric acid were produced when organic substances were burned (43).

Measurement of the body's heat production, also known as calorimetry, is an indication of the overall metabolic rate. Heat production can be measured directly (direct calorimetry) or it can be estimated from the oxygen consumed or from the carbon dioxide and water produced (indirect calorimetry). The ultimate source of energy for metabolic and physical work is the combustion of food, i.e., oxidation of nutrients. Measurement of the oxygen consumed by the body provides a measure of the energy expenditure of the body. The units for the measurement of oxygen uptake can be expressed in absolute (e.g., liters per minute) or relative (e.g., mL/kg per minute) terms.

Oxygen uptake units can be transferred into heat units such as the gram-calorie (cal) or the kilogram-calorie (kcal). The gram-calorie is the amount of heat necessary to raise the temperature of 1 g of water 1 degree C, whereas the kilocalorie is the amount of heat necessary to raise the temperature of 1 kg of water 1 degree C. Expressing oxygen uptake in kilocalories allows comparison among nutrient energy, metabolic energy, and mechanical energy.

In discussing metabolic energy expenditure, it is desirable to use the same units. However, this is not always feasible. In calculations that involve measurements of speed (m per minute) it is preferable to express energy expenditure in cal/kg per minute; however, kilocalories per hour, kilocalories per minute, and gram-calories per kilogram per minute body weight have also been used.

When dealing with mechanical energy levels and work, joules (J) are the preferred units. For work rate, the units are watts (W). Horse power (hp) is used occasionally in reference to work rate. Table 5-1 lists some commonly used conversion relationships.

In 1949, Weir (113) determined a method for expressing energy expenditure in units of kilocalories and calories. Using Weir's mathematical analysis, Passmore and Draper (79) recommend the use of the following relation between energy expenditure (E) in kilocalories per minute and the oxygen percentage concentration of expired air (0_e):

$$E = \frac{4.92\,V}{100}(20.93 - 0_e)$$

Where V is volume of expired air in liters per minute. This can be simplified to the following conversions:

5 kcal per minute = 1 liter oxygen per minute

5 cal per minute = 1 mL oxygen per minute

As a somewhat more complex translation of oxygen values into calories, consider the following equation relating oxygen consumption in milliliters per minute ($V0_2$) per kilogram body weight to speed of walking (v) in meters

per minute.

$$V0_2/kg = 5.9 + 0.0011\,v^2$$

Multiplying by the conversion factor 5 yields:

$$cal/kg \text{ per minute} = 29.5 + 0.0055\,v^2$$

LYING, SITTING, AND STANDING

It is important, particularly when dealing with the effects of various types of disabilities, to compare the energy demand of walking with that of an immobile (or relatively immobile) state, such as lying, sitting, or quiet standing.

Lying

The "basal metabolic rate" is frequently referred to as though, in the words of Durnin and Passmore, "it is a fundamental biological property of the individual or species" (29). It is preferable to refer to a resting rate, measured 3 to 4 hours after an ordinary meal. This measurement does not significantly differ from a basal rate, requires no special standardization of environmental and other conditions, and, most importantly, does not assume that a "fixed minimum metabolism on which life depends" is involved. Resting metabolism has been shown to be indistinguishable from basal metabolism (29). This is demonstrated in Table 5-2.

Column 5 of Table 5-2 is the predicted value of the resting metabolic rate, according to tables from Durnin and Passmore (29), for average male and female subjects. These authors divided subjects into four categories (thin, average, plump, and fat) corresponding to percent fat of 5, 10, 15, and 20% for males and 15, 20, 25, and 30% for females. These authors also show that the differences between male and female subjects in the values of the basal and resting metabolic rates are eliminated when lean body mass is used instead of total body mass in the presentation of metabolic values.

Column 6 of Table 5-2 is the predicted value of metabolic rates as calculated from Kleiber's (43) equation:

$$metabolic\ rate\ (kcal/hr) = 3\,(w)^{3/4}$$

where w is gross body weight (kg). For female subjects, the coefficient is scaled down to 2.775 from 3, which is proportionally the same as the coefficients 37 and 40 for the values given in column 5 of Table 5-2.

Column 7 of Table 5-2 is the value for the basal metabolic rate as predicted by the Mayo Foundation Normal Standards (12) based on body surface area for young males.

$$basic\ metabolic\ rate = 40\ kcal/m^2/hr$$

The coefficient is 37 kcal/m²/hr for females.

TABLE 5-1 Common Conversion Relationships

To Change	To	Multiply By
cal	J	4.186
kcal	J	4186
kcal	kg-m	427
kcal/hr	W	1.16
W	cal/min	14.33
hp	W	746

▶ **TABLE 5-2 Predicted Resting Values Compared with Experimental Values for Quiet Standing**

Subject	Sex	Height (m)	Weight (kg)	Durnin and Passmore[a]	Kleiber[b]	Mayo[c]	Mean Resting (kcal/hr) (Predicted)[d]	Standing (kcal/hr) (Experimental)[e]	Standing: Resting
1	M	1.74	69	71.8	71.9	73.0	72.2	86.9	1.20
2	M	1.72	64	67.7	68.0	70.2	68.6	87.0	1.27
3	M	1.80	64	67.7	68.0	72.5	69.4	96.3	1.39
4	M	1.70	67	70.1	70.5	71.0	70.5	89.8	1.27
5	M	1.70	66	69.2	69.8	70.6	69.9	79.0	1.13
6	M	1.73	63	66.2	67.3	70.1	67.9	82.4	1.21
7	M	1.96	87	85.4[f]	85.5	87.8	86.2	126.1	1.46
8	M	1.72	68	70.9	71.0	71.9	71.3	96.2	1.35
9	M	1.89	83	82.6[f]	82.5	83.8	83.0	97.5	1.17
10	M	1.82	79	79.7	79.5	79.9	79.7	115.2	1.45
11	M	1.68	62	66.2	66.3	68.0	66.8	89.8	1.34
12	M	1.79	80	80.4	80.2	79.3	80.0	101.8	1.27
13	M	1.80	84	83.3[f]	83.2	81.3	82.6	99.6	1.21
14	M	1.79	71	73.4	73.4	75.4	74.1	92.8	1.25
15	M	1.79	79	79.7	79.5	78.9	79.4	94.2	1.19
16	M	1.87	69	71.8	71.8	76.9	73.5	92.7	1.26
17	M	1.84	75	76.8	76.5	78.8	77.4	101.1	1.31
Means		1.78	72	74.3	74.4	75.8	74.9	95.8	1.28
18	F	1.71	61	59.6	60.6	63.3	61.2	72.6	1.19
19	F	1.68	59	58.0	59.1	61.6	59.6	77.0	1.29
20	F	1.64	68	65.2	65.7	64.3	65.1	70.3	1.08
21	F	1.73	78	73.3	72.8	70.8	72.3	79.1	1.09
22	F	1.72	64	62.2	62.8	64.9	63.3	69.1	1.09
23	F	1.77	67	64.4	65.0	67.5	65.6	78.8	1.20
24	F	1.70	64	62.2	62.8	64.3	63.1	79.3	1.26
25	F	1.64	57	56.3	57.6	59.6	57.8	76.3	1.32
26	F	1.78	73	69.1	69.3	70.3	69.6	86.8	1.25
27	F	1.66	62	60.5	61.3	62.4	61.4	72.4	1.18
28	F	1.59	53	52.9	54.5	56.5	54.6[g]	49.4[g]	0.90[g]
29	F	1.62	56	55.4	56.8	58.7	57.0	79.9	1.40
30	F	1.70	59	58.0	59.1	62.1	59.7	66.4	1.11
31	F	1.65	70	66.6	66.9	65.2	66.2	78.3	1.18
Means		1.69	64	61.7	62.5	63.7	62.6	75.6	1.20

[a]Durnin and Passmore (1967), page 31. Values refer to "average" physique.
[b]Kleiber equation (1961). Coefficient 3 for males scaled down to 2.775 for females.
[c]Mayo Foundation standards (Boothby et al., 1936). Coefficient 40 for males and 37 for females.
[d]Mean of three preceding columns.
[e]Some experimental data from Molen and Rozendal (1967).
[f]Extrapolated. Other values are either direct or interpolated.
[g]Values are obviously incompatible and are unexplained. Not used in calculation of mean ratio.

It makes little difference in the results whether the values for metabolic rate are calculated according to Durnin and Passmore (29), Kleiber (43), or Boothby et al. (12). Not only is the claim by Durnin and Passmore that basal and resting metabolic rates are virtually indistinguishable fully justified, but the Durnin and Passmore table also provides a means of expressing metabolic rates in terms of lean body mass, which is a notable improvement over earlier predictive tables. Column 8 of Table 5-2 is the average value of columns 5 through 7. These values, recalculated as cal/kg per min, will be compared later in this chapter with the values of sitting and standing.

Table 5-3 shows resting metabolic rates for 10 male subjects, measured in our laboratory, compared with values predicted by Durnin and Passmore (29). Except for subject 1, the agreement is well within acceptable limits of prediction. The discrepancy in the case of Subject 1 is due, at least in part, to age.

Sitting

Durnin and Passmore (29) measured the energy expenditure of seated men and women while they were engaged in activities such as reading and watching television. The

▶ **TABLE 5-3** **Experimental Values of Resting Metabolism in 10 Male Subjects Compared with Values Predicted by Durnin and Passmore (1968)**[a]

Subject	Age (yr)	Weight (kg)	Experimental (kcal/min)	Predicted (kcal/min)	Ratio
1	53	70.9	0.89	1.17	1.31
2	45	77.7	1.28	1.32	1.03
3	31	87.7	1.24	1.41[a]	1.14
4	26	58.6	1.04	1.07	1.03
5	23	72.7	1.21	1.25	1.03
6	22	70.5	1.33	1.22	0.92
7	22	64.3	1.25	1.13	0.90
8	18	68.2	1.05	1.18	1.12
9	17	62.3	1.19	1.10	0.92
10	18	80.9	1.38	1.35[a]	0.98
Means			1.19	1.22	1.04

[a]Extrapolated values. Other values in this column are direct or interpolated.

measurements were made at various times of day and were unrelated to food intake. Table 5-4 shows the average results recalculated to express energy expenditure.

Their average values, which range from 19.5 to 21.4 cal/kg/min, are substantially higher than the average values for resting metabolism, derived from column 8 of Table 5-2, that equal 17.2 cal/kg per minute for males and 16.4 cal/kg per minute for females. As will be seen below, their sitting values are practically the same as the figures for quiet standing derived from column 9 of Table 5-2. This probably reflects the rather "active" sitting engaged in by the subjects. If males and females are combined, the ratio of active sitting to resting metabolism is about 1.22.

Standing

Molen and Rozendal (65) studied 10 males and 10 females under conditions of quiet standing in the laboratory. Their results were virtually identical with those obtained by Ralston on seven males and four females and are combined, therefore, with the data from Ralston for the 17 males and 14 females shown in Table 5-2, column 9. The average value

▶ **TABLE 5-4** **Sitting Energy Expenditure Based on Data by Durnin and Passmore (1967)**

Age Range (years)	Sex	Mean ± SD (cal/kg/min)	SD/Mean
20–39	M	21.4 ± 3.85	0.18
20–39	F	20.9 ± 5.09	0.24
40–64	M	21.1 ± 4.46	0.21
40–59	F	19.5 ± 3.45	0.18
65+	M	19.8 ± 3.85	0.19
60+	F	19.8 ± 5.64	0.28

± SD for males is 22.1 ± 1.68 cal/kg per minute and for females 19.9 ± 2.60, with the ratio of means being 1.11.

Molen and Rozendal (65) noted the lower energy demand of standing in females and indicated that this influenced the finding that the cost of walking was slightly less in females than in males. However, the difference is so small that Molen and Rozendal (65) combined men and women in formulating the regression equation relating energy expenditure to speed.

Note that the difference in energy cost of standing for males compared with females is eliminated if lean body weight instead of gross body weight is used. The results in this case using the values given by Durnin and Passmore (29) for body fat content become 24.5 cal/kg per minute for males and 24.8 cal/kg per minute for females.

The ratio of standing to resting is 21.0:16.8 (i.e., 1.25) if males and females are combined and values expressed as calories/kilogram per minute, derived from Table 5-2, columns 8 and 9. This ratio is similar to that for resting to active sitting (1.22). The low cost of standing reflects low activity of the postural muscles during standing, a finding corroborated by electromyography.

ENERGY EXPENDITURE OF WALKING

A modest increase in energy expenditure, on the order of 25%, occurs when a subject assumes a quiet standing position compared with a supine position. As soon as an individual beings to walk, a great increase in energy expenditure occurs, reflecting the metabolic cost to the muscles of moving the body against gravity and of accelerating and decelerating the various body segments.

Relation between Energy Expenditure and Speed in Level Walking

Ralston (84) showed that a quadratic equation:

$$E_w = b + mv^2$$

adequately predicted the energy cost of walking for adults at speeds up to ~100 m per minute (Fig. 5-2). E_w is energy expenditure in cal/kg per minute, v is speed in m per minute, and b and m are constants. In deriving this equation, Ralston used data from various investigators. Since that time, other investigators have found that an equation of the same form provides an acceptable basis for predicting energy-speed relations (11,22,24,90). Combining their equations, using weighted averages of the constants according to number of subjects (86 total: 57 males, 29 females), yields a grand average equation:

$$E_w = 32 + 0.005v^2 \qquad (1)$$

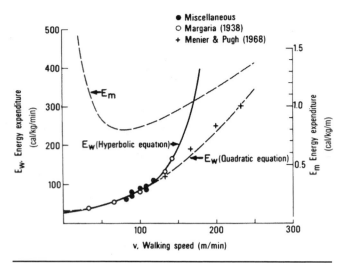

FIGURE 5-2. Energy expenditure during walking. *Top curve,* E_m (cal/kg/m), calculated from Equation 4; *middle curve,* E_w (cal/kg per minute), calculated from Equation 3; *bottom curve,* E_w (cal/kg per minute, calculated from Equation 1. (Adapted with permission from Zarrugh MY, Todd FN, Ralston HJ. Optimization of energy expenditure during level walking. *Eur J Appl Physiol* 1974;33:293–306).

Note that for a 70-kg adult male, the increase in energy expenditure of walking at 80 m/min (Table 5-5) over resting values (derived from Table 5-2, column 4) is ~ 3.7. This increase is more than three times the ratio of active sitting or quiet standing over resting values.

The previously mentioned studies included walking on treadmill, floor, firm path, and grass surfaces. There was no indication of systematic differences for the various walking surfaces. In such studies, however, close attention must be paid to the nature of the footwear. A heavy boot or slippery sole, for example, may alter the energy demand of walking.

Durnin and Passmore (29) provide a table for relating weight of subject, speed, and energy expenditure over a range of 55–110 m/min (2–4 miles/hr). Table 5-5 shows the

▶ TABLE 5-5 Energy Expenditure during Level Walking as Predicted by Equation 1 and by Durnin and Passmore (1967)

m/min	km/hr	mile/hr	$E_w = 32 + 0.0050v^2$	Durnin and Passmore (1967)
25	1.50	1.0	35	
40	2.40	1.5	40	
55	3.30	2.0	47	46
70	4.20	2.5	56	55
80	4.80	3.0	64	64
90	5.40	3.5	73	74
110	6.60	4.0	93	85

predicted values from Equation 1 and average values from Durnin and Passmore. Because the quadratic Equation 1 implies that the energy cost is proportional to body weight, Wyndham et al. (120) examined this relation in detail and found that any error involved in such a relation was not significant in the case of walking.

It is clear that over the range of 55 to 90 m per minute, the predicted results in the last two columns of Table 5-5 are virtually identical. At 110 m per minute, the Durnin and Passmore figures underestimate the average experimental values ($E_w = 93$) by 11%, whereas Equation 1 is still in good agreement with observed results (Fig. 5-2). At still higher speeds, up to about 145 m/min, which is about the top speed for natural walking, Equation 1 also fails.

Zarrugh et al. (118) deduced a more general, hyperbolic equation for predicting energy expenditure during walking, which considers step length and step rate:

$$E_w = \frac{E_o}{\left(1 - \dfrac{S^2}{S_\mu^2}\right)\left(1 - \dfrac{n^2}{n_\mu^2}\right)} \quad (2)$$

where s is step length in meters, n is step rate in steps/min, E_o is the value of E_w when $s = n = 0$ (resting), S_u is the upper limit of s as E_w approaches infinity, and n_u is the upper limit of n as E_w approaches infinity.

In natural walking, where the subject adopts his own natural cadence for a particular speed, it can be shown that Equation 2 reduces to

$$E_w = \frac{E_o}{(1 - v/v_u)^2} \quad (3)$$

where v is speed and v_u is upper limit of v, equal to $n_u s_u$ (Fig. 5-2).

E_o has an average value of ~28 cal/kg per minute and V_u an average value of ~240 m per minute. Thus, for a top natural speed of 145 m per minute,

$$E_w = \frac{28}{(1 - 145/240)^2} = 179 \text{ cal/kg/min}$$

which is in good agreement with average experimental values.

Up to speeds of about 100 m per minute, Equations 1 and 3 predict virtually identical values. Therefore Equation 1 may be used for most cases of natural walking.

Rather unexpectedly, Equation 1 predicts energy cost within about 10% for competitive race walking, which is quite unlike natural walking. Menier and Pugh (63) provide data on four male Olympic race walkers studied during treadmill walking at an altitude of 1800 m. They state that their findings agree with studies made at sea level by other investigators.

At a speed of 14 km/hr (233 m per minute) the walkers clustered closely ~ 60 mL oxygen/kg per minute, corresponding to 300 cal/kg per minute. Equation 1 predicts:

$$E_w = 32 + 0.005 \ (233)^2 = 303 \text{ cal/kg per minute}$$

which is within 1% of the observed value.

At a speed of about 135 m per minute, the walkers clustered about a value of ~ 25 mL oxygen/kg per minute, corresponding to 125 cal/kg per minute. Equation 1 predicts:

$$E_w = 32 + 0.005 \ (135)^2 = 123 \text{ cal/kg per minute}$$

which is within about 2% of the observed value.

Morgan et al. (71) recently developed a generalized equation to predict oxygen uptake (mL/kg per minute) while walking in children age 6 to 10 that takes into account both age and walking speed:

$$VO_2 = 24.9 + .0032(v)^2 - .995(\text{age}) - .263(v)$$

where v is walking speed (m per minute) and age is in years. In their longitudinal study, the children received extensive accommodation to treadmill walking on an annual basis. Nearly all of the prediction errors associated with estimating VO_2 across a wide range of speeds (40.2 to 107.2 m per minute) were less than 1 MET (3.5 mL/kg per minute). Moreover, it was demonstrated that use of adult or adolescent prediction equations to estimate walking energy expenditure would result in an underestimation of childrens' VO_2 values. In adolescents, Walker and colleagues (107) developed and cross-validated generalized equations for predicting relative VO_2 (mL/kg per minute) and caloric expenditure (kcal/kg per minute) during horizontal walking and running. Their data indicated that in adolescents the association between walking speed and VO_2 was curvilinear for speeds varying from 67 to 134 m per minute.

Significance of Constant = 28 in Equation 3

At speed $v = 0$, Equation 3 yields $E_w = 28$ cal/ kg per minute. This is much higher than the value for resting or quiet standing. Ralston (84) found that the value for extremely slow walking, in five subjects, averaged 28.6 cal/kg per minute. He concluded that the constant represented the cost of maintaining the body in motion at a barely perceptible speed.

It is clear, therefore, that calculating the "net" cost of walking, based on oxygen uptake, i.e., subtracting the resting value or the quietly standing value from the gross value, is neither theoretically nor practically justified. It is of added interest that use of net values for energy expenditure during walking does not permit formulation of Equation 2 and its derivative, Equation 3, which appear, thus far, to be the only equations successfully predicting energy expenditure throughout the entire range of natural walking speeds.

Age

None of the previously mentioned studies found a systematic effect of age on the energy expenditure of natural walking, at least within an age range of 20 to 59 years, when expressed per unit body weight.

Waters et al. (108) compared the energy expenditure of self-paced walking in young adults aged 20 to 59 years and seniors aged 60 to 80 years. They found no significant difference in oxygen uptake (mL/kg per minute) with age, although self-selected walking speed was slower in the seniors.

Blessey (9) found that in adults, the energy expenditure of walking did not vary significantly with age. However, walking represented a higher percent of maximal capacity in older adults aged 50 to 59 years (43%) compared with young adults aged 20 to 29 years (36%). This was because of the decrease in maximal oxygen uptake per kilogram that occurs with age in adults.

Martin et al. (61) examined the effects of age and physical activity on walking economy in young (18 to 28 years) and older (66 to 86 years) men and women who were sedentary or physically active. Results from their study indicated that older subjects showed an 8% higher mean walking VO_2 (mL/kg/km) compared to younger subjects. Interestingly, physical activity levels did not have an influence on walking economy. Although speculative, the authors suggested that the higher walking energy expenditure observed in the older adults may be linked to declines in the force-generating capacity of aging muscle that may require increased motor unit recruitment and the use of less-economical fast-twitch fibers.

Malatesta et al. (55) compared self-paced walking in adults aged 65 to adults aged 80. While they found no significant differences in oxygen uptake at their preferred walking speed for the older group, the preferred walking speed was significantly slower and walking at the preferred speed required a higher fraction of the oxygen uptake corresponding to the ventilatory threshold. Malatesta et al. (54) compared oxygen uptake during walking on a treadmill at a range of walking speeds in adults aged 65 compared to adults aged 80. Across the different walking speeds, they found higher oxygen uptake values and greater gait instability in the older group. However, no significant correlation was found between gait instability and higher energy expenditure.

Waters et al. (109) compared energy expenditure of self paced walking in children and adolescents and found that oxygen uptake (mL/kg per minute) was significantly higher for children (15.3) than for adolescents (12.9), and the walking speed was slightly but significantly slower for children (70 vs. 73 m per minute).

Morgan et al. (70) examined age-related changes in energy expenditure of walking in children. They studied a range of walking speeds in children age 6 to 10 years and found that for all walking speeds, oxygen uptake decreased yearly from age 6 to 8 years. When averaged across speeds, oxygen uptake was 27% higher for 6-year-olds compared to 10-year-olds. In a more recent article, Morgan et al. (74) noted that in young children, changes in walking VO_2 with age occurred in a fairly uniform manner. This finding suggests that in a group of typical healthy children, a trend towards good, average, or below-average walking economy is manifested and generally maintained during a time period characterized by marked increases in body size and varied exposure to a wide spectrum of physical activity choices.

McCann and Adams (49) studied 184 children, adolescents, adults, and seniors walking on a treadmill at a range of walking speeds. They observed that at each walking speed, oxygen uptake per kilogram was higher in children than in the older groups. They found that the higher mass-specific metabolic cost of children was explained by differences in standing metabolism and stature. Similarly, DeJaeger et al. (27) reported that standing energy expenditure was higher in children and was, on average, 43% lower in young adults compared to children age 3 to 4 years.

Skinner et al. (98) compared the energy expenditure of children and adolescents walking on a treadmill at speeds of 83 to 100 m per minute and inclines of 10% to 17.5%. He found that oxygen uptake per kilogram decreased with age for a given workload. Higher oxygen uptake in children may be explained by their increased resting metabolic rate, small step length and higher step rate at a given workload; walking may represent a higher percent of maximum oxygen uptake in children than in adolescents or adults.

Astrand and Rodahl (4) compared children and adolescents walking and running on a treadmill at various speeds. He found that a typical 8-year-old running at 180 m per minute was working at 90% of maximum oxygen uptake and that a 16-year-old walking at the same speed worked at 75% of maximum oxygen uptake. Astrand reported that an 8-year-old can increase basal metabolic rate only 9.4 times in a maximal run of 5 minutes, but that a 17-year-old boy can attain an aerobic power that is 13.5 times the basal metabolic rate.

Bar-Or (7) reported that children operate at a higher percent of maximal oxygen uptake for a given workload and that the higher energy cost in children cannot be explained merely by a difference in resting metabolism that is only ~1 to 2 mL/kg per minute, but rather by their relatively "wasteful" gait. Similarly, Astrand and Rodahl (4) noted that small bodies are more metabolically active per unit body weight than larger ones. However, they also indicate that the child's lower efficiency can partly be explained by their high step rate that is energy-expensive per unit time.

In a comprehensive review of existing data, Morgan (68) concluded that children are less metabolically economical

than adults, with the magnitude of differences in economy varying markedly among studies. His analysis also indicated that younger children are less economical than older children and adolescents, with economy differences becoming larger as age-group comparisons become more pronounced. In this review, a number of potential factors were identified that may help explain child-adult differences in relative walking energy costs. These include: (1) less efficient ventilation, (2) faster stride rates, (3) immature gait patterns, (4) larger surface area to body mass ratios, (5) shorter stature, (6) an imbalance between body mass and leg muscle contraction speed, (7) more distal distribution of mass in the lower extremities, (8) a greater reliance on fat as a metabolic substrate, and (9) a reduced ability to use anaerobic energy sources.

Taken together, these studies demonstrate that the energy expended to walk per kilogram does not change significantly with age for adults until older age is attained. The energy expended to walk expressed per unit body mass, however, decreases with age for children and adolescents.

Weight

The aerobic demand of walking is typically expressed relative to total body mass, since this mass must be supported by the lower extremities and accelerated and decelerated with each step. This ratio-scaling method of adjusting for body mass, however, has been questioned by some investigators who have suggested that regression or allometrically-based scaling methods may be more appropriate for normalizing ambulatory energy demands (89,114). In allometric scaling, VO_2 is expressed as a mathematical function of a specific body dimension, such as body mass, according to the formula:

$$y = a(x^b)$$

where y is the dependent variable (VO_2), x is the independent variable (body mass), b is the allometric coefficient (or scaling factor), a is a proportionality coefficient, and a and b are derived by linear regression after logarithmic transformation of x and y variables to yield the following equation:

$$\log y = \log a + b(\log x)$$

While allometric scaling has been used to determine the relationship between body size and aerobic power, the validity of this approach is reduced when small sample sizes are studied. Moreover, the consistency of scaling factors derived using this technique has not been high (56) Although the question of how best to adjust for variation in body size has yet to be resolved, ratio scaling continues to enjoy widespread support because it is a method of adjusting for variation in body size that is easy to understand and interpret and involves simple mathematical computations.

For the measurement of resting and maximal metabolic rate, lean body mass (LBM) is more highly correlated to oxygen uptake than total body weight (TBW) (4,29). Herfenroeder and Schoene (35) studied the effect of body composition on maximum oxygen uptake in adolescents and found the correlation between oxygen uptake and TBW to be $r = 0.71$ and for oxygen uptake and LBM, $r = 0.84$. Katch (40) reported a correlation of 0.71 between TBW and oxygen uptake at basal and maximal metabolic rates. He notes that the use of the VO_2-to-kilogram ratio implies a correlation of $r = 1.0$ and direct proportionality between VO_2 and body weight and should be corrected for when extrapolating energy expenditure from oxygen uptake in units per body weight.

Although LBM is highly correlated with aerobic capacity, most studies show that for submaximal activities such as walking, TBW correlates more highly with oxygen uptake than LBM (64,94). Similarly, Volpe and Bar-Or (106) studied lean and obese adolescents matched for TBW and found that TBW, and not adiposity, was the main predictor of walking energy cost.

Datta et al. (26) found that it was the total weight moved by subjects carrying loads of 0-50 kg on their head that correlated most highly with oxygen uptake, provided the load was not excessive or carried in an awkward position. Goldman and Iampietro (32) measured oxygen uptake in five subjects with various combinations of treadmill speeds and grades and backpack loads. They found that at a given speed and grade, the energy cost per unit weight (kcal/kg per minute) was similar regardless of the distribution of total weight between body weight and load weight within a range of 1-30 kg. Robertson et al. (88) also found this to be true when oxygen uptake was expressed per kilogram total weight moved for subjects walking and carrying loads up to 15% of body weight.

Turrell et al. (103) and Bloom and Eidex (10) compared the energy expenditure of walking for lean and obese subjects. Although energy expenditure per unit time (l per minute) was greater for the obese subjects, dividing by TBW (mL/kg per minute) gave a similar value. Bloom and Eidex (10) and Turrell et al. (103) compared lean subjects carrying weight with obese subjects with a similar total weight. They found that it was the total weight that was most highly correlated with oxygen uptake. For example, Bloom and Eidex (10) measured the energy cost of an obese 250-pound subject and a lean 150-pound subject carrying a 100-pound backpack. Dividing by total weight moved gave essentially the same energy cost in all cases. Alternatively, Myo-Thein et al. (77) found that predicting energy expenditure for trunk loads based on body weight led to overestimation of energy expenditure.

Most studies of the effects of TBW and/or obesity on the energy cost of walking have been cross-sectional, i.e., comparing obese subjects with lean individuals at one point. However, Hansen (34) studied the energy cost of treadmill walking in male volunteers under four conditions: 1) control on a balanced diet, 2) 14% to 16% weight gain via fat supplements to a balanced diet for 11 weeks, 3) 18% to

20% weight gain over 16 weeks, and 4) return to normal diet for 5 months with subject wearing backpack weight to equal weight lost over 5 months. Oxygen uptake when expressed in liters per minute increased with the total weight moved, but when expressed per unit weight moved, the value was relatively constant for a given work level.

These studies indicate that for walking, it is the total weight moved that correlates most highly with energy expenditure. However, the effects of loading the body depend on the nature of the loading (44). It has been shown that the relative increase in the absolute cost of running per kg of added mass is about 1% for added mass to the trunk, 3.5% for added mass to the thighs, and 7.0% for added mass to the feet (60). Lloyd and Cooke (46) found that oxygen uptake while walking was 5% lower using a backpack that allowed the load to be distributed between the back and front of the trunk during uphill walking.

Loads placed on the distal segments, especially the foot, have a much greater effect than loads attached to the trunk, because of the large inertial effects associated with acceleration and deceleration of the limb. Figure 5-3 shows the effect of 2 kg on each foot on the metabolic cost of walking at +2°, 0°, and –2°. At 0°, the value of E_w (cal/kg per minute) is increased by ~30%, with similar results at +2° and −2°. Contrast this to the very small effect of 5 kg attached to the trunk, where in seven subjects, the mean increase in E_w was only 4%.

A comparable experiment on lower leg loading is shown in Figure 5-4. Unfortunately, this type of experiment is not

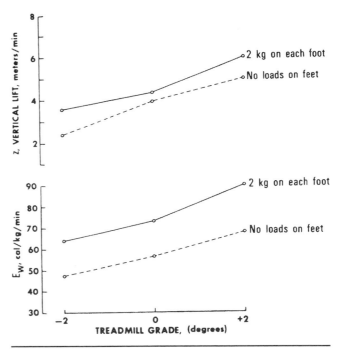

FIGURE 5-3. Effects of loading foot during walking at several grades. *Bottom*, effect on energy expenditure; *top*, effect on vertical motion of body.

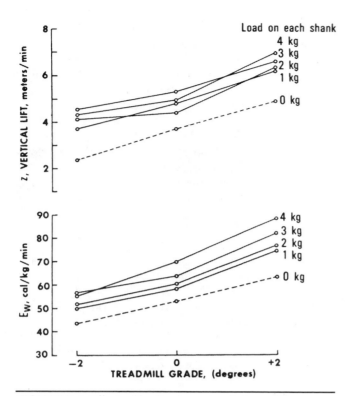

FIGURE 5-4. Effects of loading lower leg during walking at several grades. *Bottom*, effect on energy expenditure; *top*, effect on vertical motion of body.

entirely clearcut because, unexpectedly, the vertical motion of the body is also increased by loads on the limbs (as a result of greater step length), as shown in Figures 5-3 and 5-4. As a consequence of this, both inertial and gravitational effects are involved when the limbs are loaded.

The metabolic cost of trunk loading in quiet standing is practically zero. As stated in "Lying, Sitting, and Standing," the E_w for quiet standing in the young male adult is about 22 cal/kg per minute. In an experiment on a young male subject weighing 64 kg, the E_w of quiet standing was not measurably altered by attaching 20 kg uniformly around the trunk.

Laursen et al. (45) found that loads of more than 10% to 15% body weight resulted in higher energy expenditure and longer recovery from raised blood pressure. Similarly, in children, Hong et al. (37) found that loads of more than 10% body weight caused significant increases in energy expenditure and longer recovery from raised blood pressure. Given the relatively heavy loads that are often carried in a typical school backpack, further investigation of these physiologic effects is warranted.

Gender

Booyens and Keatinge (13) found significantly lower values of energy expenditure for women than for men at speeds of 91 and 107 m per minute, and the equation of Cotes et al. (24) predicts lower values for women than for men. The authors attributed this to a smaller step length in women. Recent studies, however, indicate that a smaller step length increases energy expenditure (4). Ralston (84) did not find a significant gender difference in locomotor energy cost.

Durnin and Passmore (29) stated that gender is not a factor in walking energetics. Molen and Rozendal (65) found a small difference in favor of the female when gross energy expenditure was measured, but not when net energy expenditure (i.e., gross cost minus cost of quiet standing) was used. It has been shown that the cost of quiet standing is slightly (but significantly) lower in the female than in the male. It might be expected that at lower speeds, this would explain a slight difference between males and females. Corcoran and Brengelmann (22) and Ralston (84) found a somewhat higher value for females than for males during floor walking, but were in agreement with Molen and Rozendal (65) that the difference was not important enough to justify use of different equations for males and females.

Blessey (9) found that the rate of energy expenditure did not vary with gender and that male and female adults walk at an equal percent of maximal VO_2 (39%). Similarly, Waters et al. (108) measured oxygen uptake per kilogram in young adults and seniors during free level walking and found no difference between males and females in either group. Walking speed was significantly slower in female compared with male young adults. No difference in walking speed was found between male and female seniors.

Waters et al. (109) also measured oxygen uptake per kilogram body weight in 114 children and adolescents during level walking. While they reported no difference between male and female adolescents, they did find a small but significant decrease in oxygen uptake in female children compared to male children. Walking speed was not different between males and females in either group.

In related work, Morgan et al. (72) documented gender differences in running economy in 6-year-old boys and girls. Results from their investigation revealed that absolute and mass-related values of gross and net VO_2 were significantly greater in boys compared to girls, but gross VO_2 expressed relative to fat-free mass was not different between sexes. This finding suggests that the higher locomotor VO_2 demand displayed by the boys was related to the presence of a greater muscle mass.

Leg length and body height are generally greater in males compared with females, but may explain only small differences in energy expenditure. Increased leg length may decrease the energy requirements of walking at a given speed. Brockett et al. (14) demonstrated a small but significantly higher correlation in the regression of energy cost on TBW and leg length (r = 0.77) than in the relationship between energy cost and TBW alone (r = 0.75). Van Der Walt and Wyndham (105) found a negligible relationship between leg length and oxygen uptake (r = −0.073). Workman and Armstrong (119) found that body height had a small but consistent effect on the predicted value of oxygen uptake while walking. According to their predictions, short people use more oxygen to walk than tall people of the same body weight at all walking speeds.

It may be concluded that most studies have found no consistent differences in oxygen uptake per kilogram while walking in adults of different age, weight, and gender, whereas for children and adolescents, some differences occur with age and possibly gender. When interpreting the effect of age, weight, or gender on energy expenditure, it is important to distinguish whether oxygen uptake is expressed per unit time, per unit kilogram/time, or per lean body mass and whether the person is walking at a speed associated with a percent of maximum workload (e.g., % VO_2max, % of maximal heart rate, or % maximal walking speed), a self-selected speed or a set speed. In considering the latter two conditions, it is important to recognize that a U-shaped relationship exists between walking speed and VO_2 when VO_2 is expressed relative to distance traveled (e.g., mL/kg/km or mL/kg/m). Self-selected walking speeds are often used when evaluating therapeutic interventions with an individual patient or within a group. However, because VO_2 measured under this condition is not independent of speed, strong consideration should be given to having individuals walk at a set speed if group comparisons in walking economy are being made or the impact of therapy to reduce locomotor energy cost is being evaluated. Clearly, the units in which oxygen uptake are expressed and the condition under which VO_2 is assessed can lead researchers and clinicians to different interpretations and conclusions.

WORK POWER AND EFFICIENCY

Energy efficiency can be calculated using values of mechanical energy levels (kinetic and potential) of the various segments of the body during successive moments of the walking cycle along with measurements of energy expenditure. Ralston and Lukin (86) originally used a direct method of measuring such energy levels that was suitable for certain motions of the body at moderate walking speeds up to ~100 m per minute, corresponding to cadences up to ~130 steps per minute.

The technique utilized cords that were attached to the principal segments of the body: head, arms, and trunk (HAT); thigh, shank, and foot. The attachments to thigh and shank were at the center of mass of each segment, placed according to the specifications of Dempster (28). The attachment to the foot was at the heel, and the attachment to the HAT at approximately the level of the second sacral vertebra. The cords attached to the thigh, lower leg, and foot ran horizontally backward and drove potentio-

metric transducers. Two cords were attached to the trunk, one horizontal and one vertical, and drove transducers that recorded motions of the HAT in both horizontal and vertical directions.

This method ignores certain motions that are of relatively small magnitude, such as rotational motions of the HAT and limb segments and arm swing. Earlier investigators similarly ignored such second-order effects (19). According to Winter (117), who extended this type of study to include rotational motion, only in the case of the shank does the rotational kinetic energy have significant value, contributing ~ 10% of the lower leg energy. More recently, computerized motion analysis has been used to obtain similar measurements, including rotational motion.

Masses of the body segments were determined from the volumes of water displacement and from values of the specific gravities provided in the literature. From the motions and masses, potential (gravitational) and kinetic (inertial) energy levels of the body segments were calculated for intervals of 0.02 sec during the walking cycle.

Figure 5-5 shows the changes in mechanical energy levels of the various body segments, as labeled, of a young woman of 58.6 kg, 169 cm, walking at a speed of 73.2 m per minute. Limb motion during walking enables a smooth forward progression of the body with minimal displacement of the center of gravity. At the beginning of the gait cycle, during initial stance, the HAT elevates over the lower limb generated by forward kinetic energy. In mid-stance as the HAT reaches maximal vertical elevation, the forward kinetic energy is converted into potential energy of HAT elevation. This potential energy is reconverted into forward kinetic energy in late stance as the HAT passes in front of the foot and enables energy transfer to the next step, maintaining approximately constant total mechanical energy level for HAT during most of the gait cycle.

The significant features of these data are: 1) the approximate mirror imaging of the HAT potential and HAT horizontal kinetic curves, 2) the flatness of the HAT total curve during about two-thirds of each step, 3) the disturbance of the HAT total curve during transition from stance to swing phase, which, on the basis of electromyographic evidence, coincides with the major muscle activity during the walking cycle, 4) the large channel in energy level of the swinging leg, due almost entirely to velocity (kinetic energy) changes in the limb segments, and 5) the large positive work peak in the total body after heel contact.

The positive work per step, measured by the increase in the total body work level, averaged 29.85 J (7.13 cal). The subject walked at an average cadence of 100 steps per minute, so the positive work per minute = 100 × 29.85 or 2985 J per minute (49.7 W, 713 cal per minute, 0.067 hp). Such a value for mechanical work rate is in good agreement with the results of Cavagna and Kaneko (18), who used a cinematographic method in their studies.

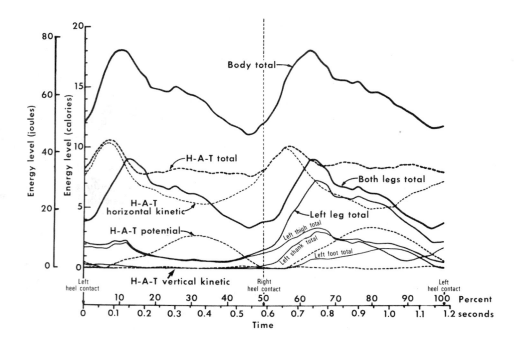

FIGURE 5-5. Energy levels of body segments and whole body of a 19-year old woman walking at 73.2 m per minute. (Adapted with permission from Ralston HJ, Lukin L. Energy levels of human body segments during level walking. *Ergonomics* 1969;12:39–46.)

The burst of positive work in each step occurred during an average interval of 0.19 sec. Hence, 29.85 J/0.19 = 157 W (2250 cal per minute, 0.21 hp) was the maximal positive power output during each step.

Wilkie (115) deduced that in single movements lasting <1 s, the usable "external power output" of the body is limited to a value somewhat less than 6 hp. In brief bouts of exercise of ~6 seconds, he gives the value 2 hp, and for long-term work lasting all day, 0.2 hp. Wilkie's figures are based on exercise by champion athletes, and he states that ordinary healthy individuals can produce less than 70% to 80% as much power. Even so, it is evident that the power expenditure in the female subject (0.21 hp) walking at a natural rate of 73.2 m per minute is much below her maximal capability. It may be concluded that there is a large margin of tolerance in the power demand of normal walking.

Statements regarding the "efficiency" of biological processes are notoriously confusing. As noted by Spanner (101), "The notion of efficiency with which a process involving energy transformation is carried out is one which comes up fairly frequently. However, the word is not always employed in precisely the same sense, and this is apt to cause some confusion." Spanner was referring to relatively straightforward chemical processes. Human walking, on the other hand, is vastly more difficult.

Clarification of the use of the terms "external work" and "internal work" may prevent this confusion. Fenn (30) referred to the elevation of the center of mass as "part of the external work" of running. Muller (75) referred to work against external resistance as external work. Snellen (99) stated that the external work in level walking is negligible and described external work as that work involved in climbing a hill. Wilkie (115) referred to work in overcoming air resistance as external work; work associated with raising and lowering the center of mass and with changes in kinetic energy of the limbs he called work that was "dissipated internally." He evidently regards the work done in climbing a hill as external work.

Cavagna et al. (19) referred to external work during locomotion as that associated with displacement of the center of mass of the body and to internal work as work not leading to a displacement of the center of mass. Ralston and Lukin (86) defined "total external positive work" as work measured by increases in the sum total of the energy levels of the body segments.

During walking, the reaction forces at the ground can do no work because the points of application of the forces are fixed (it is assumed that no slippage occurs such as when walking in sand). Thus, under conditions of level walking on the treadmill, no external work is done. The ground reaction forces can cause only acceleration of the center of mass of the body. Conversely, the forces produced by the muscles of the body can cause no acceleration of the center of mass but are responsible for the changes in energy level of the body, both kinetic and potential. Consequently, the internal work during walking is that done by muscles, while there is no external work unless one considers work done by the body on the environment (as in pushing molecules of air out of the way) or by the environment on the body.

In describing the efficiency of human walking, it is desirable to refer to work done on the environment as external work (as in pushing molecules of air out of the way). Consequently, in the case of normal walking on terrain (rather than simply level walking on the treadmill), the overall efficiency would be appropriately defined as the sum of the external work plus the internal work divided by the metabolic expenditure. This definition was used by Winter (118).

Under conditions of level walking on the treadmill, when virtually no external work is done, we shall use a definition of efficiency that is unambiguous and that we have found to be of considerable practical usefulness, especially in the comparison of work done by normal and disabled human subjects during walking.

Gross efficiency is defined as the total positive work per minute, determined from the total energy level of the body segments (Fig. 5-5) divided by the total metabolic expenditure per minute. For the female subject in Figure 5-5, the positive work, expressed in metabolic units, was 713 cal per minute, and the metabolic energy expenditure was 3010 cal per minute. The gross efficiency therefore is 713/3010 or 0.24. For the female subject walking slowly at 48.8 m per minute, the total positive work, expressed in metabolic units, was 350 cal per minute, and the total metabolic expenditure was 2544 cal per minute or 0.14.

Cavagna and Kaneko (18), who used net rather than total metabolic expenditure in calculating efficiency, obtained similar results when total expenditure was used in the calculation. This value is consistent with values of efficiency in the literature for various kinds of work, such as cycling on an ergometer. The data of Silverman et al. (97) for cycle ergometer exercise yield values of efficiencies very close to those found by Ralston and Lukin (86) for normal walking speeds, which commonly ranged from 0.20 to 0.25. Paulsen and Asmussen (81) calculated net efficiency from 23 experiments of arm vs. leg work on the ergometer and found arm work efficiency was 15.8% compared with 21.9% for leg work.

Ralston and Lukin (86) compared normal subjects with patients who had motor disability. Two below-knee amputees, wearing conventional prostheses, were studied with the techniques described previously. The subjects could walk comfortably only at lower speeds of up to 50 m per minute. As would be expected, the gross efficiencies were relatively low, ranging from ~ 0.08 to 0.14. However, 0.14 is about the same as that for the normal female subject, described previously, when walking at 48.8 m per minute. It may be concluded that one factor involved in the low value of the gross efficiency is simply the low speed, apart from the lack of normal muscle coordination associated with the disability.

As is usual in cases of motor disability, the energy expenditure per step or per meter was high compared with normal subjects, whereas the energy expenditure per minute was moderate, as a result of the low speeds used. It is the moderate energy cost per minute that is linked to moderate changes in heart rate, blood pressure, and pulmonary ventilation.

As previously mentioned, many authors have used a net energy value in calculating efficiency. Such a net value is obtained by subtracting a resting energy value from the energy expenditure or by subtracting an extrapolated value from the energy expenditure. Such a procedure can lead to very misleading conclusions. It has already been noted that use of a net value for mathematical formulation of the relation between walking speed and energy expenditure is unproductive.

Wilkie (116), in speaking of human muscular exercise, said: "The usual procedure of subtracting the resting oxygen consumption from the total does not correspond to any clear hypothesis about what is being estimated. In order to determine the efficiency of the working muscles themselves one should also subtract the extra oxygen used by heart, respiratory muscles, etc. . . . ."

Energy of Expenditure Per Unit Distance Walked

The measurement of energy efficiency is not feasible in most research and clinical laboratories. The term efficiency implies that the total amount of work performed by the body was calculated. The measurement of energy expenditure per distance walked provides a quantitative measure of energy economy, much the same as fuel economy is measured in the automobile.

Many authors have discussed the energy cost of walking expressed per unit body weight per unit distance. The curve of such energy cost, plotted against speed, is concave upward, and although fairly flat over a wide range of speeds (65–100 m per minute), the curve still exhibits a minimal value (Fig. 5-6, top). Ralston (84) showed that the mathematical form of such a curve could be deduced from the following equation:

$$E_m = \frac{E_w}{v} = \frac{32}{v} + 0.0050\,v \qquad (4)$$

where E_m is expressed in cal/kg/m and E_w is expressed in cal/kg per minute.

Differentiating E_m with respect to v (speed), and equating to zero, yields a minimal E_m of 0.80 cal/kg/m, corresponding to an optimal speed of 80 m per minute.

Similarly, Zarrugh et al. (121) proposed the following equation.

$$E_m = \frac{E_o}{v(1 - v/v_u)^2} \qquad (5)$$

where E_o is value of E_w when step length and step rate approaches zero and V_u is the upper limit of walking speed. Differentiating E_m with respect to v and equating to zero yields an optimal speed,

$$v_{opt} = v_u/3 = 240/3 = 80 \text{ m per minute} \qquad (6)$$

as in the case of Equation 4.

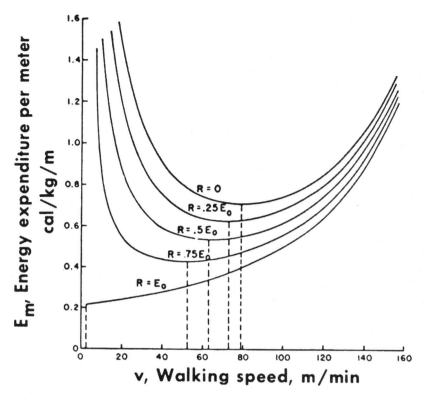

FIGURE 5-6. Gross energy expenditure per meter as function of walking speed v for typical subject walking naturally at different speeds. *Lower curves,* as increasing amounts of energy (R) are subtracted from gross energy expenditure per minute, the optimal speed corresponding to minimal E_m becomes smaller. (From Ralston HJ. Energetics of Human Walking. In: Herman RM, Grillner S, Stein PSG, Stuart DG, eds. *Neural Control of Locomotion.* New York: Plenum; 1976.)

As shown by Ralston (84), a person walking in a natural self-selected manner tends to adopt a speed close to the optimal speed. This finding was confirmed by Corcoran and Brengelmann (22) in a study of 32 subjects during floor walking. These authors found a natural average speed of 83.4 m per minute, differing from the above theoretical value of 80 m per minute by only 4%. Rose et al. (91) found a similar curve based on oxygen uptake per meter for children and adolescents walking on a treadmill with an optimal walking speed of 84 m per minute, ranging from 64 to 91 m per minute. Similarly, Morgan and associates (73) reported no significant difference in the freely-chosen walking speed (1.03 +/− 0.14 m per second) and the most economical walking speed (1.06 +/− 0.13 m per second) in six children with cerebral palsy.

Waters et al. (108,109) measured oxygen uptake per kilogram per meter in children, teenagers, and adults walking at self-selected slow, comfortable, and fast walking speeds and found a significant decrease in oxygen uptake per meter with age.

Walking speed equals steps per minute multiplied by step length. Thus, an energetically-optimal walking speed must be based on a choice of step rate and step length that yields a minimal energy cost. This is an example of a fundamental feature of human motor behavior that applies to many activities in addition to walking. In a freely chosen rate of activity, a rate is chosen that represents minimal energy expenditure per unit task. In the case of natural walking, where the unit task is traversing 1 m of ground, a speed is adopted such that each meter is covered as efficiently, from an energy standpoint, as possible.

This principle is analogous to a biological conservation of energy law. The French physiologist E. J. Marey (1895), one of the pioneers in the study of animal locomotion, anticipated the statement of this principle over a century ago (58). Commenting on the applications of measuring various gait parameters he stated, "The data afforded by these measurements may be put to practical use, for they indicate, according to the object in view, the best way of utilizing muscular force in walking or running: whether it be to traverse the greatest distance with the least expenditure of energy, or whether it be to cover a certain distance in the least possible time. There is then, for each pace, an optimum rate of steps per minute, which corresponds to the point at which the velocity increases proportionately faster than energy is expended."

Only the use of gross energy values leads to Equations 5 and 6, which establish an optimum condition of economy for free walking patterns and predict an experimentally verifiable optimal speed. The top curve of Figure 5-6 shows the gross energy expenditure per meter as a function of walking speed *v* for a typical subject when walking naturally at different speeds. The lower curves show that if increasing amounts of energy (*R*) are subtracted from the gross energy expenditure per minute, the optimal speed corresponding to minimal E_m becomes smaller and smaller. It becomes essentially zero when an amount equal to E_o is subtracted. It is not very enlightening to find that the best way to avoid energy cost during walking is not to walk! It is suggested that in other types of exercise, the gross rather than the net energy expenditures may be the fundamental energy parameter.

Energy Expenditure Per Step

Minimal energy expenditure per meter traversed per kilogram body weight (E_m) occurs at a speed of 80 m per minute. The relations will now be considered between speed (v), step rate (n), step length (s), energy expenditure per kilogram per minute (E_w), and energy expenditure per kilogram per step (E_n).

The relevant data from Zarrugh et al. (121) are shown in Table 5-6, based on studies of 10 normal males and 10 normal females ranging 20 to 55 and 20 to 49 years, respectively. E_w values are calculated from Equation 1.

The difference in the value of s/n at the higher speeds in males and females is highly significant. For example, at $v = 73.2$ m per minute, the odds against the difference being due to chance are better than 1000 to 1. Even at 48.8 m per minute, the odds are 4 to 1. The smaller values of s and s/n in females reflect the shorter average leg lengths in women compared with men, although this may not be the only factor involved.

The values shown in Table 5-6 do not strictly correspond to those of a natural walk, since the treadmill imposed the speeds. However, 73.2 m per minute is fairly close to the optimal speed (80 m per minute) and therefore should yield values of s/n close to those of natural walk.

Molen and Rozendal (66) studied 309 males and 224 females walking along pavement and path. At an average speed of 83.4 m per minute, the average value of s/n for males was 0.0072, in good agreement with the values of 0.0070 and 0.0072 at speeds of 73.2 and 97.6 m per minute in Table 5-6. At an average speed of 76.2 m per minute, the average value of s/n for females was 0.0060, in excellent agreement with the value of 0.0061 at 73.2 m per minute in Table 5-6.

The near constancy in the value of s/n in walking has physiologic significance. Not only does the value of s/n characterize the walk of the male and female, but it is also fundamental in determining the optimal speed of walking. At any given speed, imposition of an unnatural step rate (or step length) for that speed results in a higher than normal value of the energy expenditure per unit distance traversed (5,75,96,121).

Shields (96) measured the time to reach 88% of age-predicted maximum heart rate in adults walking at 90 m per minute. She found that normal step length was 72% of leg length and that this resulted in significantly better performance than a step length of 60% of leg length, but resulted in a significantly poorer performance than a step length of 80% of leg length.

In the following mathematical treatment, the average values of $s/n = 0.007$ and $s/n = 0.0064$ (Table 5-6) will be used for males and females, respectively.

In a manner similar to that followed in the preceding section, Equation 1 can be used to determine the step rate corresponding to minimal energy expenditure per step:

Since $v = sn$, and $s = 0.007n$ in males, $v = 0.007n^2$. Substituting in Equation 1

$$E_w = 32 + 0.0050v^2 = 32 + 0.0050\,(0.007n^2)^2$$
$$E_n = \frac{E_w}{n} = \frac{32}{n} + 0.005\,(0.007)^2\,n^2$$
$$= \frac{32}{n} + 2.45 \times 10^{-1}n^2$$

Differentiating E_n with respect to n and equating to zero, E_n (minimum) occurs at $n = 81.2$ steps per minute.

After interpolating from Table 5.6, this would correspond to a speed of about 46 m per minute, which is not the speed (80 m per minute) corresponding to minimal energy expenditure per meter.

▶ **TABLE 5-6   Average Values of *v, n, s, s/n, E_w*, and *E_m* for 10 Male and 10 Female Subjects[a]**

	v (m/min)	*n* (steps/min)	*s* (m)	*s/n* (m/steps/min) (S.D.)	*E_w* (cal/kg/min)	*E_n* (cal/kg/step) = *E_w/n*
Males	24.4	59.5 ± 4.33	0.41 ± 0.025	0.0069 ± 0.00065	35.0	0.59
	48.8	84.4 ± 6.48	0.59 ± 0.041	0.0070 ± 0.00072	43.9	0.52
	73.2	102.2 ± 5.43	0.72 ± 0.056	0.0070 ± 0.00066	58.8	0.58
	97.6	116.3 ± 3.13	0.84 ± 0.020	0.0072 ± 0.00026	79.6	0.68
Mean				0.0070 ± 0.00120		
Females	24.4	60.0 ± 3.95	0.41 ± 0.029	0.0068 ± 0.00065	35.0	0.58
	48.8	86.7 ± 7.26	0.57 ± 0.037	0.0066 ± 0.00070	43.9	0.51
	73.2	109.0 ± 5.49	0.67 ± 0.037	0.0061 ± 0.00045	58.8	0.54
	97.6	126.8 ± 8.98	0.77 ± 0.031	0.0061 ± 0.00050	79.6	0.63
Mean				0.0064 ± 0.00120		

[a]Values are means ± SD. From Zarrugh MY, Todd FN, Ralston HJ. Optimization of energy expenditure during level walking. Eur J Appl Physiol 1974;33:293–306.

By using the value $s/n = 0.004$ for females, E_n (optimum) occurs at $n = 85$ steps per minute. Interpolating from Table 5-6, this would correspond to a speed of about 47 m per minute, again representing an undesirable method of walking.

Clearly, the optimal step rate for minimal energy per step does not represent a desirable method of walking, at least in normal subjects.

The significance of this conclusion is addressed in "Work, Power, and Efficiency" concerning disability, where the inability to walk at higher speeds causes the energy expenditure per step to greatly exceed normal values. In such cases, the energy expenditure per minute is kept low because of low step rate.

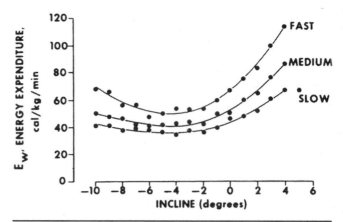

FIGURE 5-7. Effect of grade on energy expenditure of a normal young male while walking at three speeds.

Terrain

Passmore and Durnin (80), in their review of energy expenditure, state, "The type of surface may have a slight effect on the energy cost of walking. However, unless the surface is markedly rough, the effect will probably not exceed 10% more than walking on a flat surface." Haisman and Goldman (33) found that energy expenditure of walking with a 20-kg backpack was 10% higher when walking on grassland compared with blacktop at walking speeds of 53 and 80 m per minute. Passmore and Durnin (80) reported an increase of ~ 35% in oxygen uptake for a subject walking at a speed of 90 m per minute on plowed field compared with asphalt road. Strydom et al. (102), in a study of 11 young men, observed that the metabolic cost of walking at ~ 80 m per minute with loads of 23 kg was 80% greater on loose sand then on a hard surface.

In the latter two cases cited, the walking speed was fairly brisk, and therefore the results might not be relevant to the effect of loose soil at lower speeds. However, is clear that the nature of the terrain must always be considered in anticipating the metabolic demand of walking.

Terrain coefficients were developed to correct for the type of surface traversed (78). Single coefficients were found to fit all measured walking surfaces except for snow (76). The coefficient for soft snow was found to increase as the snow footprint depth increased.

Slope Walking

Figure 5-7 presents the essential metabolic features of slope walking. A normal young adult male walked on the treadmill at speeds of 48.8, 73.2, and 97.6 m per minute and at grades ranging from + 4° to −10° (+ 7% to −18%). The metabolic cost rapidly increased with increasing grade. Also noted is the more modest decrease in cost at grades in the range of 0 to −4° (0% to −7%). The experimental points are fitted by fourth-degree polynomial functions (smooth curves), all of which exhibit minima close to −4°. At lower

grades, the metabolic cost increases as a result of postural changes and the use of muscles in "braking" action.

Several investigators have developed equations relating energy expenditure to speed and grade. Formulas for estimating the energy requirements of walking at various speeds and grades have been published by the American College of Sports Medicine (1). Montoye et al. (67) validated these formulas and found that the formulas are accurate for estimating the mean oxygen requirements in 6% to 18% grade walking in adult males. In horizontal walking and walking at 3% grade, the formulas underestimate oxygen uptake in all age groups.

In boys younger than 18 years, the formulas underestimate the energy requirement in walking at all grade levels. Montoye et al. (67) concluded that when applied to adults, the formulas provide a reasonable estimate of the actual oxygen requirement of steady-state treadmill walking.

Table 5-7 shows representative data, such as those provided by McDonald (51), based on experiments by Margaria (59) on three normal adult males. The calculated values of E_w (cal/kg per minute) and E_w (cal/kg/m) have been added, based on a body weight of 72 kg.

As has been noted earlier, during level walking, a person tends to adopt a speed such that energy expenditure per unit distance is minimized. From Table 5-7, it is evident that minimal values of E_m occur at slopes of + 10 to −20% at speeds of 80 to 100 m per minute. Therefore, it may be expected that persons will adopt such speeds at those grades. Above + 10%, and below −20%, E_m minima do not occur within the range of speeds shown.

While the subject of Figure 5-7 exhibited minimal values of E_w at a slope of about −7% (−4°), the minimal value of E_w in Table 5-7 occurs at a slope of about −10%. Similarly, Pivarnik and Sherman (83) found the minimal values of Ev occurred at grades of −5 to −10% at walking speeds of 80 m per minute. Above these grades, E_w increased significantly with increasing grades of 0, 5, and 10%.

▶ **TABLE 5-7** **Estimates of E_w (cal/kg/min) and E_m (cal/kg/m) at Various Speeds and Grades**[a]

Grade		40 m/min		60 m/min		80 m/min		100 m/min		120 m/min	
%	Degrees	E_w	E_m	E_w	E_m	E_w	E_m	E_w	E_m	E_w	E_m
−40	−21.8	54	1.35	70	1.17	85	1.06	98	0.98	106	0.88
−35	−19.3	47	1.18	60	1.00	72	0.90	84	0.84	93	0.78
−30	−16.7	46	1.15	56	0.93	67	0.84	79	0.79	90	0.75
−25	−14.0	44	1.10	53	0.88	63	0.79	74	0.74	87	0.73
−20	−11.3	41	1.03	46	0.77	53	0.66	63	0.63	77	0.64
−15	−8.5	33	0.83	37	0.62	44	0.55	54	0.54	69	0.58
−10	−5.7	30	0.75	35	0.58	43	0.54	54	0.54	70	0.58
−5	−2.9	32	0.80	38	0.63	48	0.60	61	0.61	82	0.68
0	0	41	1.03	49	0.82	62	0.78	81	0.81	110	0.92
5	2.9	59	1.48	74	1.23	95	1.19	125	1.25	167	1.39
10	5.7	69	1.73	93	1.55	121	1.51	155	1.55	193	1.61
15	8.5	82	2.05	114	1.90	150	1.88	187	1.87		
20	11.3	98	2.45	140	2.33	185	2.31				
25	14.0	114	2.85	170	2.83						
30	16.7	133	3.33	204	3.40						
35	19.3	153	3.83								
40	21.8	174	4.35								

[a](Modified from McDonald I. Statistical studies of recorded energy expenditure of man. Part II. Expenditure on walking related to weight, sex, age, height, speed and gradient [abstract]. *Nutr Abstr Rev* 1961;31:739–762.)

Immobilization

The effects of restricting motion at various joints such as the ankle, knee, hip, and the spine on the metabolic cost of walking were studied by Ralston (85) using immobilization with a brace (ankle) or plaster casts (knee, hip,

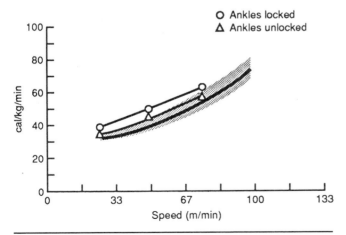

FIGURE 5-8. Effects of immobilization of both ankle joints on average energy expenditure, as a function of speed, for three subjects walking. *Heavy line,* average values for 12 normal subjects; *stippled area,* scatter of normal values. (From Ralston HJ. Effects of Immobilizations of Various Body Segments on the Energy Cost of Human Locomotion. *Ergonomics* 1965;(suppl):53.)

spine). The energy expenditure of three subjects walking with both ankle braces locked and unlocked was compared with normal values (Fig. 5-8). Normal male subjects of average physique tend to adopt a walking speed of ~80 m per minute. At this speed with both ankles immobilized, the energy expenditure was 9% above average. With one ankle immobilized, the increase was 6%.

Knee restriction at 0, 15, and 30 degrees produced only minimal increased energy needs (Fig. 5-9). At a walking speed of 74 m per minute, locomotor energy demand was significantly elevated at 45 degrees knee flexion, with energy expenditure being 19% higher than with a 0° knee flexion angle and 37% higher than with the knee unrestricted. Correction of leg length by use of a shoe lift did not significantly alter this result. Hip restriction at an angle of 60 degrees was 28% higher than at 30 degrees and 39% higher than with the hip unrestricted at a walking speed of 57 m per minute (Fig. 5-10). Hip immobilization at 30 degrees consistently resulted in the lowest values of all the angles studied, with 0 degrees being intermediate in results. Correction of leg length by use of a shoe lift did not materially alter this result. Trunk restriction increased energy expenditure by 10% over a wide range of speeds (Fig. 5-11). Restriction of arm motion in seven subjects, over a wide range of speeds, had no significant effect on the energy cost of walking.

Similarly, Mattsson and Brostrom (62) found that in adults walking at self-selected comfortable speeds, immobilization of the knee resulted in a 23% increase in oxygen

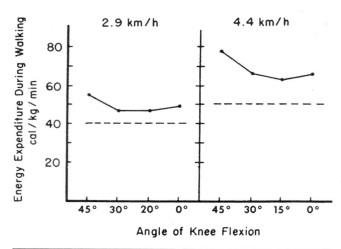

FIGURE 5-9. Effect of angle of immobilization of knee on average energy expenditures of eight subjects during walking. *Broken lines,* mean values for normal walking. (From Ralston HJ. Effects of Immobilizations of Various Body Segments on the Energy Cost of Human Locomotion. *Ergonnomics* 1965;(suppl):53.)

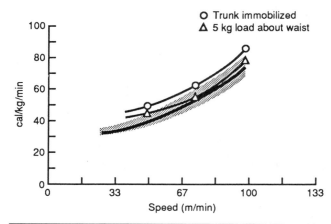

FIGURE 5-11. Effect of restriction of trunk motion on average energy expenditure, as a function of speed, of seven subjects with and without restriction of shoulder, spine, and pelvic motion. *Panel B: heavy line,* average values for 12 normal subjects; *stippled area,* scatter of normal values. (Modified with permission, from Ralston HJ. Effects of immobilization of various body segments on the energy cost of human locomotion. Ergonomics 1965;(suppl):53.)

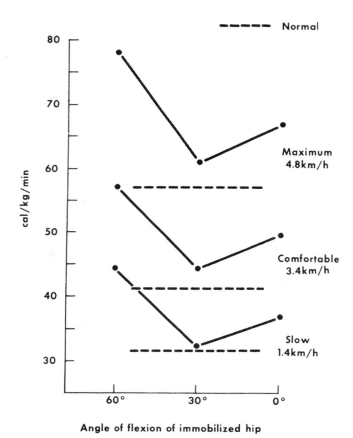

FIGURE 5-10. Effect of angle of immobilization of hip on average energy expenditures of four subjects during walking. Broken lines, mean values for normal walking. (From Ralston HJ. Effects of Immobilizations of Various Body Segments on the Energy Cost of Human Locomotion. *Ergonnomics* 1965;(suppl):53.)

uptake per meter walked (0.156 vs. 0.196 mL/kg per minute). Walking speed decreased from 79 to 60 m per minute. Waters and Mulroy (111) compared the effect of restriction of the ankle, knee and hip on oxygen cost (mL/kg/m) during walking and found a progressive rise in the rate of energy cost caused by the loss of joint motion progressing from the ankle, to the knee and to the hip. Oxygen cost during walking increased slightly (13%) with ankle fusion, to a greater degree (33%) with knee immobilization with a cylinder cast and still higher with hip fusion (46%). Waters and Lunsford (110) found that the energy cost of walking with the knee flexed increased progressively with the position of knee flexion. Immobilization of the knee flexed 15 degrees resulted in increased oxygen cost of 13% compared to an increase of 45% with the knee flexed 45 degrees.

Disability

Measuring the energy expenditure of walking in persons with a disability provides objective documentation of the degree of disability and the effect of treatment such as surgery, physical therapy, ambulatory aids, and prosthetics. Bard and Ralston (6) measured oxygen uptake and calculated calories/kilogram per minute in an amputee walking with three different combinations of prosthetics and/or crutches. They found that when the patient walked at a comfortable walking speed (74 m per minute) with his usual suction-socket prosthesis with a SACH foot, the energy expenditure was only 20% above normal. When using a pylon instead of his usual prosthesis, the

▌ **TABLE 5-8 Average Values of Energy Expenditure of Normal and Hemiplegic Subjects during Normal Stair Climbing Using Alternate Gait**[a]

Experimental Conditions	Steps/min		Energy Expenditure				
			cal/kg/min		cal/kg/step		
	Normal	Hemiplegic	Normal	Hemiplegic	Normal	Hemiplegic	
Rest (sitting)			18.9	15.6			
Low stairs	72	47	53.3	49.1	0.74	1.04	
High stairs	70	44	70.3	61.5	1.00	1.40	

[a]From Hirschberg GG, Ralston HJ. Energy cost of stair-climbing in normal and hemiplegic subjects. *Am J Phys Med* 1965;44:165.

energy expenditure increased sharply at speeds above 60 m per minute. Energy expenditure was highest when using forearm crutches for all walking speeds. When expressed in calories/kilogram/meter, the optimal energy expenditure with crutches was 30% higher than with the usual prosthesis, whereas the optimal walking speed was 20% less.

In a comprehensive review of the energy cost of walking with disability, Waters and Mulroy (111) note that while there are a substantial number of studies on the energy expenditure of walking for persons with lower-extremity amputation, a direct comparison of the results of the different studies is difficult because young individuals with amputations, which are usually traumatic, are not consistently distinguished from older persons with amputations, which are usually vascular. Yet, there are significant differences between these two groups with respect to gait performance. In addition, Waters and Mulroy (111) note that use of upper-extremity assistive devices, prosthetic fit and experience using the prosthesis influence the results but are not well-controlled for. They noted that research has shown that there is a higher oxygen cost of walking for persons with lower limb amputations; however, whether the increased cost resulted from a slower walking speed or a higher rate of oxygen uptake depended on the level of amputation and physical fitness of the individual.

Hirschberg and Ralston (36) compared normal and hemiplegic subjects climbing stairs with low (10 cm) and high (19 cm) risers using alternating gait (Table 5-8). As might be expected, the energy expenditure per step was much greater, on the order of 40% higher, in the hemiplegic subjects compared to the normal subjects. The energy expenditure per minute is not very different in the two types of subjects, because hemiplegic patients adopt a low step rate. Note that such physiologic variables as heart rate, blood pressure, and respiratory rate are linked to the metabolic rate per minute rather than to the metabolic rate per meter or per step. These physiologic variables, while slightly higher in the hemiplegic than in the normal subjects, were still within acceptable limits.

Not shown in Table 5-8, but worthy of note, is the fact that alternating gait required 28% to 30% less metabolic demand per step than unilateral leading gait in both normal and hemiplegic subjects. Also, high stairs elicited a greater physiologic demand, per minute and per step, than low stairs, in both normal and hemiplegic subjects.

McBeath et al. (47) measured oxygen uptake in normal men walking with loftstrand and axillary crutches. They found that walking with crutches or canes resulted in significantly higher energy expenditure and that the comfortable walking speed of assisted ambulation was significantly slower than normal. With both loftstrand and axillary crutches, the oxygen uptake per meter walked was greater than normal for the three-point partial weight-bearing and the two-point alternating gaits, but not as great as the costs for the three-point non-weight-bearing and the swing-through gaits.

Corcoran et al. (23) studied hemiplegic subjects walking with plastic and metal braces. They found that use of a brace significantly decreased oxygen uptake per meter, but there were no differences between plastic versus metal braces. Rose et al. (92) measured oxygen uptake in children with cerebral palsy walking at progressively increasing speeds on a treadmill. Oxygen uptake at rest and at a maximal walking speed were not different from normal values. However, maximal walking speed averaged only 56 m per minute for cerebral palsy subjects compared with 122 m per minute for normal subjects. Oxygen uptake per meter walked averaged 280% greater for children with cerebral palsy compared with normal controls (92). Oxygen uptake per meter at the most economical walking speed was 0.48 mL/kg/m compared with 0.17 mL/kg/m for normal subjects. Diplegic subjects had significantly higher values than hemiplegic subjects.

Unnithan and colleagues (104) reported that children with cerebral palsy exhibited substantially higher treadmill walking energy costs compared to a control group of able-bodied children. Similarly, Morgan et al. (73) demonstrated that children with spastic hemiplegic CP demonstrated higher walking V0$_2$ values (mL/kg per minute) while walking at 1.5, 2, and 2.5 mph compared to a matched group of able-bodied children. However, only V0$_2$

comparisons at the two highest speeds were significantly different between groups. Campbell and Ball (17) measured oxygen uptake (mL/kg per minute) in children with cerebral palsy walking at a single comfortable speed. They found that oxygen uptake values varied widely but were higher than normal for all children with cerebral palsy. In non-disabled children, oxygen uptake at the normal walking speed decreases with age. The opposite trend occurred in the children with cerebral palsy, in that oxygen uptake values increased with age. This may reflect increased size and decreased relative strength with age in cerebral palsy, causing walking to become more difficult because of increases in body mass and adiposity that are not matched by commensurate gains in leg muscle strength. From a practical standpoint, an increase in walking energy costs, when combined with lower values of maximal aerobic power (38,73,104), results in a higher relative exercise intensity at any given walking speed. This, in turn, can lead to greater levels of fatigue, decreased community walking activity, and increased reliance on wheelchair use.

In order to accurately determine the impact of clinical treatments aimed at reducing locomotor energy cost in youth with cerebral palsy, it is important to consider within- and between-day variability in walking VO_2. Limited data (42,57) suggest that fairly stable ambulatory oxygen uptake values can be achieved if testing is preceded by a short period (5 to 15 minutes) of treadmill accommodation.

HEART RATE AS AN ESTIMATE OF ENERGY EXPENDITURE

The rate of oxygen uptake can be used to assess the energy expended while walking, but the instrumentation is cumbersome to wear and is unavailable in most clinical settings. Conversely, heart rate is an easily measured parameter and has been found to be an accurate and convenient estimate of energy expenditure during steady-state submaximal work in normal and disabled adults engaged in walking and cycling (4,50,81) and in normal and disabled children walking (92) and exercising on a cycle ergometer (7,21).

Limitations exist for the use of heart rate as an estimate of energy expenditure. At very rapid rates of walking, the relationship is unpredictable between heart and oxygen uptake (4). Heart rate may be affected by factors other than oxygen uptake, such as anxiety or anticipation, particularly at rest and low levels of activity (4,7). Ganguli and Datta (31) state that the effect of anxiety is usually overcome quite readily by habituation after the first or second test in an investigation that constitutes a series of tests. Furthermore, the importance of anxiety lessens as the intensity of exercise is increased.

Heart rate is also affected by climatic stress, dehydration, fever, various diseases, and medications (4,7). At a given workload, heart rate increases with the use of a smaller active muscle mass such as with upper-extremity work (6). Paulsen and Asmussen (81) compared heart rate and oxygen uptake and found the relationship to be linear, but the slope of the relationship was increased for upper-extremity work compared with lower-extremity work. The increase in heart rate at a given level of oxygen uptake is inversely proportional to the size of muscle mass being used.

Despite the aforementioned limitations, heart rate is a clinically-useful estimate of energy expenditure. Because of its marked sensitivity to any increase or decrease in conditioning, heart rate is a valuable gauge for determination of fitness and compliance to exercise programs. The slope of the relationship between heart rate and oxygen uptake is used to assess fitness level. With training, heart rate decreases for a given level of oxygen uptake or workload (4). Saltin et al. (95) found that the slope of the relationship between heart rate and oxygen uptake (liters per minute) increased with bed rest and decreased with training.

During steady-state submaximal workloads, heart rate has been found to be a reliable estimate of energy expenditure. Astrand and Rodahl (4) found that in adults, oxygen uptake and heart rate increase linearly throughout a wide range of submaximal workloads on the cycle ergometer. The relationship was unpredictable at maximum levels of exercise. Cooper et al. (21) found that a linear relationship existed between oxygen uptake (liters per minute) and heart rate in 107 children performing on a cycle ergometer. The mean correlation was 0.68, but the mode fell between 0.8 and 0.9, with the lowest correlation coefficients occurring in the youngest ages owing to a greater influence of noise on a smaller range of oxygen uptake. The younger subjects also started and stopped during the protocol, resulting in increased variation of heart rate. They found that the slope (0.33) of the relationship, when normalized for body weight, did not significantly change with age or weight, but the mean slope was significantly greater for boys (0.37) than for girls (0.29).

Rose et al. (92) investigated the relationship between heart rate and oxygen uptake for 18 children who were nondisabled and 13 children with cerebral palsy walking on a treadmill (Fig. 5-12). The relationship was linear between heart rate (beats per minute) and oxygen uptake (mL/kg per minute) in the nondisabled children and children with cerebral palsy. The mean correlation within an individual was very high (nondisabled, 0.98, cerebral palsy, 0.99). Within the normal and cerebral palsy groups, the correlation was also high (nondisabled, 0.83, cerebral palsy, 0.84). The linear relationship between heart rate and mass-related oxygen uptake existed throughout a wide range of walking speeds (22-131 m per minute). The slope of the relationship between heart rate and oxygen uptake was not significantly different for the normal

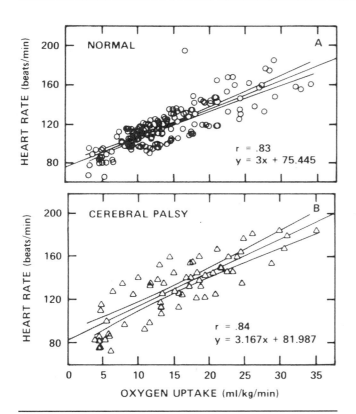

FIGURE 5-12. Scatterplot and linear regression line with 95% confidence limits around the mean for heart rate vs. oxygen uptake for 18 non-disabled children (**A**) and 13 children with cerebral palsy (**B**). (From Rose et al. *J Pediatr Orthop* 1989;9:276–279).

subjects (0.30) compared to children with cerebral palsy (0.32) and did not differ significantly with age.

Age

Astrand and Rodahl (4) reported that adult heart rate does not change with age for a given workload (100 W). Waters et al. (108) found no difference in heart rate between adults (20–59 years) and seniors (60–80 years) walking at a self-selected comfortable walking speed. However, walking speed was significantly slower in the seniors (73 m per minute) compared with young adults (80 m per minute). Conversely, Bassey et al. (8) reported that during self-paced walking, heart rate was approximately 10 beats per minute lower in subjects aged 20 to 29 compared with 60 to 69 years when body fat was considered.

A given heart rate may represent a higher percent of maximal capacity in older adults because maximum heart rate decreases with age in adults (4). Astrand and Rodahl (4) studied 350 subjects aged 25 to 60 working at 50% VO_2 max. They reported that heart rate was 110 beats per minute for a typical 65-year man compared with 130 beats per minute for a 25-year man. Thus, in the typical 65-year-old, walking may represent a higher percent of maximal

capacity. Similarly, Blessey (9) found that in adults aged 20 to 29, walking represented 36% of maximal oxygen uptake compared with 43% of maximal oxygen uptake for adults aged 50 to 59.

Waters et al. (109) found that heart rate was higher in children (114 beats per minute) than in adolescents (97 beats per minute) walking at a comfortable self-selected speed. Walking speed was slightly, but significantly, higher in the adolescents (73 m per minute) compared with the children (70 m per minute). Similarly, Bar-Or (7) concluded that submaximal heart rate declined with age in children performing the same absolute exercise task. He noted that some of this difference can be explained by variations in relative exercise intensity, i.e., given the level of oxygen uptake or percent maximal oxygen uptake. As previously mentioned, Cooper et al. (21) and Rose et al. (92) found that the slope of the relationship between heart rate and oxygen uptake per kilogram did not differ significantly with age for children and adolescents. It may be concluded that the age-related decrease in heart rate in children and adults while walking is related to the difference in relative exercise intensity.

Gender

Waters et al. (108) found that during self-paced walking, heart rate was slightly but significantly higher in young female adults (104 beats per minute) and seniors (106 beats per minute) compared with male young adults (94 beats per minute) and seniors (97 beats per minute). Walking speed was significantly slower in female young adults (76 beats per minute) compared with male young adults (84 m per minute). Bassey et al. (8) found that women had walking heart rates that are 4.4 beats per minute higher, even when stature and weight are controlled for. Gender differences disappeared when percent fat and fat-free mass were controlled.

Waters et al. (109) found that heart rate during self-paced walking was significantly higher in female children (118 beats per minute) and adolescents (103 beats per minute) compared with male children (111 beats per minute) and adolescents (90 beats per minute).

Bar-Or (7) also found that female children and adolescents have a higher heart rate than males at a given workload. He suggested that the higher heart rates may be related to decreased stroke volume or to lower levels of habitual activity.

Although the relative influence of body weight, age and gender on heart have not been completely resolved, heart rate is an accurate and reliable estimate of energy expenditure. More specifically, heart rate is an indication of the cardiovascular demands of a given activity. Paulsen and Asmussen (81) stated: "While the caloric output estimated from the pulse rate thus may be overestimated when compared to the actual metabolism, it nevertheless gives an

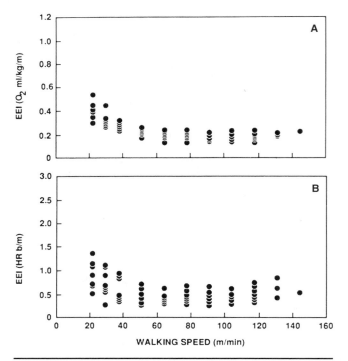

FIGURE 5-13. EEI based on oxygen uptake (**A**) and heart rate (**B**) as a function of walking speed for 18 non-disabled children. (From Rose et al. *Dev Med Child Neurol* 1990;32:333–340.)

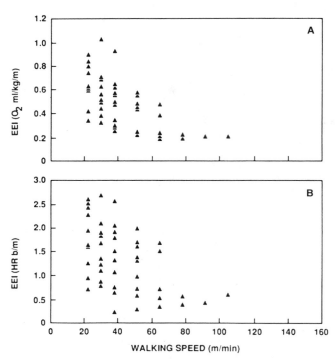

FIGURE 5-14. EEI based on oxygen uptake (**A**) and heart rate (**B**) as a function of walking sped for 13 children with cerebral palsy. (From Rose et al. *Dev Med Child Neurol* 1990;32:333–340.)

expression of the total load put on the organism during the work."

Heart Rate Per Distance Walked

Heart rate expressed per distance walked provides information on energy economy, as does oxygen uptake expressed per distance walked. Because resting heart rate is known to increase with decreased body size and level of fitness, the resting heart rate is subtracted from the walking heart rate, and this value is divided by the walking speed. The following calculation of an energy expenditure index (EEI; beats per minute) can be made:

$$\text{EEI} = \frac{\text{walking heart rate} - \text{resting heart rate}}{\text{walking speed}}$$

Rose et al. (90) compared oxygen uptake and heart rate per meter walked in 12 children with cerebral palsy and 18 normal controls walking at progressively faster speeds on a treadmill (Figs. 5-13 and 5-14). The curve generated by the heart rate per meter walked was similar to the curve generated by the oxygen uptake per meter walked for both cerebral palsy and normal subjects.

Optimal walking speed averaged 75 m per minute for nondisabled subjects and 50 m per minute for subjects with cerebral palsy. EEl values for cerebral palsy subjects averaged 3.3 times higher than values for normal subjects.

The diplegic cerebral palsy subjects' EEl values averaged three times higher than the hemiplegic subjects.

MacGregor (52) had previously calculated this index for 73 normal adults walking at self selected walking speed and found that 99% of the values for normal adults fell between 0.11 and 0.51 beats per minute. MacGregor referred to this index as the physiologic cost index. MacGregor (52) studied an adult polio patient and a nondisabled adult walking on the floor at slow, fast, and self selected speeds. He found that heart rate per meter walked was higher for the polio patient (0.5–0.9) than for the nondisabled adult (0.35). Furthermore, the rate increased for the polio patient when the brace was removed or unlatched.

Butler et al. (16) used this index to measure 72 children aged 3 to 12 years at a single self-selected speed and found the mean value to be 0.4 beats per minute. No change with age was found. They also compared four children with physical disability, two with cerebral palsy, and two with spina bifida, with and without their usual orthotic. They found that the four disabled children had higher values compared with the nondisabled children, but use of the orthotic decreased the index value. Children with spina bifida decreased from 6.9 and 5.8 beats per minute to 3.8 and 3.2 beats per minute and children with cerebral palsy decreased from 1.5 and 1.6 beats per minute to 0.98 and 0.7 beats per minute.

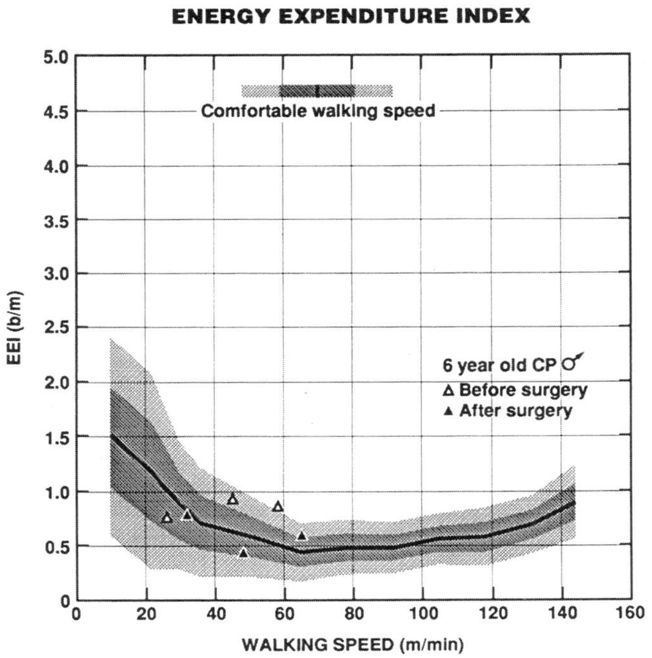

ENERGY EXPENDITURE INDEX

FIGURE 5-15. EEI based on heart rate as a function of walking speed. *Shaded,* EEI (mean ± 2 SD). *Bar,* range of comfortable walking speeds (mean ± 2 SD) for 103 non-disabled children and adolescents. (From Rose et al. *J Pedatr Orthop* 1991;11:571–578.) Preoperative and postoperative EEI values for self-selected slow, comfortable, and fast values for a 6-year-old boy with spastic diplegic cerebral palsy (CP) who underwent bilateral split tibialis posterior tendon transfer and tendoachilles lengthening.

Rose et al. (91) reported normal values for the EEI based on heart rate obtained from 103 children and adolescents aged 6 to 18 walking on the floor at self-selected slow, comfortable, and fast speeds and walking on the treadmill at progressively increasing speeds (Fig. 5-15). A plot of these values generates a curve showing that the lowest EEI value and optimal energy economy occurred at the self-selected comfortable walking speeds. EEI values for the self-selected fast walking speeds are significantly lower than EEI values for the self-selected slow walking speeds. The average self-selected comfortable floor walking EEI

value for the 102 subjects was 0.47 beats per minute (Table 3-9). This value was similar to the most economical EEI (heart rate) value of 0.41 beats per minute for 18 normal children walking on the treadmill who were previously studied. These values for children averaged slightly higher, but fell within the normal range of values for adults reported by MacGregor (52).

The average self-selected comfortable floor walking EEI decreased slightly with age, but the differences were not statistically significant (Table 5.9). The comfortable walking speed was significantly slower for the younger age group compared with the older three age groups, but there was no significant difference in walking speed between the three older age groups. The self-selected comfortable EEl for all males (0.45 beats per minute) and females (0.49 beats per minute) was not significantly different. In the oldest age group, females displayed slight but significantly higher EEI values. Figure 5-16 shows data from a 6-year-old boy with spastic hemiplegic cerebral palsy who was tested before and after a bilateral split tibialis posterior tendon transfer and tendoachilles lengthening. He walked independently at self-selected slow, comfortable, and fast walking speeds. The three self-selected walking speeds were slightly faster after surgery (32, 48, 65 m per minute) compared with before surgery (26, 45, 58 m per minute). The comfortable and fast EEI values were lower after surgery (0.78,0.42, and 0.59 beats per minute compared with before surgery (0.74, 0.91, and 0.85 beats per minute).

While documentation of heart rate per distance walked provides an easily-measured index of energy expenditure and assessment of degree of walking impairment, data from a recent study by Keefer et al. (41) of 13 children with hemiplegic CP revealed no association between EEI and gross VO_2 during treadmill walking at 0.67, 0.89, and 1.12 m per second. Similarly, a lack of relation between EEI and net VO_2 was evident at the two slowest walking speeds. Interestingly, analysis of individual data showed an unmatched response pattern between EEI and net VO_2 in a majority of subjects. Taken together, results from this investigation suggest that caution should be applied when using EEI to estimate walking energy expenditure in

▌**TABLE 5-9 Self Selected Walking Speeds and Corresponding EEI for Each Age Group**[a]

	Floor Walking Speed (m/min)			*EEI (beats/min)*		
Age (yr)	*Slow*	*Comfortable*	*Fast*	*Slow*	*Comfortable*	*Fast*
6–8	35 ± 9.9	65 ± 8.4	93 ± 13.1	0.75 ± 0.36	0.48 ± 0.15	0.60 ± 0.20
9–11	39 ± 11.0	70 ± 11.1	105 ± 12.0	0.69 ± 0.32	0.47 ± 0.11	0.61 ± 0.18
12–14	37 ± 11.0	76 ± 11.8	106 ± 11.6	0.69 ± 0.27	0.47 ± 0.11	0.58 ± 0.14
15–18	35 ± 11.2	75 ± 8.7	107 ± 11.2	0.70 ± 0.36	0.45 ± 0.14	0.57 ± 0.15

[a]Values are means ± SD. From Rose J, Gamble JG, Lee J, Lee R, Haskell WL. The energy expenditure index: A method to quantitate and compare walking energy expenditure for children and adolescents. J Pediatr Orthop 1991; 11:571–578.

children with cerebral palsy. Because resting heart rate is used to determine EEI, and can be influenced by a variety of factors, including anxiety, it is possible that an adjusted EEI measure that does not incorporate resting heart rate may more directly reflect walking energy profiles in children with CP. Along these lines, preliminary analysis of individual data from the Keefer et al. data set (41) has revealed a much more coherent response between gross VO_2 and a modified EEI value (gross HR/meter). Given this promising initial finding, a reexamination of the association between VO_2 and a modified expression of EEI is warranted in children with CP in order to develop a protocol to assess exercise heart rate during free walking and treadmill walking. Such research could prove useful in providing a simple-to-use field method of describing locomotor energy profiles or quantifying changes in walking energy cost following medical intervention and rehabilitation.

REFERENCES

1. American College of Sports Medicine. *Guidelines for Graded Exercise Testing and Exercise Prescription*. 7th edition, Lippincott Williams & Wilkins; 2006;286–299.
2. Armstrong N, Welsman JR. Assessment and interpretation of aerobic fitness in children and adolescents. *Exer Sport Sci Rev* 1994;22:435–475.
3. Ashkin A, Schutze K, Dziedzic JM, Euteneuer U, Schliwa M. Force generation of organelle transport measured in vivo by an infrared laser trap. *Nature* 1990;348:346–348.
4. Astrand PO, Rodahl K. *Textbook of Work Physiology*. New York: McGraw and Hill, 1970:9, 59, 153, 166, 306–308, 330–338, 361,413.
5. Atzler E, Herbst R. Arbeitsphysiologische Studien. *Pfliigers Arch* 1927;215:291–291.
6. Bard G, Ralston HJ. Measurement of energy expenditure during ambulation, with special reference to evaluation of assistive devices. *Arch Phys Med Rehab* 1959;40:415–420.
7. Bar-Or O. Pediatric sports medicine for the practitioner: From physiologic principles to clinical applications. New York: Springer-Verlag; 1983;4–10,22–23.
8. Bassey EJ, MacDonald IA, Patrick JM. Factors affecting the heart rate during self paced walking. *Eur J Appl Physiol* 1982;48:105–115.
9. Blessey R. Energy cost of normal walking. *Ortho Clin North Am* 1978;9:356–358.
10. Bloom WI, Eidex MD. The comparison of energy expenditure in the obese and lean. *Metabolism* 1967;16:685–692.
11. Bobbert AC. Energy expenditure in level and grade walking. *J Appl Physiol* 1960;15:1015–1021.
12. Boothby WM, Berkson J, Dunn HL. Studies of the energy of metabolism of normal individuals: A standard for basal metabolism, with a nomogram for clinical application. *Am J Physiol* 1936;116:468–484.
13. Booyens J, Keatinge WR. The expenditure of energy by men and women walking. *J Physiol (Lond)* 1957;138:165–171.
14. Brockett JE, Brophy EM, Konish F, et al. Influence of body size, body fat, nutrient intake and physical fitness on the energy expenditure of walking. *Army Med Nutr Lab Rep 177*. Fitzsimmons Army Hospital, Denver, 1956.
15. Brooks GA, Fahey TD. *Exercise Physiology: Human Bioenergetics and its Applications*. New York: John Wiley; 1984:39–54.
16. Butler P, Engelbrecht M, Major RE, Tait JH, Stallard J, Patrick JH. Physiologic cost index of walking of normal children and its use as an indicator of physical handicap. *Dev Med Child Neurol* 1984;26:607–612.
17. Campbell J, Ball J. Energetics of walking in cerebral palsy. *Orthop Clin North Am* 1978;9:374–377.
18. Cavagna GA, Kaneko M. Mechanical work and efficiency in level walking and running. *J Physiol (Lond)* 1977;268:647–681.
19. Cavagna GA, Saibene FP, Margaria R. External work in walking. *J Appl Physiol* 1963;18:1.
20. Cooke R. Force generation in muscle. *Curr Opin Cell Biol* 1990;2: 62–66.
21. Cooper DM, Weiler-Ravell D, Whipp BJ, Wasserman K. Growth-related changes in oxygen uptake and heart rate during progressive exercise in children. *Pediatr Res* 1984;18:845–851.
22. Corcoran PI, Brengelmann GL. Oxygen uptake in normal and handicapped subjects, in relation to speed of walking beside velocity-controlled cart. *Arch Phys Med Rehabil* 1970;51:78–87.
23. Corcoran PI, Jebsen RH, Brengelmann GL, Simons BC. Effects of plastic and metal leg braces on speed and energy cost of hemiparetic ambulation. *Arch Phys Med Rehab* 1970;51:69–77.
24. Cotes JE, Meade F. The energy expenditure and mechanical energy demand in walking. *Ergonomics* 1960;3:97–119.
25. Cotes JE, Meade F, Wise ME. Standardized test exercise. *Fed Proc* 1957;16:25–26.
26. Datta SR, Chatteyee BB, Roy BN. The relationship between energy expenditure and pulse rates with body weight and the load carried during load carrying on the level. *Ergonomics* 1973;16: 507–513.
27. DeJaeger D, Willems PA, Heglund NC. The energy cost of walking in children. *Eur J Physiol E-Pub* 11/23/2000.
28. Dempster WT. Space requirements of the 'seated operator: Geometrical, kinematic, and mechanical aspects of the body with special reference to the limbs. Wright Air Development Center. Technical Report 55-159. Wright-Patterson Air Force Base, Ohio, 1955.
29. Durnin JVGA, Passmore R. *Energy, Work, Leisure*. London: Heinemann Educational Books, 1967.
30. Fenn WO. Work against gravity and work due to velocity changes in running: Movements on the center of gravity within the body and foot pressure on the ground. *Am J Physiol* 1930;93:42–43.
31. Ganguli S, Datta SR. A new method for prediction of energy expenditure from heart rate. *Inst Engineer* 1978;58:57–61.
32. Goldman RF, Iampietro PF. Energy cost of load carriage. *J Appl Physiol* 1972;17:675–676.
33. Haisman MF, Goldman RF. The effect of terrain on the energy cost of walking with back loads and handcart loads. *J Appl Physiol* 1974;36:545–548.
34. Hansen JS. Exercise responses following production of experimental obesity. *J Appl Physiol* 1973;35:587–591.
35. Herfenroeder AC, Schoene RB. Predicting maximum oxygen uptake in adolescents. *Am J Dis Child* 1989;143:673–677.
36. Hirschberg GG, Ralston HJ. Energy cost of stair-climbing in normal and hemiplegic subjects. *Am J Phys Med* 1965;44:165.
37. Hong Y, Li JX, Wong ASK, Robinson PD. Effects of load carriage on heart rate, blood pressure and energy expenditure in children. *Ergonomics* 2000;43:717–727.
38. Hoofwijk M, Unnithan V, Bar-Or O. Maximal treadmill performance of children with cerebral palsy. *Pediatr Exerc Sci* 1995;7:305–313.
39. Houston ME. *Biochemistry Primer for Exercise Science, in Human Kinetics*. 2nd edition. Champaign, IL 2001:65–70.
40. Katch VL. Use of the oxygen/body weight ratio in correlational analysis: Spurious correlations and statistical considerations. *Med Sci Sports* 1973;5:253–257.
41. Keefer DJ, Tseh W, Caputo JL, et al. Comparison of direct and indirect measures of walking energy expenditure in children with cerebral palsy. *Dev Med Child Neurol* 2004;46:320–324.
42. Keefer DJ, Tseh W, Caputo JL, Apperson K, McGreal S Morgan DW. Within- and between-day stability of treadmill walking VO2 in children with hemiplegic cerebral palsy. *Gait Posture*, 2005;21:80–84.
43. Kleiber M. The fire of life. *An Introduction to Animal Energetics*. Huntington NY: Robert E. Krieger; 1975:3–4,214.
44. Knapik JJ, Reynolds KL, Harman E. Soldier load carriage: historical, physiologic, biomechanical and medical aspects. *Mil Med* 2004;169:45–56.
45. Laursen B, Ekner K, Simonsen EB, Viogt M, Sjogaard G. Kinetics and energetics during uphill and downhill carrying of different weights. *Appl Ergon* 2000;31:159–166.

46. Lloyd R, Cooke CB. The oxygen consumption associated with un-loaded walking and load carriage using two different backpack de-signs. *Eur J Appl Physiol* 2000;81:486–492.

47. McBeath AA, Bahrke M, Balke B. Efficiency of assisted ambula-tion determined by oxygen consumption measurement. *J Bone Joint Surg* 1974;56A:994–1000.

48. McArdle, WD, Katch FI, Katch VL. *Exercise Physiology*. 5th ed. Bal-timore: Lippincott Williams & Wilkins; 2001, p. 39,147.

49. McCann DJ, Adams WC. A dimensional paradigm for identifying the size-independent cost of walking. *Med Sci Sports Exerc* 2002; 34:1009–1017.

50. McCardle WD, Magel JR, Lesmes GR, Pechar GS. Metabolic and cardiovascular adjustment to work in air and water at 18°, 25°, and 33°C. *J Appl Physiol* 1976;40:85–90.

51. McDonald I. Statistical studies of recorded energy expenditure of man. Part II. Expenditure on walking related to weight, sex, age, height, speed and gradient [abstract]. *Nutr Abstr Rev* 1961;31:739–762.

52. MacGregor J. The objective measurement of physical performance with long-term ambulatory physiologic surveillance equipment. (L.A.P.S.E.). In: Scott FD, Rafferty EB, Goulding L, eds. *Third Inter-national Symposium on Ambulatory Monitoring*. London: Academic, 1980:29–38.

53. MacGregor J. Rehabilitation ambulatory monitoring. In: Kenedi RM, Paul JP, Hughes J, eds. *Disability*. London: MacMillan; 1979; 159–172.

54. Malatesta D, Simar D, Dauvilliers Y, et al. Energy cost of walk-ing and gait instability in healthy 65- and 80-yr-olds. *J Appl Physiol* 2003;95:2248–2256.

55. Malatesta D, Simar D, Dauvilliers Y, et al. Aerobic determinants of the decline in preferred walking speed in healthy, active 65-and 80-year olds. *Pfluger Arch* 2004;447:1915–21 (e-pub Dec. 10, 2003).

56. Malina RM, Bouchard C, Bar-Or O. Growth, Maturation and Phys-ical Activity. In: *Human Kinetics*.2nd ed. Champaign, IL, 2004, p. 72.

57. Maltais D, Bar-Or O, Pierrynowski M, Galea V. Repeated treadmill walks affect physiologic responses in children with cerebral palsy. *Med Sci Sports Exerc*, 2003;35:1653–1661.

58. Marey EJ. Movement. Translated by E. Pritchard. New York: Apple-ton, Century, Crofts, 1895.

59. Margaria R. Sulla fisiologia e specialmente suI consumo energetico della marcia e della corsa a varie velocita ed inclinazioni del terreno. vol 7 Atti Reale Accad. Naz Lincei Giovanni Bardi, Rome, 1938.

60. Martin PE. Mechanical and physiologic responses to lower ex-tremity loading during running. *Med Sci Sports Exerc* 1985;17:427–433.

61. Martin PE, Rothstein DE, Larish DD. Effects of age and physical activity status on the speed-aerobic demand relationship of walking. *J Appl Physiol* 1992:73:200–206.

62. Mattsson E, Brostrom LA. The increase in energy cost of walking with an immobilized knee or an unstable ankle. *Scand J Rehab Med* 1990;22:51–53.

63. Menier DR, Pugh LGCE. The relation of oxygen intake and ve-locity of walking and running, in competition walkers. *J Physiol* 1968;197:717–721.

64. Miller AT, Blyth CS. Influence of body fat content on the metabolic cost of work. *J Appl Physiol* 1955;88:139–141.

65. Molen NH, Rozendal RH. Energy expenditure in normal test sub-jects walking on a motor-driven treadmill. *Proc Kon Ned Akad Wet Ser C* 1967;75:192.

66. Molen NH, Rozendal RH. Fundamental characteristics of human gait in relation to sex and location. *Proc Kon Ned Akad Wet Ser C* 1972;75:215.

67. Montoye HS, Ayer T, Nagler F, Howley ET. The oxygen requirement for horizontal and grade walking on a motor-driven treadmill. *Med Sci Sport Exer* 1985;17:640–645.

68. Morgan DW. Economy of locomotion. In: *Paediatric exercise science and medicine*. Armstrong N, Mechelen WV, eds. Oxford: Oxford Uni-versity Press;. 2000:183–190.

69. Morgan DW, Boblett K, Caputo J, et al. Comparison of freely-chosen and energetically-optimal walking speeds in children with cerebral palsy. *Pediatr Exerc Sci* 1999;11:181–182.

70. Morgan DW, Tseh W, Caputo JL, et al. Longitudinal profiles of oxy-gen uptake during treadmill walking in able-bodied children: the locomotion energy and growth study. *Gait Posture* 2001;15:230–235.

71. Morgan DW, Tseh W, Caputo JL, et al. Prediction of the aerobic demand of walking in children. *Med Sci Sports Exerc*, 2002;34:2097–2102.

72. Morgan DW, Tseh W, Caputo JL, et al. Sex differences in run-ning economy of young children. *Pediatr Exerc Sci* 1999;11:122–128.

73. Morgan DW, Keefer DJ, Tseh W, et al. Walking energy use in children with spastic hemiplegia. *Pediatr Exerc Sci* 2005;17:91–92.

74. Morgan DW, Tseh W, Caputo JL, et al. Longitudinal stratification of gait economy in young boys and girls: the locomotion energy and growth study. *Eur J Appl Physiol* 2004;91:30–34.

75. Muller EA. Der Wirkungsgrad des Gehens. *Arbeitsphysiologie* 1950;14:236.

76. Myer MJ, Steudel K. Effect of limb mass and its distribution on the energetic cost of running. *J Exp Biol* 1985;116:363–373.

77. Myo-Thein , Lammert O, Garby L. Effect of trunkload on the energy expenditure on treadmill walking and ergometer cycling. *Eur J Appl Physiol* 1985;54:122–124.

78. Pandolf KB, Haisman MF, Goldman RF. Metabolic energy expen-diture and terrain coefficients for walking on snow. *Ergonomic* 1976;19:683–690.

79. Passmore R, Draper MH. Energy Metabolism. In: Albanese A, ed. *Newer Methods of Nutritional Biochemistry*. New York: Academic; 1965.

80. Passmore R, Durnin JVGA. Human energy expenditure. *Physiol Rev* 1955;35:801.

81. Paulsen E, Asmussen E. Energy requirements of practical jobs from pulse increase and ergometer test. *Ergonomics* 1963;5:33–36.

82. Perry J. The mechanics of walking in hemiplegia. *Clin Orthop Rel Res* 1969 63:23–31.

83. Pivarnik JM, Sherman NW. Responses of aerobically fit men and women to uphill versus downhill walking and slow jogging. *Med Sci Sports Exerc* 1990;22:127–139.

84. Ralston HJ. Energy-speed relation and optimal speed during level walking. *Int Z Angew Physiol* 1958;17:277.

85. Ralston HJ. Effects of immobilization of various body segments on the energy cost of human locomotion. *Ergonomics* 1965; (suppl):53.

86. Ralston HJ, Lukin L. Energy levels of human body segments during level walking. Ergonomics 1969;12:39–46.

87. Ralston HJ. Energetics of human walking. In: Herman RM, Grillner S, Stein PSG, Stuart DG, eds. *Neural Control of Locomotion*, New York: Plenum; 1976.

88. Robertson RJ, Caspersen CJ, Allison TB, Skrinar GS, Abbott RA, Metz KF. Differentiated perceptions of exertion and energy cost of young women while carrying loads. *Eur J Appl Physiol Occup Physiol* 1982;49:69–78.

89. Rogers DM, Turley KR, Kujawa KI, Harper, KM, Wilmore JH. Allo-metric scaling factors of oxygen uptake during exercise in children. *Pediatr Exerc Sci* 1995;7:12–25.

90. Rose J, Gamble JG, Burgos A, Medeiros J, Haskell WL. Energy ex-penditure index of activity for normal children and for children with cerebral palsy. *Dev Med Child Neurol* 1990;32:333–340.

91. Rose J, Gamble JG, Lee J, Lee R, Haskell WL. The energy expen-diture index: A method to quantitate and compare walking en-ergy expenditure for children and adolescents. *J Pediatr Orthop* 1991;11:571–578.

92. Rose J, Gamble JG, Medeiros JM, Burgos SA, Haskell WL. En-ergy cost of walking in normal children and in those with cerebral palsy. Comparison of heart rate and oxygen uptake. *J Pediatr Orthop* 1989;9:276–279.

93. Ross J, Schell M. Thermodynamic efficiency in nonlinear biochem-ical reactions. 1987;16:401–421.

94. Rush PJ, Pierson WR. The relationship of body surface area, mass and indices of energy expenditure. *Rev Can Biol* 1962;21:1–6.

95. Saltin B, Bloomquist G, Mitchell JH, Johnson Jr RL, Wildenthakk, Chapman CB. Response to submaximal and maximal exercise after bed rest and training [abstract]. *Circulation* 1968;38(suppl 7).

96. Shields ST. The effect of varying lengths of stride on performance during submaximal treadmill stress testing. *J Sports Med* 1982;22:66–72.

97. Silverman L, Lee G, Plotkin T, Sawyers LA, Yancey AR. Air flow measurements on human subjects with and without respiratory resistance at several work rates. *Arch Industr Hyg Occup Med* 1951; 3:461.

98. Skinner JS, Bar-Or O, Bergesteinova V, et al. Comparison of continuous and intermittent tests for determining maximal oxygen intake in children. *Acta Paediatr Scand* 1971;217(suppl):24–28.

99. Snellen JW. External work in level and grade walking on a motor-driven treadmill. *J Appl Physiol* 1960;15:759.

100. Soule RG, Goldman RF. Energy cost of loads carried on the head, hands or feet. *J Appl Physiol* 1969;27:687–690.

101. Spanner DC. *Introduction to Thermodynamics*. New York: Academic; 1965.

102. Strydom NB, Bredell GAG, Genade AJS, Morrison JG, Viljoen JH, van Graan CH. The metabolic cost of marching at 3 m.p.h. over firm and sandy surfaces. *Int Z Angew Physiol* 1966;23:166–171.

103. Turrell DJ, Austin RC, Alexander JK. Cardiorespiratory responses of very obese subjects to treadmill exercise. *J Lab Clin Med* 1964;64:107–116.

104. Unnithan BB, Dowling JJ, Frost G, Bar-Or O. Role of cocontraction in the O_2 cost of walking in children with cerebral palsy. *Med Sci Sports Exerc* 1996;28:1498–1504.

105. Van Der Walt WH, Wyndham CH. An equation for prediction of energy expenditure of walking and running. *J Appl Physiol* 1973; 34:559–563.

106. Volpe AB, Bar-Or O. Energy cost of walking in boys who differ in adiposity but are matched for body mass. *Med Sci Sports Exerc* 2003; 35:669–674.

107. Walker JL, Murray TD, Jackson AS, Morrow JR, Michaud TJ. The energy cost of horizontal walking and running in adolescents. *Med Sci Sports Exerc* 1999;31:311–322.

108. Waters RL, Hislop HJ, Perry J, Thomas L, Campbell J. Comparative cost of walking in young and old adults. *J Orthop Res* 1983;1: 73–76.

109. Waters RL, Hislop HJ, Thomas L, Campbell J. Energy cost of walking in normal children and teenagers. *Dev Med Child Neurol* 1983;25:184–188.

110. Waters RL, Lunsford BR. Energy expenditure of normal and pathological gait: application to orthotic prescription. In: *Atlas of Orthotics*. St Louis: C.V. Mosby Co; 1985.

111. Waters RL, Mulroy S. The energy expenditure of normal and pathologic gait. *Gait and Posture* 1999;9:207–231.

112. Wassermann K, Hansen JE, Sue DY, Whipp BJ. *Principles of Exercise Testing and Interpretation*. Philadelphia: Lea and Febiger; 1986:4–5.

113. Weir JB de V. New methods for calculating metabolic rate with special reference to protein metabolism. *J Physiol (Lond.)* 1949;109:1.

114. Welsman JR, Armstrong N, Nevill AM, Winter EM, Kirby BJ. Scaling peak VO_2 for differences in body size. *Med Sci Sports Exerc* 1996;28:259–265.

115. Wilkie DR. Man as a source of mechanical power. *Ergonomics* 1960;3:1.

116. Wilkie DR. The efficiency of muscular contraction. *J Mechanochem Cell Motil* 1974;2:257–267.

117. Winter DA. Analysis of instantaneous energy *of* normal gait. *J Biomech* 1976;9:253–257.

118. Winter DA. A new definition of mechanical work done in human movement. *J Appl Physiol* 1979;46:79–83.

119. Workman J, Armstrong BW. Metabolic cost of walking: Equation and model. *J Appl Physiol* 1986;61:1369–1374.

120. Wyndham CH, vander Walt WH, van Rensburg AJ, Rogers GG, Strydom NB. The influence of body weight on energy expenditure during walking on a road and on a treadmill. *Int Z Angew Physiol* 1971;29:285–292.

121. Zarrugh MY, Todd FN, Ralston HJ. Optimization of energy expenditure during level walking. *Eur J Appl Physiol* 1974;33:293–306.

Chapter 6

Muscle Activity During Walking

Jennette L. Boakes and George T. Rab

Muscles provide the power for human locomotion. Their anatomic, molecular, and chemical structures provide a biologically efficient source of power that is controlled by an equally exquisite organization of central and peripheral nerves with diverse sensors and feedback loops. Muscles and motor control are easy to take for granted since the system works so effortlessly. Advances in the fields of molecular biology, ultrastructural anatomy, histology, and physiology in recent decades have allowed a much better understanding of this complex neuromuscular system. Muscles produce active movement by conversion of metabolic energy into muscle fiber contraction, using both oxidative and glycolytic metabolism. In the human, muscle structure varies with the functional demand: smooth muscle produces peristaltic contraction in the bowel and sets vascular tone; cardiac muscle powers the contraction of the heart; and skeletal muscle produces motion of the joints. Skeletal muscle will be considered in detail here.

MUSCLE STRUCTURE

The skeletal muscle system is the largest single organ of the body. It can be subdivided into muscle groups, which all perform similar actions, such as knee flexors or knee extensors. Muscle groups are further subdivided into specific muscles. Each muscle is composed of individual cells, called muscle fibers, which are grouped together into muscle fascicles. Each fascicle has its own blood supply and its own fibrous sheath called the perimysium (Fig. 6-1), and the entire muscle is covered by the epimysium (23).

Skeletal muscle cells are roughly cylindrical with a diameter of 10–100 μm and are up to 20 cm long. The muscle cells contain elements common to every cell in the body, such as a cell membrane, mitochondria for oxidative metabolism, and all of the machinery necessary for protein synthesis and cell replication. Muscle cells are multinucleated and densely packed with contractile proteins and energy stores. A complex network of supporting cells and proteins, which are responsible for the growth and repair

of the muscle fiber, surrounds each cell. A closer look at the muscle fiber reveals that it is elegantly designed to generate force beginning at the molecular level with a series of chemical reactions.

Although the gross appearance of individual muscles varies widely, all skeletal muscles have a common microstructure composed of similar macromolecules. Viewed through a light microscope (Fig. 6-2), skeletal muscle has a regular pattern of lines or striations clearly visible (thus the term striated muscle). These striations correspond to the basic functional unit of all skeletal muscle, the sarcomere, which contains the contractile proteins actin and myosin (Figs. 6-1, D–E). Sarcomeres join in a longitudinal series to form myofibrils of 1 to 2 μm in diameter. At each end of the sarcomere is the Z disk, from which emanates a group of parallel thin proteins called actin; the free ends of the actin face the center of the sarcomere. Here, a second disk (which corresponds to the M line) anchors parallel thick myosin molecules that interdigitate with the actin groups (Fig. 6-3) (17,23,27). Myosin has globular projections that can cross link with the actin molecule; once this link has been formed, the globular chains undergo stearic alteration and bend toward the M line, pulling the actin strands closer to the center of the sarcomere (14,15). The process repeats as the cross-link is broken, the globular chain straightens, and a new cross-link is formed. Thus, the two Z disks are pulled closer together by the bending of multiple projections of the myosin, a process that has been compared with the movement of oars. The distance between the Z disks is defined as the sarcomere length.

EXCITATION-CONTRACTION COUPLE

A group of reservoir-like membranes, the sarcoplasmic reticulum, and an excitable membrane, the sarcolemma, surround the sarcomere. The sarcolemma extends into the sarcomere with transverse extensions called T-tubules. These membranes convert the electrical signals from the

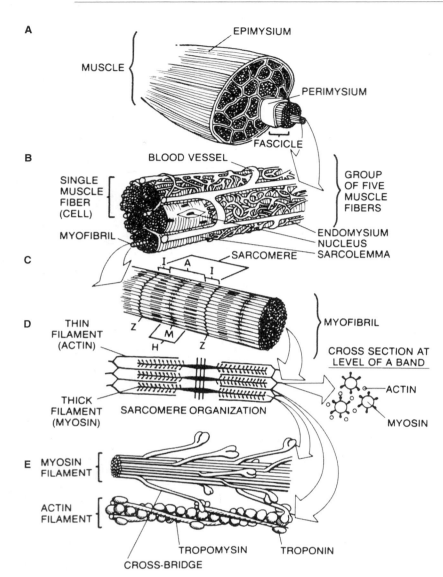

FIGURE 6-1. Basic structural organization of muscle tissue from macroscopic to molecular. **A:** muscle; **(B)** muscle fiber; **(C)** myofibril; **(D)** sarcomere; **(E)** molecular level. (From Nordin M, Frankel VH. *Basic Biomechanics of the Musculoskeletal System,* 2nd ed. Philadelphia: Lea & Febiger; 1989.)

nervous system into a mechanical contraction of muscle to generate force. This process is termed the excitation-contraction couple. In order for effective force production to occur, contraction must be excited along the entire length of the fiber simultaneously. Motor nerve axons from the brainstem or the spinal cord branch distally and form motor end plates, which allow electrochemical transmission between the nerve ending and muscle fibers (Figs. 6-2 and 6-4). The motor end plate contains microscopic vesicles at the axon terminal that release the neurotransmitter acetylcholine. Acetylcholine diffuses and binds with a receptor site on the muscle and initiates the action potential in the sarcolemma. The signal is spread rapidly through the sarcolemma by electrical depolarization. This signals the rapid release of calcium ions from the sarcoplasmic reticulum. The change in intracellular calcium concentration causes the molecular interaction of actin and myosin described above. The contraction subsides as a calcium pump, powered by ATP, returns calcium to the sarcoplasmic reticulum.

MOTOR UNIT

The motor unit is the functional and anatomic grouping of all the muscle fibers connected to a single motor axon. It represents the smallest number of fibers that can contract in a muscle. Each individual axon can supply 3 to 200 muscle fibers, depending on the physiologic function of the muscle. The number of muscle fibers per motor unit is low in the extraocular muscles, where fine control is necessary; it is high in leg muscles, where power is more important. All fibers of a motor unit must necessarily contract together. The fibers, however, tend to be distributed throughout a fascicle, so they may not physically touch, although they are neurologically connected. Motor unit

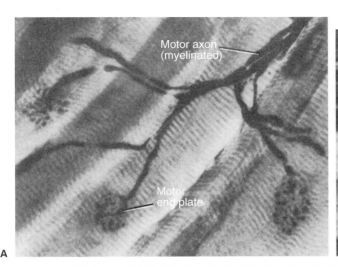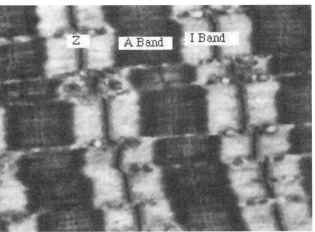

FIGURE 6-2. (**A**) Skeletal muscle showing striations and the motor axon with associated end plates. (From Cormack DH, ed. *Ham's Histology*, 9th ed. Philadelphia: JB Lippincott, 1987:398). (**B**) A myofilament shows several distinct bands, each of which has been given a special letter. The lightest (least electron dense) band is known as the I band and consists mostly of actin. The wide, dark band, known as the A band, is composed primarily of myosin. In the center of the I band is the Z-line. In the middle of the A band is another dense line known as the M line. (Courtesy of R. Lieber.)

contraction is initiated by an action potential in the motor axon. When a single action potential reaches a muscle fiber, there is a brief latent period followed by a contraction of that fiber. As the brain's signal for contraction increases, it recruits more motor units and increases the 'firing frequency' of the units already recruited. The duration of contraction and the tension generated is precisely controlled by varying the number of motor units that are recruited simultaneously.

Types of Muscle Fibers—Physiologic and Histologic Properties

Four motor unit types have been described based on the contractile properties of the motor units such as force, velocity, and fatigability (5). Some muscle fibers have a slow twitch (60–120 msec) and generate a relatively low peak tension. Slow-twitch fibers (often called type I) have many capillaries and contain large quantities of myoglobin and mitochondria; they are fatigue resistant and rely on aerobic (oxidative) metabolism. Other muscle fibers have a fast twitch (10–50 msec) and generate a relatively high peak tension. Some fast-twitch fibers have few mitochondria and are unable to maintain high tensions for more than a few contractions without rest; they rely on anaerobic (glycolytic) metabolism and are called type IIB, fast fatigable (FF) or fast glycolytic (FG) fibers. Some of the fibers with faster contraction times are able to maintain force production even after a large number of contractions. They tend to have both oxidative and glycolytic enzymes and thus are called fast oxidative-glycolytic (FOG) fibers or type IIA. Because they differ in metabolic enzymes, slow-twitch and fast-twitch fibers can be distinguished from each other by various histochemical staining for ATPase and other enzymatic activity (8) (Fig. 6-5). The characteristics of muscle fiber types are summarized in Table 6-1.

All fibers in a single motor unit are of the same fiber type. The recruitment of motor units is determined by the movement required. Most human muscles contain all fiber types in varying proportions. Because slow-twitch (type I) fibers are fatigue resistant, they are likely recruited when skeletal muscles are performing activities where great strength is not a requirement but activity for several hours is. Fast-twitch (type II) fibers generate high forces, and more of these are recruited when muscles are used for short bursts of great strength.

Skeletal muscle is one of the most adaptable tissues in the body. With training, muscle fibers will increase in size and strength or increase their oxidative capacity or both depending on the type of training. Chronic electrical stimulation provides one of the purest experimental models of

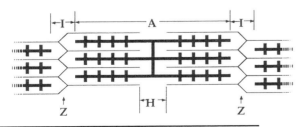

FIGURE 6-3. Diagrammatic structure of sarcomere.

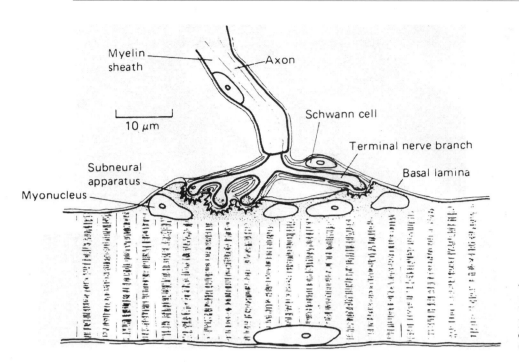

FIGURE 6-4. Line drawing of ultrastructure of a motor end plate. (From Walton J. *Disorders of Voluntary Muscle*. Edinburgh: Churchill Livingstone; 1988:6.)

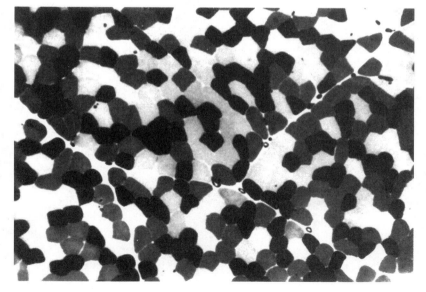

FIGURE 6-5. Variation in fiber types in normal human muscle is demonstrated in this cross section stained for ATPase activity (pH 4.6). Slow-twitch fibers stain darker, and fast-twitch stain lighter (×64). (From Filipe MI, Lake BD. *Histochemistry in Pathology*. London: Churchill Livingstone; 1983:93.)

▶ **TABLE 6-1 Characteristics of Muscle Fiber Types**

Type	Fiber Color	Diameter	Speed of Contraction	Fatigue Resistance	Myosin ATPase Activity	Vascularity	Metabolism
I	Red	Small	Slow	More	Lower	Higher	Oxidative
IIA	White	Medium	Fast	Less	Higher	Lower	Oxidative glycolytic
IIB	White	Large	Fast	Less	Higher	Lower	Glycolytic

muscle adaptation to 'controlled exercise.' When chronic, low-frequency stimulation similar to the activity of a 'slow' muscle is imposed on a predominantly 'fast' muscle, the muscle fibers undergo a predictable progression of transforming their metabolic and contractile properties into a 'slow' muscle (19). Conversely, the absence of normal electrical innervation, as in spinal cord injury, induces a transformation from slow-twitch to fast-twitch fiber type (18). However, in humans exercise alone without a change in the neural input does not produce fiber type transformation (1); rather, the proportion of each fiber type recruited changes depending on the type of training.

Motor Control

A complex system of motor control allows voluntary and involuntary muscle activity. Motor signals originate in the cortex of the brain and pass through deeper cerebral centers and the spinal cord before they reach muscle. Specialized sensor cells continuously feed information about joint and muscle position and movement back to the brain and spinal cord, where the motor signal can be modified to produce smooth, coordinated muscle contractions necessary for complex movement.

Even the simplest voluntary movement of muscle is the result of exceptionally complex central nervous system activity. Cell networks in the cerebral cortex first conceive of the movement and communicate with cells in the motor cortex. There, under monitoring and direction of other cortical and subcortical cell groups, an electrochemical membrane potential is generated; this action potential travels in the motor neuron axon through the brainstem and spinal cord along the pyramidal tracts to synapse with a second motor cell (the anterior horn cell) in the spinal cord. Action potentials from the anterior horn cell travel through axons in the peripheral nerve (α-motor neuron) to the motor end plate, and stimulate muscle contraction as described above. At each level, feedback and modification (both inhibitive and facilitative) of the cells can occur. Many extra neural cells (interneurons) are involved in the process and assist in integrating and coordinating complex movement (27).

Variations in muscle contraction depend on feedback from specialized sensory receptors within the muscle. A single action potential in an α-motoneuron results in a twitch of the muscle fibers in the motor unit. Skeletal muscle contraction is maintained by asynchronous activity of many α-motoneurons that make up the motoneuron pool innervating each muscle. Increasing the force of muscle contraction is achieved by increasing the firing rate of α-motoneurons and by recruitment (activation of more and larger diameter motor units). A given amount of motoneuron activity produces a given level of tension; however, a given tension results in different degrees of contraction depending on the load on the muscle. Feedback is needed to assure that the intended contraction occurs. This feedback is provided by highly specialized neural and muscle fibers that provide information about muscle and tendon length, tension, and contraction velocity to the central nervous system.

The muscle spindle and Golgi tendon organ are two receptors particularly important to motor control. Muscle spindles are located throughout the muscle belly and lie parallel to the skeletal muscle fibers; they provide feedback regulation of muscle length and static stretch. The Golgi tendon organs are connected in series with the tendon at the musculotendinous junction and are sensitive to dynamic changes in length of the muscle (by responding to active tension of contraction). These sensors combine with joint position receptors as a "feedback loop" in a complex system of motor control that results in the normal motion of walking.

A simple schematic diagram of motor control (typical of many theoretical models) is shown in Figure 6-6.

WHOLE MUSCLE STRUCTURE

Not only is skeletal muscle highly organized microscopically, it is also highly organized at the macroscopic level. Muscle architecture refers to the arrangement of muscle fascicles relative to the line of force generation. Muscles with fibers oriented parallel to the line of force have *parallel* architecture with muscle length roughly equal to fiber length. Muscles with fibers that are oriented at a single angle relative to the line of force are called *unipennate*. Most muscles, however, are *multipennate* with muscle fibers oriented at differing angles relative to the line of force generation (Fig. 6-7). Muscle fibers of parallel architecture can be much longer than pennate muscle fibers. Longer

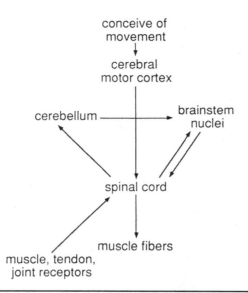

FIGURE 6-6. Simplified diagram of basic functional neural relationships and feedback activities of motor control.

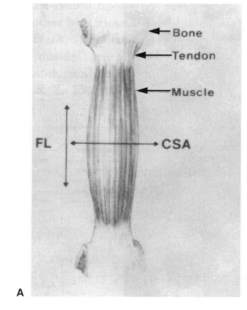

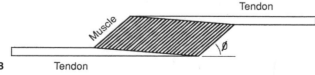

FIGURE 6-7. Gross appearance of two different muscles demonstrates variation associated with differing functions. A strap muscle (**A**) provides high contractile velocity, whereas bipennate (**B**) muscles generate increased force at the expense of shortening velocity. FL, average fiber length; CSA, average fiber cross-sectional area. (From Lieber RL. Skeletal muscle adaptability. I. Review of basic properties. *Dev Med Child Neurol* 1986;28:390–397.)

fibers allow greater excursion and can contract much faster. A pennate architecture allows more fascicles to be packed next to each other in a small space compared with a parallel architecture, increasing the physiological cross-sectional area (PCSA) of the muscle. PCSA is the sum of the cross-sectional areas of all the muscle fibers within the muscle and is directly proportional to the amount of force a muscle can generate. Greater pennation allows a muscle to generate more force at the expense of decreasing overall excursion. Older anatomy books almost made a "science" of the different shapes of individual muscles, but neither fiber length nor PCSA can be easily determined by the gross appearance of the muscle (12).

Mechanical Properties of Muscle

The mechanical behavior of muscle has been studied at the whole muscle, isolated muscle fiber, and myofibril levels (4,10,12,17,27). The relationships among the muscle length and generated tension, the speed of contraction, and the balance between elastic and contractile structures at each level influence muscle biomechanics during human motion. If the muscle shortens while it is contracting, it is termed a concentric contraction; eccentric contraction occurs when muscle is lengthening while contracting. When muscle generates tension but neither shortens, nor lengthens, and no movement occurs, it is termed an isometric contraction.

Length and Tension Relationships

An intact mammalian muscle contains contractile elements (sarcomeres) and elastic components (fascia and tendons), both of which affect tension in the muscle. Gordon, Huxley, and Julian (10) defined the sarcomere length-tension relationship that forms the basis for understanding muscle force generation (Fig. 6-8). Muscle force varies as a function of initial sarcomere length, based upon the amount of myofilament overlap. On the ascending limb of the length-tension curve, actin filaments from opposite sides of the sarcomere touch or overlap (Fig. 6-8A). The overlap interferes with the formation of cross-bridges with myosin, so that force generation is impaired. As sarcomere length increases, so does force generation, until a plateau is reached (Fig. 6-8B). The plateau occurs because the myosin molecule contains a "bare region" where no further cross-bridges with actin can form. Therefore, changes in sarcomere length do not increase force production on the plateau. The plateau region is considered the "optimal sarcomere length" for force generation. Increasing sarcomere length beyond the optimal length results in less myofilament overlap and forces production decreases (Fig. 6-8C).

The behavior of whole muscle can be predicted based on knowledge of the microscopic mechanics. Figure 6-9 models a whole muscle exhibiting maximal isometric

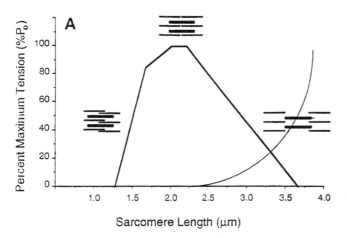

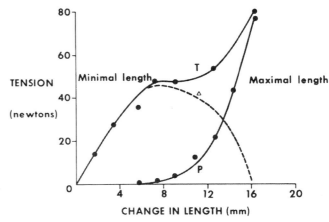

FIGURE 6-8. The sarcomere length-tension curve for isolated frog skeletal muscle fibers. Thick line represents muscle maximum tetanic tension and schematic sarcomeres represent the relative overlap of actin and myosin filaments in the various portions of the length-tension curve: (**A**) ascending limb, (**B**) plateau, (**C**) descending limb. Thin line represents muscle passive tension. (Modified from Gordon AM, Huxley AF, Julian FJ. The variation in isometric tension with sarcomere length in vertebrate muscle fibers. *J Physiol* 1966;184:170–192.)

FIGURE 6-10. Measured isometric length-tension relationship in forearm flexor muscles of an amputee. Note similarity to theoretical curve. T, total tension curve; P, passive tension curve; Δ, contribution of contractile elements. See text. (From Ralston et al., *Am J Physiol* 1947;151:612.)

contraction. (It is generating tension without a change in total muscle length.) The force developed by the muscle during isometric contraction varies with its starting length. Note that there is an optimal length (L_o) at which a muscle can generate maximal active contraction. Below L_o, the elastic components of muscle are slack, but as the muscle elongates passively there is a nonlinear increase in passive elastic tension. The sum of these active and passive tensile components is the overall length-tension relationship.

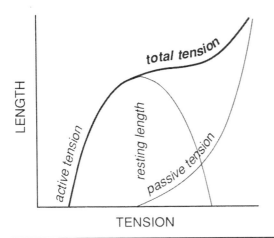

FIGURE 6-9. Theoretical isometric length-tension relationship of a whole muscle. Active tension (from contraction) and passive tension (from viscoelastic structures) combine to give total tension (*heavy line*). At the optimal resting length of muscle, the passive viscoelastic tension drops to zero.

Experimental laboratory measurements correspond closely to the theoretical model. Figure 6-10 shows actual length-tension relationships in an amputee who had a skin tunnel created through the flexor muscles of the forearm. The active component of the contractile element (Δ) is derived by subtracting the passive tension curve from the total tension curve.

In most muscles used in walking, there is an optimal length corresponding to a position where that muscle must act with strength and efficiency. When posture deviation changes that length, the ability of the muscle to generate tension drops (Fig. 6-11), offering a practical illustration of the active length-tension relationship of muscle. Thus, mechanical behavior of the intact whole muscle is a direct result of its microstructure.

Speed of Muscle Contraction

While the isometric length-tension relationship has an anatomic basis, the force-velocity relationship does not. Muscles produce motion by concentric or eccentric contractions. The velocity of muscle contraction is dependent on the force resisting the muscle. When a muscle is activated to lift a load less than its maximum, the muscle begins to shorten. A lighter load can be lifted more quickly than a heavy load. As the load on the muscle increases beyond its maximum, the muscle can no longer shorten to lift the load and begins to elongate while still maximally contracting—an eccentric contraction. The absolute tension generated in the muscle during an eccentric contraction is very high in part because the elastic components in addition to the contractile components in muscle act to resist lengthening. It is important to understand the concept of eccentric contraction, because much of the muscle activity during gait occurs while it is actively lengthening.

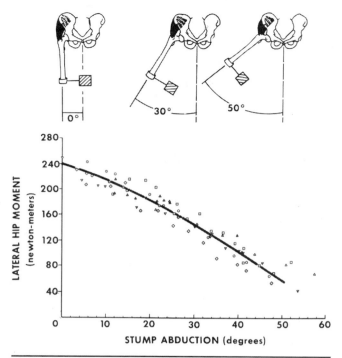

FIGURE 6-11. Hip moment vs. hip abduction plotted for maximal strength of hip abduction in three above-knee amputees. Note rapid decrease hip moment caused by muscle shortening with progressive abduction.

BIOMECHANICS OF MUSCLE

Most muscles originate proximally in a broad attachment to either periosteum (the membrane on the surface of bone) or fascial sheets. Insertions at the distal end are thinner tendinous attachments to bone. By convention, we usually think of the origin as immobile and the insertion as moving. In the case of the brachialis muscle powering elbow flexion, this may be accurate; in other cases, such as the gastrocnemius and soleus group raising a subject on tiptoe, neither end of the muscle is truly immobile.

Muscles produce movement of a joint by generating linear force at a distance from the center of the joint. This is known as a torque or moment. The moment is calculated as the product of force and the distance from the muscle insertion to the center of joint movement. The farther the tendon of a muscle lies from the joint center, the greater the moment will be (23). The ability of a muscle to produce torque results from the interaction of muscle properties and joint biomechanics (13,20,21). As a joint moves, the muscles crossing the joint change in length; this alters their ability to generate tension at each given joint angle. The effective lever arm of the muscle also changes (Fig. 6-12). In some joints, such as the knee, the center of rotation moves as the knee joint rotates; this characteristic contributes further to the variation in muscle moment during motion.

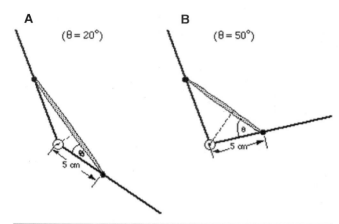

FIGURE 6-12. Schematic example of moment arm change with joint angle. At small joint angles, the moment arm (*dotted line*) is relatively small. At larger joint angles, moment arm increases considerably. (From Lieber RL. *Skeletal Muscle Structure and Function*. Williams & Wilkins, 1992:122.)

Muscles do not generate maximum forces throughout the entire range of motion and may not even generate maximum force in the midrange of muscle motion. Studies of torque production in animals and humans have shown that the joint angle where the muscle generates maximal force is not the same angle where the moment arm is maximum (13,20,21). In fact, in many cases, muscle force is maximized at the extreme end of the range of motion.

Thus, during normal joint rotation, both moment arm and muscle force are constantly changing. The degree of joint motion depends on both the excursion of the muscle and the distance of its lever arm from the joint center. The excursion a muscle allows is proportional to its fiber length. If two muscles have the same fiber length, the one with the smaller lever arm will cause the joint to move through a greater arc but will require more force to do so.

Muscles that span two joints (such as the hamstrings) have a more complex mechanical role since the lever arms may continually vary (in different ways) at each end of the muscle as it acts on two separate joints. Also, changes in the lever arm at one end of a two joint muscle can change its length, thus affecting length-tension properties at the other end. Two joint muscles often allow transfer of energy between joints, and they are important to human walking.

An important concept in biomechanics of muscle is work. Positive work is performed when a muscle is concentrically contracting—the biceps brachii performs positive work when a weight is lifted while the elbow is flexing. Negative work is performed when a muscle is eccentrically contracting; an example of this would be the activity of the hamstrings as they contract at the end of swing phase to decelerate the leg before foot strike. These definitions of work come from mechanics, where they are analogous to what one would expect from a spring acting on a weight (28). Note that these are not metabolic terms; contracting muscles consume energy whether they are producing

▶ **TABLE 6-2 Muscle Actions during Gait Cycle**[a]

Phase of Gait	Mechanical Goals	Active Muscle Groups	Examples
Stance phase			
Initial contact	Position foot, begin deceleration	Ankle dorsiflexors, hip extensors, knee flexors	Anterior tibialis, gluteus maximus, hamstrings
Loading response	Accept weight, stabilize pelvis, decelerate mass	Knee extensors, hip abductors, ankle plantarflexors	Vasti, gluteus medius, gastrocnemius
Midstance	Stabilize knee, preserve momentum	Ankle plantarflexors (isometric)	Gastrocnemius, soleus
Terminal stance	Accelerate mass	Ankle plantarflexors (concentric)	Gastrocnemius, soleus
Preswing	Prepare for swing	Hip flexors	Iliopsoas, rectus femoris
Swing phase			
Initial swing	Clear foot, vary cadence	Ankle dorsiflexors, hip flexors	Anterior tibialis, iliopsoas, rectus femoris
Mid swing	Clear foot	Ankle dorsiflexors	Anterior tibialis
Terminal swing	Decelerate shank, decelerate leg, position foot, prepare for contact	Knee flexors, hip extensors, ankle dorsiflexors, knee extensors	Hamstrings, gluteus maximus, anterior tibialis, vasti

[a]Modified and derived from Ref. 11.

positive or negative work. However, electromyographic (EMG) activity is less in eccentric contraction than in concentric contraction and requires less motor unit activity.

Normal human walking is an energy-efficient activity, and it is not surprising that much of the muscle activity during walking is isometric or eccentric. This negative work allows the limbs to absorb energy while resisting the pull of gravity, yet remains metabolically efficient. Positive work of muscles during walking allows acceleration of limbs and powers such activities as push-off and extension of the hip after foot strike. Negative work holds us upright, and positive work moves us forward!

PHASIC ACTION OF MUSCLES IN HUMAN WALKING

Many muscles are active primarily in stance phase or primarily in swing phase. This phasic contraction defines the role of that muscle in producing normal walking activity. Contraction that is prolonged or out of phase during walking may characterize abnormalities of motor control, such as stroke or cerebral palsy. Out of phase muscle contractions can cause abnormal movements, or they can occur while antagonist muscles are trying to produce normal walking patterns, leading to co-contraction. This obviously affects both the mechanical and metabolic efficiency of walking.

In normal walking, muscles contract and relax in a precise, orchestrated fashion. EMG studies of muscles have been coupled with accurate three-dimensional measurement of gait movements to clarify the sequence of muscle recruitment necessary for walking to occur (9,26). Level walking at a comfortable pace is a natural place to study phasic activity of muscle groups (Table 6-2). As the walking cycle progresses, muscle action becomes primarily isometric or eccentric, which is a more energy efficient

form of contraction. Most muscles responsible for these contractions have a high proportion of fatigue-resistant type I fibers. Shortening contractions, which use more energy, are used only in brief bursts in normal walking.

At initial foot contact (Fig. 6-13), the limb begins to decelerate the body as it reaches the floor. This is

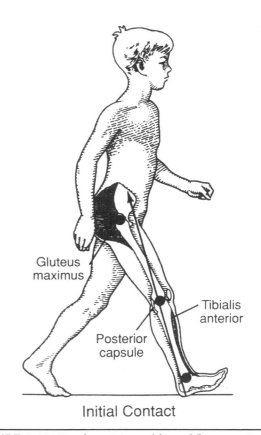

Gluteus maximus

Tibialis anterior

Posterior capsule

Initial Contact

FIGURE 6-13. Muscle activity and line of floor reaction force at initial foot contact. (From Gage JR. An overview of normal walking. *Instr Course Lect* 1990;39:294.)

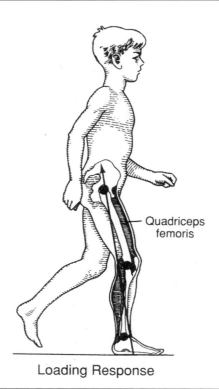

Loading Response

FIGURE 6-14. Muscle activity and line of floor reaction force during loading response. (From Gage JR. An overview of normal walking. *Instr Course Lect* 1990;39:297.)

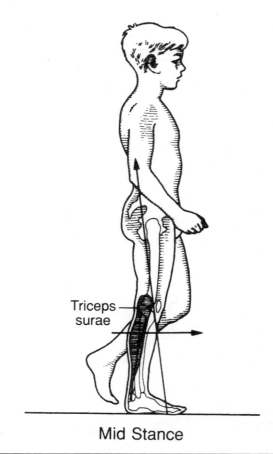

Mid Stance

FIGURE 6-15. Muscle activity and line of floor reaction force at midstance. (From Gage JR. An overview of normal walking. *Instr Course Lect* 1990;39:294–297.)

accomplished by simultaneous activity of the knee extensor and flexor muscles to stabilize and position the knee in space. Hip extensor contraction decelerates the thigh and aids in knee extension and foot placement. At the same time, the anterior tibialis begins a lengthening contraction to gradually "ease down" the foot and keep it from slapping down on the floor.

Now the limb begins its loading response (Fig. 6-14) in which it accepts the weight of the body by contracting the knee extensors (vasti). The knee bends slightly and begins extending under the shortening contraction of the knee extensors, acting much like a spring. This knee extension is aided by plantarflexion of the ankle (eccentric contraction), which tends to move the contact point of the limb forward and shift the reaction force of the body anteriorly at the knee, inducing it to straighten. The gluteus medius contracts isometrically and stabilizes the pelvis in the frontal plane.

At midstance (Fig. 6-15), the center of gravity of the body has reached its highest point and is carried forward by momentum. As long as the knee remains extended, this can be accomplished with very little energy by keeping the foot on the floor and allowing the body mass to "fall forward" in the line of walking progression. Lengthening contraction of the soleus muscle keeps the forefoot pressed against the floor, creating a force couple or linkage that

allows the knee to remain extended without the need for muscle action of the quadriceps.

At terminal stance (Fig. 6-16), the knee extension-ankle plantarflexion force couple continues to keep the knee passively extended, but now the ankle plantar flexors begin a shortening contraction that accelerates the body forward. This burst of energy is responsible for most power generation that keeps the body moving forward in normal gait (29). There may be a small burst of iliopsoas activity to lead into the unloading response of preswing.

Preswing (Fig. 6-17) begins after the opposite limb has reached the floor and begins to accept weight. In this phase, ankle plantar flexors are no longer active, and the hip flexors (iliopsoas and rectus femoris) begin to lift the limb and swing it forward, generally by concentric contraction. Since the limb behaves like a passive pendulum for much of the swing phase, the energy consumed in preswing muscle activity is efficiently brief, setting the stage for the largely passive events of the following cycle of gait.

Initial swing sees the end of iliopsoas and rectus femoris activity. The exact duration of swing and length of stride

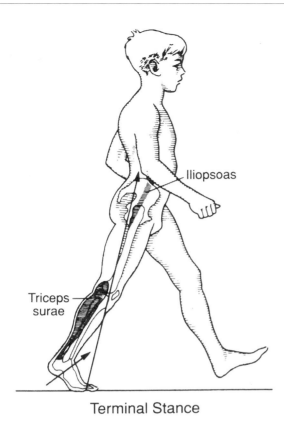

Terminal Stance

FIGURE 6-16. Muscle activity and line of floor reaction force at terminal response stance. (From Gage JR. An overview of normal walking. *Instr Course Lect* 1990;39:297–298.)

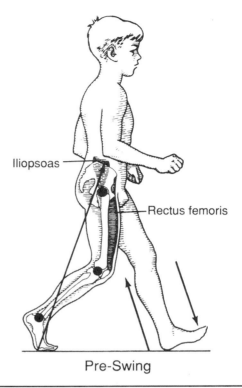

Pre-Swing

FIGURE 6-17. Muscle activity and line of floor reaction force at preswing. (From Gage JR. An overview of normal walking. *Instr Course Lect* 1990;39:297–299.)

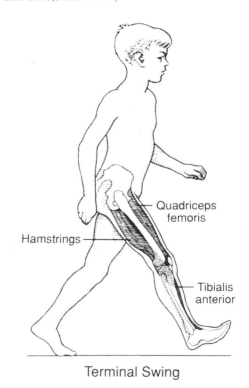

Terminal Swing

FIGURE 6-18. Muscle activity and line of floor reaction force during terminal swing. (From Gage JR. An overview of normal walking. *Instr Course Lect* 1990;39:300.)

depend on the length of the freely swinging leg (pendulum) and the dynamic friction of the knee joint and its associated tissues (thigh muscles, etc.). Prolongation of swing phase activity of the hip or knee flexors, or premature contraction of the hamstrings, can change the geometry of the freely swinging leg. For level walking, each person tends to self-select the optimum speed for individual leg length and energy efficiency. At the ankle (which was plantarflexed at preswing), the ankle dorsiflexors begin a shortening contraction to allow the foot to clear the floor.

Midswing sees continuation of the passive pendulum action of the leg. Foot clearance is continued by activity of the anterior tibialis muscle.

At terminal swing (Fig. 6-18), the limb begins active deceleration by contracting the hamstrings eccentrically or isometrically. This efficiently slows both hip flexion and knee extension. The knee prepares to accept weight by early quadriceps activity. The tibialis anterior continues its activity but switches to an isometric or elongating contraction as it gently "floats" the foot over the floor immediately before foot contact. As the foot touches the floor, the cycle repeats itself.

During level human walking, muscle contraction is controlled to produce maximum energy efficiency with appropriate forward movement. Many muscles responsible for walking contract isometrically, or while lengthening, to allow maintenance of upright posture against gravity or transfer and storage of energy between limb segments. Brief bursts of more energy-expensive shortening contraction of muscle are added when needed to provide power for forward motion.

Many investigators have studied the electrical activity responsible for phasic contraction of muscles. The actual length of phasic EMG activity of individual muscles will depend on walking speed, age, body size, and the many technical issues involved in EMG collection. For instance, cross talk surface electrodes but may be avoided with indwelling wire electrodes. The magnitude of EMG signals may not be directly proportional to the tension created in

a muscle that is changing length; thus, some investigators illustrate EMG activity as simple "on–off" diagrams (Fig. 6-19A). Others attempt to provide more information by normalization of the EMG linear envelope (24,29), usually to the standard of EMG activity during maximal isometric contraction (Fig. 6-19B). Much variability in reported data is caused by sensitivity of muscle phasic contractile patterns to walking velocity, but there is also evidence that normal physiologic walking strategies include some variation in muscle timing stride to stride (24). Depending on the presence or absence of neuromuscular disease, and on the specific muscle, EMG data from five to ten gait cycles may need to be averaged to obtain a representative sample (2). Examples of phasic EMG activity during walking reported by different laboratories are shown in Figure 6-19.

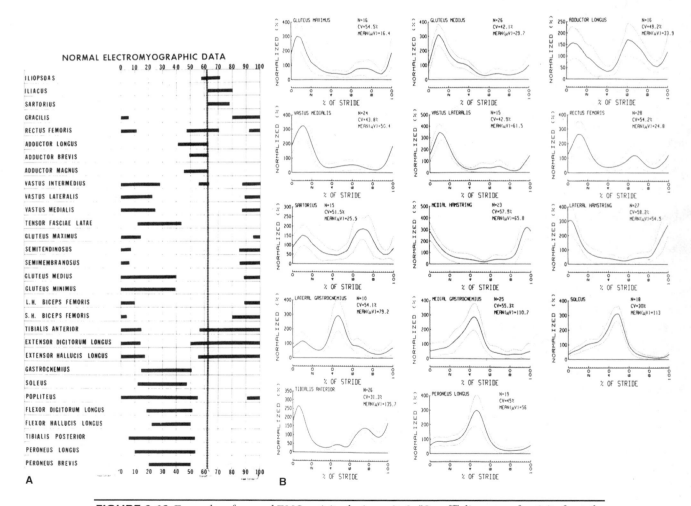

FIGURE 6-19. Examples of normal EMG activity during gait. **A:** "On-off" diagrams of activity from the University of California, San Francisco based on fine-wire EMG. (Modified from Ref. 22.) **B:** *Curves* are normalized EMG envelopes (data from University of Waterloo). (Modified from Ref. 25.) **C:** Timing of functional muscle activity with peak activity noted (data from Rancho Los Amigos Hospital.) (Modified from Ref. 24.) Differences between these types of data reflect the measure variability in phasic activity that has been observed during human walking (see text).

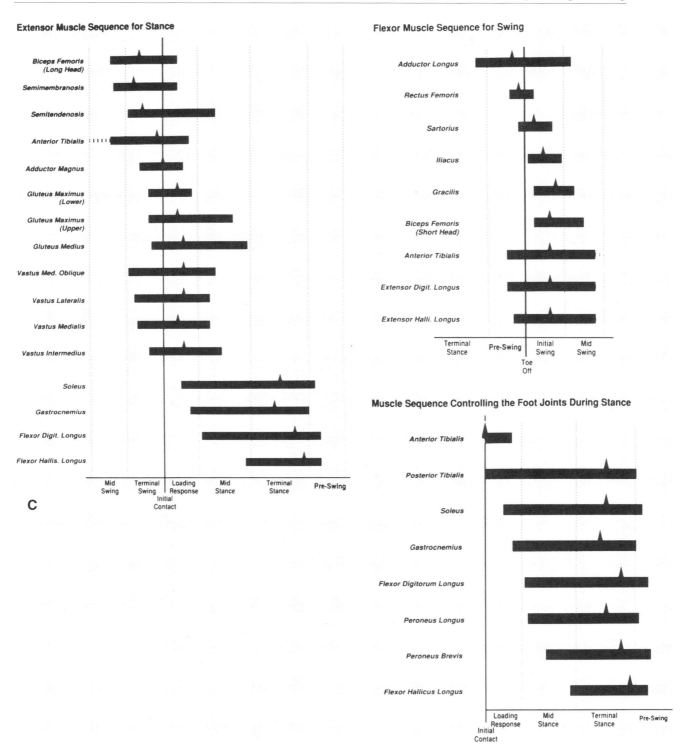

FIGURE 6-19. (*Continued*)

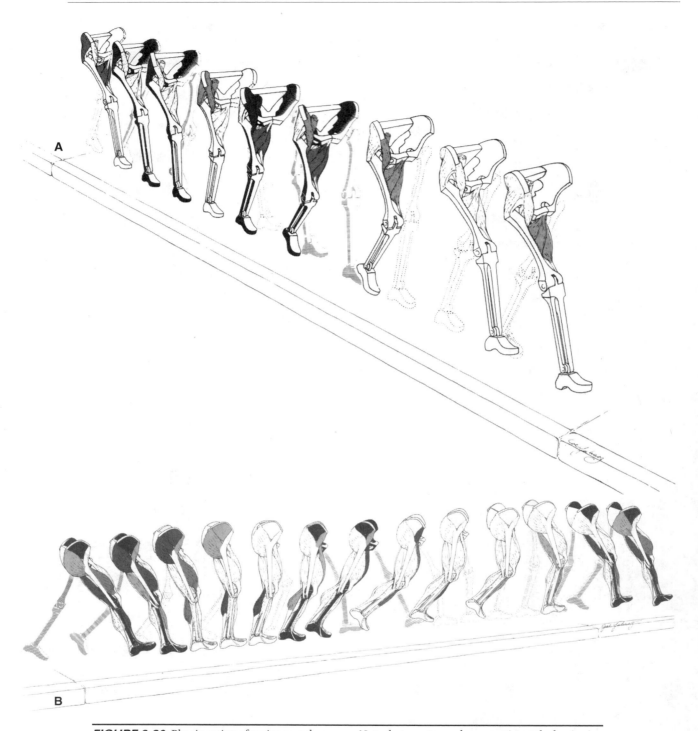

FIGURE 6-20. Phasic action of major muscle groups. Note that most muscles are active at the beginning and end of swing phase. During midstance, there is minimal muscle activity. This suggests that the main function of muscle is to accelerate and decelerate the limbs and that after weight acceptance, the metabolic demands of muscle decrease as momentum allows body weight to advance forward.

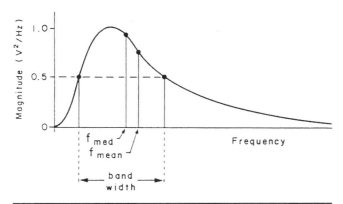

FIGURE 6-21. Frequency spectrum of an EMG signal. Median and mean frequencies and bandwidth are useful parameters for describing physiologic muscle function. (From Basmajian JV, DeLuca CJ. *Muscles Alive—Their Functions Revealed by Electromyography*, 5th ed. Baltimore: Williams & Wilkins; 1985:99.)

Estimates of phasic muscle activity and three-dimensional motion of the limbs have been pictorially combined to give an overall view of gait and muscle action (Figure 6-20).

EMG INTERPRETATION

EMG of active muscle can give information about muscle physiology and motor control beyond issues of timing during gait. Modern diagnostic EMG can identify neural injury or compression, denervated muscle, or primary pathologic processes. The EMG signal itself is a highly complex

wave form whose shape depends on the type and location of electrode, the number of motor unit action potentials detected, the spatial geometry of the motor unit itself, and filtering characteristics of muscle tissue. By processing the raw EMG signal electrically and mathematically, information about force generation, motor unit recruitment, and muscle fatigue may be extracted (3).

The EMG signal is the sum of signals from multiple motor unit action potential "trains" (MUAPT). Each MUAPT has a firing rate that depends on time and force generation. The frequency distribution of the MUAPT firing impulses can be described by the Fourier transform (frequency analysis) of the interpulse intervals. The total EMG signal, which is the sum of all MUAPTs, can similarly be analyzed by calculating the power density spectrum, which depends on force, time, and the individual firing rates of the MUAPTs (Fig. 6-21). From the power density spectrum, the mean frequency (average frequency) and median frequency (frequency that divides the spectrum into two regions of equal power) can be calculated.

As a muscle contracts continuously, it exhibits fatigue. Fatigue eventually leads to a loss in force, pain, tremor, and decline in work output (3). In addition, there are physiological and chemical changes in the muscle fiber itself, such as the increase in lactate concentration. These changes, known as "localized muscle fatigue," cause a decrease in the conduction velocity of the motor unit action potential and therefore a decrease in the frequency of the EMG signal (25). This shift of the mean or median frequency of the power spectrum means that more low frequency of the power spectrum is transmitted to the EMG signal, and this power is detected as increased EMG amplitude since the muscle tissue acts as a low-pass filter (3). This increase in

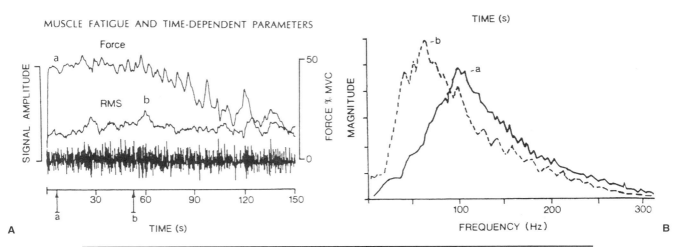

FIGURE 6-22. A: As a muscle exhibits isotonic contraction (force) over time, the EMG signal amplitude (RMS) increases; eventually (at time b) the muscle fatigues and cannot sustain force. **B:** Power spectrum of EMG undergoes a shift to lower frequency (from time a to time b) as muscle fatigue progresses and isotonic contraction is no longer possible. (From Basmajian JV, DeLuca CJ. *Muscles Alive—Their Functions Revealed by Electromyography*, 5th ed. Baltimore: Williams & Wilkins, 1985:205.)

EMG amplitude and decrease in the mean (or median) frequency can be seen during sustained muscle contraction as fatigue occurs (Fig. 6-22).

The ability to use EMG analysis to quantitate localized muscle fatigue has great importance for the study of exercise physiology, athletic training, ergonomics, physical therapy, and physical medicine (3). The noninvasive nature of this technique makes it particularly applicable to studies of muscle physiology in animals and humans.

REFERENCES

1. Always SE, MacDougall JD, Sale DG, Sutton JR, McComas AJ. Functional and structural adaptations in skeletal muscle of trained athletes. *J Appl Physiol* 1988; 64: 1114–1120.
2. Ambrosini D, VanEvery T, Kaufman KR, Sutherland DH. Averaging of electromyographic data in gait analysis of cerebral palsy patients [abstract]. *West Coast Gait Lab Conference*, Los Angeles, 1991.
3. Basmajian JV, DeLuca CJ. *Muscles Alive—Their Functions Revealed by Electromyography*, 5th ed. Baltimore: Williams & Wilkins; 1985.
4. Bourne GH, ed. *The Structure and Function of Muscle*. New York: Academic Press; 1960.
5. Burke RE, Levine DN, Tsairis P, Zajac FE III. Physiological types and histological profiles in motor units of the cat gastrocnemius. *J Physiol* 1973;234:723–748.
6. Cormack DH, ed. *Ham's Histology*, 9th ed. Philadelphia: JB Lippincott; 1987.
7. Edström L, Kugelberg E. Histochemical composition, distribution of fibers and fatigability of single motor units. *J Neurol Neurosurg Psychiatry* 1968;31:424–433.
8. Filipe MI, Lake BD. *Histochemistry in Pathology*. London: Churchill Livingstone, 1983.
9. Gage JR. An overview of normal walking. *Course Lect* 1990;39:291–303.
10. Gordon AM, Huxley AF, Julian FJ. The variation in isometric tension with sarcomere length in vertebrate muscle fibers. *J Physiol* 1966;184:170–192.
11. Hill AV. The mechanics of active muscle. *Proc Soc Lond* [Biol] 1953;141:104–117.
12. Henneman E, Olson CB. Relations between structure and function in the design of skeletal muscles. *J Neurophysiol* 1965;28:581–598.
13. Hoy MG, Zajac FE, Gordon ME. A musculoskeletal model of the human lower extremity: the effect of muscle, tendon and moment arm on the moment-angle relationship of musculotendon actuators at the hip, knee, and ankle. *J Biomechanics* 1990;23:157–169.
14. Huxley AF. Muscle structure and theories of contraction. *Prog Biophys* 1957;7:255–318.
15. Huxley HE, Hanson J. Chantes in the cross-striations of muscle during contraction and stretch, and their structural interpretation. *Nature* 1954;173:973–976.
16. Kugelberg E, Edström L. Differential histochemical effect of muscle contractions on phosphorylase and glycogen in various types of fibers. Relation to fatigue. *J Neurol Neurosurg Psychiatry* 1968;31:415–423.
17. Lieber RL. Skeletal muscle adaptability. I. Review of basic properties. *Dev Med Child Neurol* 1986;28:390–397.
18. Lieber RL. Skeletal muscle adaptability. II. Muscle properties following spinal-cord injury. *Dev Med Child Neurol* 1986;28:533–542.
19. Lieber RL. Skeletal muscle adaptability. III. Muscle properties following chronic electrical stimulation. *Dev Med Child Neurol* 1986;28:662–670.
20. Lieber RL, Boakes JL. Sarcomere length and joint kinematics during torque production in the frog hindlimb. *Am J Physiol (Cell Physiol)* 1988;23:C759–C768.
21. Lieber RL, Boakes JL. Muscle force and moment arm contributions to torque production in the frog hindlimb. *Am J Physiol (Cell Physiol)* 1988;23:C769–C772.
22. Lieber RL. *Skeletal Muscle Structure and Function*. (p. 122). Williams & Wilkins; 1992.
23. Nordin M, Frankel VH. Basic biomechanics of the musculoskeletal system, 2nd ed. Philadelphia: Lea & Febiger; 1989.
24. Perry J. *Gait Analysis-Normal and Pathological Function*. Thorofare, NJ: Slack; 1992.
25. Stulen FB, DeLuca CJ. Frequency parameters of the myoelectric signal as a measure of muscle conduction velocity. *IEEE Trans Biomed Eng* 1981;28:515–523.
26. Sutherland DH. *Gait Disorders in Childhood and Adolescence*. (p. 23–26). Baltimore: Williams & Wilkins; 1984.
27. Vander AJ, Sherman JH, Lucuano DS. *Human Physiology*. New York: McGraw-Hill; 1990.
28. Winter DA. *Biomechanics of Human Movement*. New York: John Wiley & Sons; 1979.
29. Winter DA. *The Biomechanics and Motor Control of Human Gait*. Waterloo: University of Waterloo Press; 1987.

Chapter 7

Development of Gait

Rosanne Kermoian, M. Elise Johanson, Erin E. Butler, and Stephen Skinner

Walking is the motor milestone most eagerly awaited by parents and is the hallmark of young children's emerging independence. Although gait is a complex motor skill, it begins in infancy and develops rapidly, attaining many adult characteristics by 7 to 8 years of age. This chapter summarizes the changes that occur in children's gait with age, addresses the search for mechanisms underlying the development of gait and the functional consequences of children's mobility.

FIRST FUNCTIONAL CHALLENGES

Learning to walk is a complex motor problem that is magnified by factors unique to childhood. The acquisition of postural balance during gait is made more difficult by infants' body dimensions and their rapid rate of growth (3,4,88). Relative to adults and older children, infants are top-heavy, with large heads and trunks and short legs that make them less stable during movement (88). Their short stature results in faster body sway, requiring more rapid corrections to prevent falls and their physical growth results in the need for ongoing adaptation to changes. Children's lack of experience also contributes to the difficulty of the motor challenge. Prior to taking the their first steps, for example, children rarely practice the dynamic bipedal and unipedal stance control necessary for independent ambulation (18).

Despite the magnitude of the motor problem, children typically begin to pull-to-stand and take steps while holding onto things around 8 to 10 months of age. Supported walking or "cruising" continues for 2 months, on average, with crawling continuing as a means of getting from place to place. During supported walking, children require external support to maintain balance and their movements are characterized by erratic joint motions, variable step rates and step lengths, and inconsistent timing of muscle actions (36,81,87).

The onset of independent walking typically begins around the first birthday and, as with supported walking,

is interspersed with bouts of crawling (5,83). During the first 3 to 6 months of walking, many gait characteristics such as velocity, stride length and joint motions change rapidly and are only loosely related (18,38). During the following months and up to 7 to 8 years of age, the rate of change slows, and the relation between the characteristics of gait become more predictable (17,18,83). Bril and Breniere (18) interpret this pattern of gait acquisition as reflecting a two-step process of development. During the early *integration phase*, children are learning to combine the independent elements that contribute to gait for physical growth and a wide range of environmental and task demands.

Three particularly notable features of early walking are (1) the intensity with which gait skills are practiced, (2) *en bloc* movement patterns (i.e., moving separate parts of the body as a single mechanical unit), and (3) marked variability in a given child's gait from step to step, trial to trial, and day to day.

Adolph and colleagues (3,4) have likened the practice schedules of newly walking infants to that of elite athletes and musicians. Converging evidence acquired from foot switches placed in the infant's shoes, daily checklists and telephone diaries of observations by mothers who were trained to record their children's movements show that newly walking infants are upright more than 6 hours per day, averaging between 500 and 1,500 walking steps per hour. By the end of each day infants may have taken 9,000 walking steps and traveled a distance equivalent to the length of 29 football fields (3,4).

During the first months of walking, practice is distributed throughout the day, a pattern that may be critical to maintaining the infants' motivation to practice their new gait skills and to consolidating their motor learning (3). Walking occurs in different locations and over indoor and outdoor surfaces that vary in height, rigidity, and texture (3,4). Walking occurs for a variety of purposes as diverse as attaining a desired object to following a sibling from place to place (49).

119

Early walking is characterized by *en bloc* movement patterns that can be seen in the stiff coupling of body parts (e.g., trunk and arms) and co-activation of muscle groups. These movement patterns can be observed during motor learning throughout life, as in the stiff legged posture of novice skiers. *En bloc* movement patterns are thought to simplify the motor problem by decreasing the number of biomechanical degrees of freedom that must simultaneously be controlled, thereby limiting the number of components of a new skill that must be learned at the same time (61). It has been hypothesized that *en bloc* movement patterns in early walking make it possible for infants to focus on the critical skills of maintaining an upright posture while moving forward (18).

Measurements of early walking in children are characterized by marked levels of variability that decrease with age and walking experience (18,83). This variability in the gait of newly walking children has been attributed to a number different of factors including poor motor control and interlimb coordination, inconsistent walking speed, active exploration of different movement patterns, and the challenge of obtaining accurate gait measurements from young children (18,27,32).

CHARACTERIZING CHILDREN'S GAIT

Measurements of time and distance (temporal-spatial) parameters, joint motions, muscle activation, energy cost, and ground reaction forces during walking have proved to be sensitive indicators of changes in gait patterns that occur as children increase in age and gain walking experience. Understanding the timing of the changes in these measurements and how they are linked to other neurological and behavioral events provides insight into the mechanisms underlying children's development. To date, the most comprehensive characterization of children's gait is that of Sutherland, Olshen, Biden and Wyatt (83), whose rich description of walking patterns in children ages one to seven years has provided a solid foundation for the characterization of children's gait.

Temporal-Spatial Parameters

Changes in gait that are associated with age and walking experience are described by measurements of temporal-spatial parameters: velocity, stride length, cadence, and time spent in single or double limb support. Following the first few months of walking, gait velocity, stride length, and single limb stance begin to increase while cadence and double limb support decrease (83). As leg length and height continue to increase, stride length and velocity also increase. With age, there are further developments in the temporal-spatial parameters of gait (9,83) that are associated with changes in the size of body segments. However, after 3 years of age the increase occurs at a significantly

slower rate than between 1 and 3 years of age (67,83,89,95). The principal reduction in cadence occurs between the ages of 1 and 2 years, and thereafter declines gradually until adulthood. Although cadence decreases between 3.5 and 7 years of age, it remains approximately 26% higher than the normal adult mean (83).

Velocity, stride length and cadence are only loosely related in the first few months of walking, which leads to instability and limited speed (38). By 4 to 5 years of age, velocity, stride length, and cadence become closely related and exhibit a more adultlike pattern, one in which both cadence and stride length are increased as a means to walk faster.

Kinematics

Children begin walking around 12 months of age with relatively stiff, slightly flexed hips and knees, a flat foot-strike, and a wide base of support. The arms are held away from the body in a symmetrical position for balance. They lack reciprocal arm swing (83). With age, the flexed posture of the hips and knees normalizes (6,34,81) and a well-defined heel strike at initial contact occurs. The base of support (step width) decreases and there is a lowered arm posture (34,53,83). The arm and leg movements progress from an ipsilaterally synchronous pattern to a reciprocal pattern (34,87).

Head: Head motion becomes more predictable with age, a process that may continue past 12 years of age (7,45). During the first 10 to 15 weeks of walking, lateral and anterior-posterior movement of the head and trunk decreases, a change that parallels decreases in step width and double limb support and increases in velocity and stride length (54). During the following 4 months of walking, head motion is minimized by stiff coupling of the head to the trunk so that they move as a single unit. Consequently, as the head is translated upward during initial swing, the orbital region of the eye and vestibular apparatus of the inner ear also move upward; as the head translates downward during terminal stance the position of the eyes and ears move downward.

After walking 18 months, children show some evidence of the mature pattern of head motion (18,55). In mature gait, there is greater disassociation of the head and trunk. As the head necessarily translates upward during initial swing, it tilts downward approximately the same number of degrees as the upward translation so that the position of the eyes and ears remain level. As the head translates downward during terminal stance, the head tilts upward. Compensatory head tilt in response to head translation during gait thus serves to keep the orbital region of the eye and vestibular apparatus of the inner ear at a constant height relative to the ground throughout the gait cycle. This pattern of head movement contributes to postural control during gait by providing a stable platform for the visual and vestibular sensory systems in the same way that keeping the head oriented toward a specific spot helps ballet dancers maintain their balance during a pirorette (44,66).

Trunk and upper extremities: A wide base of support and lateral motion of the trunk characterize early walking. By approximately 2.5 years of age, the base of support reduces to within the width of the pelvis and movement of the trunk is minimized (19).

During early walking, children's arms are typically held stiffly in a high-guard position (i.e., both shoulders raised in abduction and external rotation with elbow flexion). As step width decreases, the arms lower to a middle- and low-guard position (34,53). The raised and symmetrical positioning of the arms during early walking is thought to play a role in maintaining the body in an upright posture while moving forward, the arms being lowered as postural balance improves (53). Reciprocal arm swing, the mature form of arm movement during gait, in which the leg and contralateral arm move forward in synchrony, is seen in 50% of children by 1.5 years of age and 100% by 4 years of age (83). Arm swing and free moments tend to reinforce each other and act to balance the trunk torques induced by the lower limb (56).

Pelvis: During early walking the pelvis is more anteriorly tilted than in mature walking. In 1- to 2-year-old children, in the frontal plane, swing phase is accompanied by an ipsilateral pelvic hike above neutral. By age 2.5 years, the pelvis drops below neutral in swing. Changes in pelvic obliquity can be explained, in part, by the progressive narrowing of the wide base of support (83). Pelvic rotation in the transverse plane emerges approximately 4 weeks after independent walking (19), and by age 3 years there is a trend toward a lower dynamic range of pelvic rotation (83).

Hip: Early walking is characterized by increased flexion and external rotation of the hip throughout stance (83). Full hip extension during single limb support in terminal stance is normally seen by age 2 years; hip rotation throughout the gait cycle stabilizes in mature form by age 3 years (83). Hip abduction and adduction are closely linked to pelvic obliquity, with progressively less stance phase adduction observed until approximately 2.5 years of age when pelvic obliquity stabilizes in mature form (83).

Knee: The knee is flexed throughout the gait cycle when children begin to walk. This differs from the mature gait pattern in which the knee is extended throughout most of stance phase, with the exception of loading response and preswing. By age 2 years, there is an increase in knee flexion during the loading response (81,83). However, a mature knee pattern from initial contact to terminal stance is not consistently observed until age 4 years. The second phase of knee flexion during the gait cycle occurs just prior to swing (preswing) to advance the limb and is indistinguishable from the adult pattern by 2 years of age (83).

ANKLE DORSIFLEXION/ PLANTAR FLEXION

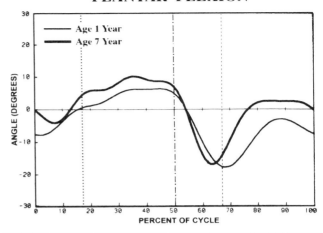

FIGURE 7-1. Ankle motion during gait at one year of age (n = 45) and seven years of age (n = 46). Note the lack of dorsiflexion at initial contact (0% gait cycle) and in terminal swing (80% to 90% gait cycle) for the one-year-olds. Dorsiflexion is increased in stance phase (35% to 50% gait cycle) for the seven-year-olds. (Adapted from Sutherland D et al. *The Development of Mature Walking,* Philadelphia: Lippincott 1988; 93, 97.)

Ankle: In early walkers, 1 to 1.5 years of age, a combination of ankle plantar flexion and knee flexion result in a flat foot at initial contact. A consistent heel strike is achieved at an average of 22 weeks after independent walking (19) or 18 months of age (83). Once heel contact is established, the ankle plantar flexes during the loading response. With age, as the body is moved over the stance limb in single limb support, the degree of ankle dorsiflexion increases. This change has been attributed to the developing strength of the calf muscles that control tibial advancement over the supporting limb (47). In general, swing phase dorsiflexion is present in early walking but increases with age until normal adult motions are achieved. The described changes in ankle motion are illustrated in Figure 7-1.

Kinetics

In a study of children ranging from 11 months to 14 years of age, Beck et al. (9) found a trend toward decreasing force amplitudes until 5 years of age, after which the vertical, fore-aft and medial-lateral ground reaction forces remained constant at all three walking speeds studied (slow, comfortable, and fast). The initial decrease in the relative magnitude of the ground reaction force was hypothesized to indicate the development of a more efficient gait, based on the assumption that a reduction in the floor reaction forces reflects a reduction in muscular effort (9). Other investigators, reporting age differences in ground reaction force, have found that children show changes in the amplitude and timing of kinetic data until 9 years of age (29,62,84). The difficulty of collecting force data in young

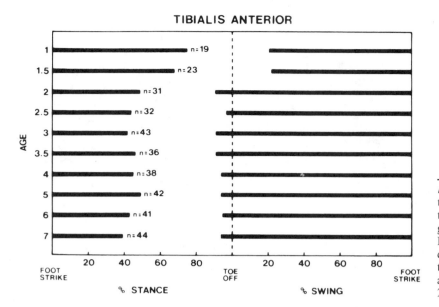

FIGURE 7-2. Average times of onset and cessation of EMG activity as measured by surface electrodes over the tibialis anterior in each of 10 age groups expressed as percentages of the gait cycle. For the one-year-olds, the activation is prolonged during stance, lasting until nearly toe off. This activity is co-contraction with the calf muscles that are also active in stance. (From Sutherland et al. *The Development of Mature Walking* 1988;155.)

children may contribute to the discrepancy in age-related changes. Walking speed may also account for the discrepancy. Stansfield et al. (78) demonstrated that normalized speed, and not age, characterized ground reaction force patterns in 5- to 12-year-old children when speed, step length, cadence, and force were normalized to unitless quantities using the method described by Hof and Zijlstra (43).

Muscle Timing

New walkers is characterized by prolonged activity in most muscle groups, resulting in co-contraction of antagonist leg muscles during the gait cycle. With age, the duration of muscle activity shortens and a reciprocal pattern is observed between agonist and antagonist muscles. This pattern is most notable in the quadriceps and hamstrings, and calf and pretibial muscle groups (83,87). In new walkers, there is nearly continuous activity in the quadriceps throughout the gait cycle, which is thought to be essential to the maintenance of an upright posture in the presence of excessive knee flexion in stance that is characteristic of early walking (83). Hamstring muscle activity is also prolonged and has similar timing to that of the quadriceps muscles, beginning in mid swing and ending at the end of single limb stance. By the age of 2 years, the hamstrings and quadriceps achieve nearly normal timing (83).

At the ankle, the pretibial muscles are active at initial contact and loading response, secondary to the flat foot contact, with prolonged activity in stance. From age 2 to 7 years, the pretibial muscles terminate activity after the beginning of single limb stance and resume their activity at initial swing, similar to that of mature walking. Figure 7-2 demonstrates the prolonged activation of the tibialis anterior during stance at younger ages. For most new walkers, the calf group is active in terminal swing as well as

in stance. With age, the swing phase activity of the calf disappears. However, approximately 25% of children from age 2 to 7 years have premature firing of the ankle plantar flexors in swing and early stance phase (83).

The observed co-contraction in newly walking children and emergence of mature patterns of muscle activation has been attributed to a number of different factors. One explanation is that co-contraction maintains the body in equilibrium in an upright position and that the integration of the stretch-reflex activity into the preprogrammed leg muscle EMG with age corresponds to an increase in gastrocnemius activity stabilizing the body during gait (11). Forssberg (36) and others (e.g., 58) attribute the emerging pattern of muscle activation to innate central pattern generators (CPGs) in the spinal cord that are hypothesized to produce both infant stepping and generate the basic locomotor rhythm in adults. Further work is needed to determine the role of the stretch reflex, supraspinal influences, and other factors in shaping and fine-tuning muscle activity during gait (35).

Effort and Energy Cost

The amount of energy required for walking is directly proportional to walking speed at all ages. Oxygen consumption measured in children walking at slow, comfortable, and fast speeds demonstrates that small children have a higher expenditure of energy during walking than teenagers or adults (92). A linear relationship between age and oxygen consumption per kilogram of body weight per minute and oxygen consumption per kilogram per meter walked has been observed, with the youngest subjects (6 years of age) having the highest values of oxygen consumption. In a study of the energy cost of walking as a function of walking speed in children from 3 to 12 years, the net cost of transport of the 3-to-4-year olds and 5-to-6-year olds was found to be 70% and 40% greater, respectively, than in adults (31).

Measurement of heart rate can also provide an estimate of the effort required for walking; at least at submaximal levels, oxygen uptake and heart rate are linearly related. Rose et al. (70), using treadmill ambulation, determined that oxygen consumption and heart rate in children were linearly related over a wide range of walking speeds (22 to 130 m per minute).

CURRENT DIRECTIONS IN CHARACTERIZING CHILDREN'S GAIT

Adaptation to Environmental and Task Demands

Flexible adaptation of gait to current conditions is the hallmark of mature walking, contributing to such critical functions as initiating gait, changing speed or direction, stepping over obstacles without interrupting ongoing gait, walking through narrow openings, and stopping before reaching an intended target of locomotion (59). Characterizing age-related changes in the way children adapt their gait to environmental and task demands is a relatively new and promising area of investigation.

Anticipatory control: Children's ability to flexibly adapt their gait in anticipation of future motor and sensory events improves with age. Data to date suggest that anticipatory control during gait develops more slowly and is more challenging than skills tapped by more traditional measures of gait. The ability to respond to external threats to balance during the gait initiation process, for example, does not emerge until 2 to 3 years of age, and children do not react efficiently to perturbation during gait initiation until after 4 to 5 years of age (99). Consistently anticipating a change in the direction of walking by turning the head prior to pivoting does not occur before 5.5 years of age and even at 8.5 years of age has not attained the adult pattern of turning the head a full second prior to pivoting the body (37). Difficulty with anticipatory control may play an important role in mild gait problems, such as those seen in children who have been identified as clumsy, and thus be more sensitive to the effects of premature birth and subtle neurologic difficulties than other measures of gait (40,94).

Mechanics of changing walking speed: Todd et al. (89) were among the first to propose that children's ability to vary their walking speed and the strategy by which they do so are sensitive measures of gait function. Their data demonstrate that children modify their speed in a predictable manner, using characteristic combinations of cadence and stride lengths.

Time and distance variables (speed, stride length, cadence) are typically recorded while children are instructed to walk at a self-selected comfortable speed. For children with disabilities, their self-selected walking speed is of-

ten reported as a percentage of walking speed for non-impaired children of the same age. Measurements of self-selected walking speed are related to children's age and height, increase with walking experience and are associated with children's lowest energy expenditure. Thus they provide a useful baseline characterization of gait in clinical settings, where the primary goal of surgical or rehabilitative therapy is often to improve children's self-selected walking speed.

In contrast, gait measurements collected while children are walking at their fastest speed reveal their ability to change speed and the strategy by which they walk faster. The normal strategy observed in mature gait is to increase both the stride length and cadence linearly. In immature gait, factors which contribute to an increase in stride length such as heel strike, hip extension in late midstance, and full knee extension in terminal swing may not yet be developed. In gait pathology, stride length can be restricted by joint contracture, spasticity, or musculoskeletal deformity leaving increased cadence as the only strategy for walking faster. Recent data collected by Abel and Damiano (1) have shown that the strategy children use to change their walking speed differentiates between the gait of children with cerebral palsy and their nonimpaired peers. Children with cerebral palsy, although able to increase their walking speed, rely more on increasing cadence than stride length to change speed.

The advantages of measuring speed, stride length, and cadence at both children's self-selected free and fast speed in clinical populations is illustrated in Figure 7-3. The plot illustrates the relation between speed, stride length, and cadence for a child instructed to walk at both self-selected and fast walking speeds. The darkened reference line indicates the expected values for a non-impaired child of the same height walking at the same speed. The data demonstrate the compromised stride length and dramatic increase in cadence in the barefoot condition when a 5-year-old child with spina bifida is asked to walk at a fast speed. When the child wears ankle-foot orthoses (braced condition) he is able to increase his walking speed by increasing both stride length and cadence.

Minimizing Variance in Gait Measurements

A serious limitation of standard gait measurements for children is that they yield a wide range of "normal" values due to unspecified factors. Much of the variability observed in the data of children who are the same age is thought to be caused by factors that are specific to childhood, such as individual differences in the rate of growth (e.g., height and limb length) and individual differences in the rate of motor skill acquisition. The extent to which children's ages are not perfectly correlated with their growth or motor skill will necessarily result in unexplained variance in measurement (91). Differences in children's self-selected walking speed

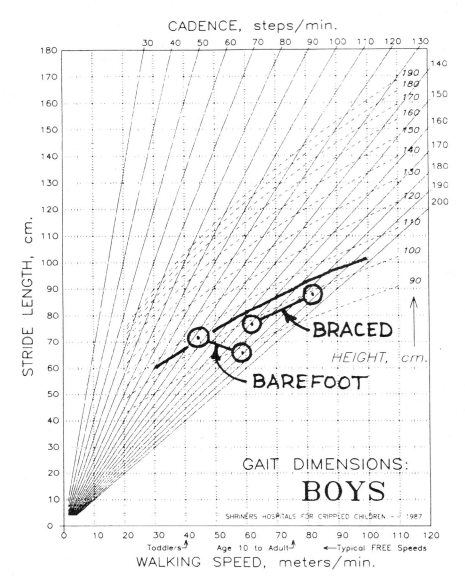

FIGURE 7-3. Speed, stride length, and cadence data from a five-year-old boy, 105 cm in height, with spina bifida can be visualized on this graph. The child was instructed to walk at his self-selected and fast speed in two conditions: braced (with orthoses) and barefoot. For each condition the self-selected and fast walking data points (*circled*) are connected by a line. The expected relationship between speed, stride length, and cadence for a typically-developing child of the same height is indicated by the solid line drawn along the dashed reference lines for height in centimeters. In the barefoot condition, he walks slower compared to the braced condition even when he is attempting to walk at his fastest speed, and he is unable to increase his stride length. In order to increase his walking speed, the child increases his cadence from 122 steps per minute to 180 steps per minute without an increase in stride length. With the braces on, his self-selected and his fastest speed are greater than his barefoot speed. The additional stability provided by the braces enabled him to increase both his stride length and cadence proportionally to achieve the faster walking speed. (From Todd FN, Lamoreux LW, Skinner SR, et al. *J Bone Joint Surg Am* 1989;71-A:196–204.)

may also increase the variability in gait data by differentially affecting temporal-spatial parameters, joint kinematics and kinetics, and muscle timing (9,78,79,90). Currently, there are a number of techniques being used to minimize the variability in children's gait data so as to better understand the mechanisms contributing to the development of gait, and to increase the comparability of data from different children or individual children followed over time.

To minimize variability in gait data owing to height, Hof and Zijlstra (43) proposed a nondimensional scaling technique in which the effect of height can be accounted for in a mechanically consistent way using a pendulum model of gait. The technique uses geometrical scaling in which leg length and acceleration caused by gravity are the only factors: The data are unitless. The assumption is made that any variability remaining in the data after these factors are accounted for must be caused by factors other than height. Stansfield et al. (78,79) and Vaughn

et al. (91) have used this technique to eliminate the effects of height to study the changes in a number of other variables including walking speed, step length, and cadence. Other techniques that have been used to eliminate variability due to height include statistical detrending with respect to two or more variables. This normalization method involves iteratively removing the trends between two or more variables, such as height and stride length. O'Malley (63), using Sutherland's data to compare several statistical methods for removing the effects of height and age, recommended simultaneous normalization when two or more variables are involved. This method has the additional benefit of retaining the original units of measurement.

To minimize variability that results from changes in walking speed as well as height, Todd et al. (89) used data from 324 non-impaired children to develop a set of equations that predict the appropriate stride length (in cm) for a child of a specific height walking at his or her chosen walking speed. Placing the emphasis on stride length rather than walking speed reduces the variability that is introduced by children voluntarily varying their self-selected speed. Normalizing stride length for height and walking speed assures that children with disabilities are not penalized merely because they are smaller in stature or walk at a slower speed than their peers.

The equations that were used to define the normal reference curves in Figure 7-3 describe the expected relation between speed, stride length, and cadence for children who are between 80 and 170 cm in height. The equations are presented in the Appendix along with two sets of constants, one for boys and one for girls. Measurements of a child's height and free walking speed are used to calculate the predicted stride length. Measurement of the child's actual stride length can be expressed as a percentage of the predicted stride length. This method can be used to express the degree of walking disability or changes in functional status over time.

THE SEARCH FOR MECHANISMS UNDERLYING THE DEVELOPMENT OF GAIT

Over the past decade, there has been a distinct shift in the study of gait development from characterizing gait in children of different ages to searching for the mechanisms that bring about developmental change. Why do infants around the world typically begin to walk between 12 and 18 months of age and look strikingly similar from the time that they begin to negotiate their first steps?

Historically, the answers to these questions were straightforward. The emergence of the major motor milestones, such as walking, and the subsequent refinement of these skills was attributed to maturation of the central nervous system (CNS). Although elegant in its simplicity, the brain-to-behavior causal link has been seriously challenged over the past decade by theory and empirical evidence, suggesting that the CNS may not always have primary status in the development of gait (85).

Peripheral factors contribute to the development of gait: Among the most powerful tests of neuromaturational explanations of gait are studies demonstrating how peripheral factors (non-CNS factors), such as the weight of the lower extremities, can determine the emergence of new motor patterns. Thelen's studies of infant stepping were among the first to demonstrate that the development of a behavior that had been attributed to the CNS could be determined by change in peripheral factors (85). Thelen hypothesized that neonatal stepping movements (the "stepping reflex") would seemingly disappear as young infants gained leg fat and subsequently reappear toward the end of the first year of life when their leg muscles became strong enough to lift their limbs against gravity. Among the most convincing data supporting this explanation are

studies in which Thelen and colleagues experimentally manipulated infants' leg weight and strength. If young infants who were still producing neonatal stepping movements had their legs weighted to simulate the leg weight gained over the first 2 months of life, they could no longer step (88). Yet, if young infants who were no longer spontaneously producing neonatal stepping movements had their legs partially submerged in a tank of water to minimize the effect of gravity, they were once again able to step (88). Furthermore, when infants were held over a motorized treadmill to augment their leg strength, they produced stepping movements throughout the first year of life, well past the time the "stepping reflex" had disappeared and prior to the time they were spontaneously producing independent stepping movements (86). Taken together, these studies show how the peripheral factors of leg weight and muscle strength can reliably alter the developmental course of one component of independent walking, that of stepping.

The search for peripheral factors contributing to gait has resulted in research on the role of experience in the development of gait. Such investigations are surprisingly diverse, ranging from the effects of prenatal movement experience (e.g., breech positioning during the third trimester results in increased likelihood of hip flexion during gait at 12 to 18 months of age [76]), to the effect of seasonal and environmental influences on motor development (e.g., bundling of Inuit children in the fall and winter results in delayed walking onset relative to spring and summer, unpublished Kaplan-Estrin, et al).

Gait is determined by interplay among factors: Although peripheral factors may independently account for some changes in gait development, it is likely that neither peripheral nor central factors function in isolation. Recent studies demonstrate how multiple factors, each operating independently, can interact in a way that either facilitates or limits the emergence of walking. In these studies, neuromaturation is typically treated as one factor among many. Work by Woollacott et al. (100) and Sienko-Thomas et al. (74), for example, provide an elegant demonstration of how central and peripheral factors jointly considered elucidate our understanding of mechanisms constraining the development of gait in children with cerebral palsy. To test the effects of abnormal lower extremity postures observed in children with cerebral palsy on muscular responses in standing and walking, non-impaired children were positioned in a crouching posture and activation patterns in the lower extremity musculature were recorded. Standing in the abnormal posture elicited muscular responses in non-impaired children that resembled that of children with cerebral palsy, including activation of muscles in a proximal to distal fashion and excessive co-contraction. These studies demonstrate one means by which CNS damage, as evidenced by muscle and joint contracture and crouched position, may affect the development of standing and gait.

FUNCTIONAL CONSEQUENCES OF MOBILITY

Physiological Change

Bone mineral density: In children, as in adults, the act of walking contributes to health by improving aerobic capacity, resting metabolic rate, body composition, and fat metabolism. Many studies on the effect of mobility on physiology address the issue of bone mineral accrual. Mechanical loading associated with physical activity increases bone mineral density in children (57). Intermittent weight-bearing, such as occurs during walking, is thought to be more effective for bone accrual than static weight-bearing (13,52,71). Not surprisingly, children with mobility deficits, such as those with cerebral palsy, have been found to be at higher risk for fractures and osteoporosis than can be predicted by their nutritional deficiencies and abnormal vitamin D metabolism from anticonvulsant medication (25,41,73). Using a number of different measures of bone mineral accrual (e.g., bone mineral density, bone mineral composition and broadband ultrasound attenuation, a measure of disruption of the microstructural parameters), findings across studies show that skeletal fragility in children is directly related to the extent of their mobility (26,77,98). Children who walk independently have the highest bone density, followed by children who walk with a mobility aid, children who are non-mobile but who regularly weight-bear in a standing frame, and children who are non-mobile and do not weight-bear. Further work is needed to determine whether there are sensitive periods during development when ambulation is most critical to bone mineral accrual. However, recent data suggest that intermittent weight-bearing may be particularly important during the two-year window of the pubertal growth spurt when human growth hormone and sex hormones surge and approximately 25% of the adult skeleton develops (65).

Increased sensitivity of the vestibular and visual sensory systems: The onset of mobility is associated with increased responsiveness of the vestibular and visual sensory systems. Both systems, although functional from a very young age, undergo prolonged postnatal development and become more finely tuned with mobility experience.

Although the vestibular system is anatomically differentiated at birth, the capacity for the CNS to utilize head movement information transmitted by the otolith and canal system of the inner ear does not reach adult-level functioning until approximately 12 years of age (64). Research on delays in postural and locomotor development associated with hypoactive or absent vestibular function suggests that the otolith system, in particular, facilitates walking because of its role as a gravitational and inertial force detector (64). Consistent with that prediction, cross-sectional and longitudinal data demonstrate that the onset of walking is associated with increased sensitivity of the otolith but not the canal system, regardless of the age at which the infants begin to walk (96,97). These findings demonstrate that development of the otolith system occurs with the onset of walking, although further work is needed to determine whether walking experience brings about changes in the otolith system or vice versa.

Mobility improves visual proprioception. Adults control their posture and perceive their direction of self-motion from the pattern of visual motion (optical flow) generated as they move (6). This coupling between posture and motion in large areas of the visual field has been demonstrated even in neonates, who make directionally appropriate compensatory movements of their heads to optical flow (46). Only after mobility onset, however, does the total amount of visual stimulation needed to control posture decrease significantly: Optical flow in the periphery of the visual field, as compared to movement of the entire visual field, is sufficient to elicit directionally appropriate postural adjustments in infants who are independently mobile but not in pre-mobile infants of the same age (12,42). Only mobile infants respond to the same illusion of movement that adults experience when seated in a stationary train that is passed by a moving train.

Neural Change

Just as the CNS plays a role in the process of learning to walk, learning to walk may in turn affect brain development. Neural change that is associated with the acquisition of complex motor skills has been attributed to neuroplasticity, the active reciprocal process of specific experience shaping neural connectivity (22). This process occurs during both development and normal learning (82). Recent data demonstrate that complex motor skill learning in adults results in selective anatomical changes in the cortex (e.g., learning to juggle increases gray matter in cortical areas that are associated with the processing and storage of complex visual motion [33]) and selective functional changes in the cortex (e.g., training in a complex finger movement task results in remodeling of the somatosensory cortex [60]). In children, the effect of neuroplasticity is thought to be even more powerful than in adults because there are more uncommitted resources in the brain and less competition for these resources among developing functional systems (51). Thus, it is reasonable to assume that the act of learning to walk has a positive effect on the structure and function of the brain.

Although this issue has not been investigated directly, data on pre-walking mobility are consistent with the hypothesis that the demands associated with learning a complex mobility skill bring about changes in cortical organization. Bell and Fox (10) found a higher degree of connectivity and synaptic elaboration, as measured by resting EEG coherence, between intrahemispheric frontal, parietal, and occipital sites in children who had been crawling 1 to 4 weeks than in pre-mobile children or children who had been crawling for more than 4 weeks. All children were 8 months of age. This pattern of findings points to the possibility that learning how to crawl results in an initial overproduction of cortico-cortical connections that is followed by subsequent pruning of unused synapses as the motor skill of crawling becomes more routine. A more efficient pattern of interconnectivity may also follow the onset of walking.

Behavioral Change

The emergence of independent mobility has widespread and enduring functional consequences for children's cognitive, perceptual, and socioemotional development (e.g., 16,20,49). Before children are mobile, they spend relatively long periods of time in one place and their play is limited to objects that are within arms' reach. Following mobility onset, they have many new opportunities. Learning how to navigate through the environment is particularly challenging. A few specific demands associated with safe and successful navigation and selected findings from studies on the effects of mobility on children's development are listed below.

- **Visual attention to the environment** is critical in order to monitor the route, and avoid collisions and falls. Wariness of heights, a skill that is essential to safe mobility, develops after mobility onset even though children can perceive heights long before they move independently (23).
- **Working memory** is needed in order to keep a destination in mind, regardless of the time it takes to get there and distractions encountered along the way. Object permanence, the ability to remember where an object has been hidden, is the hallmark of infant intelligence and a measure of working memory. Object permanence improves after mobility onset (8,10,50) and continues to improve the longer children have been independently mobile (50).
- **Strategies for remembering the route** are necessary so as to avoid getting lost. Following mobility onset infants are significantly more likely to use landmarks and environmental cues to locate objects, even when they are confined to a seated position (28,48,49).
- **The ability to remember and transfer information acquired in one setting to similar problems encountered in another setting** is essential to successful navigation in new locations. One of the many things children need to learn is that doorways, regardless of their size and shape, are the place one enters or leaves a room. Findings indicate that mobile children when compared to non-mobile children of the same age are more likely to generalize information to new settings. For example, they are more likely to activate a new toy if it works in the same way as one they saw demonstrated 24 hours before in a different location (39). This important skill underlies children's development in domains as seemingly unrelated to mobility as language learning (72).

- **The need and opportunity for children to make independent decisions** occurs constantly during mobility, teaching children that they have their own unique wishes and desires, a critical step in socioemotional development. The consequences of increased autonomy can be seen in the "testing of wills" between newly walking children and their parents. Children who are mobile are more likely to persist in their activities and express anger if their activities are thwarted than same-age peers (48). Parents, in turn, begin using the word "no" with their mobile children and expecting them to comply with their demands (24).

Converging evidence from studies using different research designs demonstrate that the dramatic changes in behavior are not merely a correlate of independent mobility but a consequence of it. In general, children of the same age who are crawling on hand-and-knees perform at higher levels than children who are not yet mobile (48,49). Children who cannot move independently, but who can move from place to place with the aid of a baby walker, behave similarly to infants who are crawling. Case studies of infants with mobility delays caused by heavy casting that prevented crawling or spina bifida (L4-5 or below) perform poorly until after they begin to move, at which time they show a spurt in performance.

Essential features of mobility: Behavioral changes associated with mobility emerge slowly over a period of weeks or months and improve concomitantly with gains in motor skill. This pattern of acquisition suggests that movement parameters such as speed, distance traveled and efficiency of movement, either separately or jointly considered, may be essential for behavioral change. A direct link between movement parameters and outcome is supported by the fact that mobility in a baby walker, a fast and efficient form of movement, is associated with behavioral change; whereas, belly crawling, a slow and effortful form of movement, is not (8,50). Walking, as compared to pre-walking mobility, results in higher movement velocity, efficiency, greater distance traveled, and total time spent moving (3,4). Studies to date suggest that walking magnifies the changes that have been documented with creeping on hands-and-knees (e.g., 2,28). The gains in biomechanical efficiency that come with upright mobility may be particularly important to behavioral and nueral change, making it possible for children to pay less attention to the act of moving and more attention to the environment.

Clinical populations: Taken together, these studies demonstrate important functional consequences of mobility. Under typical circumstances, mobility can facilitate other areas of children's development. However, it is unlikely that it is the only means by which children can learn (69). Unfortunately, few studies have examined the effect of mobility delays or disability on infants and children with orthopaedic or neuromuscular disorders. Interpretation of the findings from studies to date is limited by the possibility that the children's underlying medical condition is responsible for both learning and mobility. In addition, the studies do not capitalize on the power of experimental or longitudinal designs. The sample sizes are small and heterogeneous. Keeping these limitations in mind, the most conservative interpretation is that mobility, although not necessary for the acquisition of rudimentary skills, commonly affects the rate of acquisition and final level of skill attainment of a number of spatial and social skills (68,75,80,93). When powered mobility aids are provided, mobility has beneficial and predictable consequences, even for children with severe motor and cognitive deficits (15,21,30).

SUMMARY

The study of children's gait over the past decade has led to a more complete characterization of how gait changes with age and walking experience. To address the wide range of "normal values" found in children's gait measurements due to unexplained factors, there is an increased focus on the factors that systematically contribute to measurement variability. One technique for normalizing gait data to eliminate variability due to height and walking speed is presented in this chapter. To better address issues of gait function, research characterizing gait now encompasses studies of children's ability to adapt their gait to environmental and task demands. These skills (e.g., stepping over an obstacle without stopping) are notably poor in immature and pathological gait.

In addition to advances in characterizing gait, gait research has broadened to include studies of the mechanisms underlying age-related changes in gait and the functional consequences of mobility for other domains of children's development. Investigations of mechanisms underlying the development of gait have highlighted the importance of biomechanical and experiential factors in promoting development. Studies of the functional consequences of mobility have revealed surprisingly widespread and enduring effects of mobility for children's physiological, neural, and behavioral development.

REFERENCES

1. Abel MF, Damiano DL. Strategies for increasing walking speed in diplegic cerebral palsy. *J Pediatr Ortho* 1996;16:753–758.
2. Adolph KE. Learning in the development of infant locomotion. *Monogr Soc Res Child Dev* 1997;62:1–158
3. Adolph KE. Learning to keep balance. *Adv Child Dev Behav* 2002;30: 1–40.
4. Adolph KE, Avolio AM. Walking infants adapt locomotion to changing body dimensions. *J Exp Psychol Hum Percept and Perform* 2000;26:1148–1166.
5. Adolph KE, Vereijken B, Shrout PE. What changes in infant walking and why. *Child Dev* 2003;74:475–497.
6. Andersen GJ. Perception of self-motion: psychophysical and computational approaches. *Psychol Bull* 1986;99:52–65.
7. Assaiante C, Amblard, B. Ontogenesis of head stabilisation in space during locomotion in children: influence of visual cues. *Exp Brain Res* 1993;93:499–515.
8. Bai DL, Bertenthal BI. Locomotor status and the development of spatial search skills. *Child Dev* 1992;63:215–226.
9. Beck RJ, Andriacchi TP, Kuo KN, et al. Changes in the gait patterns of growing children. *J Bone Joint Surg Am* 1981;63:1452–1457.
10. Bell MA, Fox, NA. Individual differences in object permanence performance at 8 months: Locomotor experience and brain electrical activity. *Dev Psychobiol* 1997;31:287–297.
11. Berger W, Altenmueller E, Dietz V. Normal and impaired development of children's gait. *Hum Neurobiol* 1984;3:163–170.
12. Bertenthal BI, Bai DL. Infants' sensitivity to optic flow for controlling posture. *Dev Psychol* 1989;25:936–945.
13. Biewener AA, Bertram JE. Structural response of growing bone to exercise and disuse. *J Appl Physiol* 1994;76:946–955.
14. Biringen Z, Emde, RN, Campos JJ, Appelbaum MI. Affective reorganization in the infant, the mother, and the dyad: the role of upright locomotion and its timing. *Child Dev* 1995;66:499–514.
15. Bottos M, Bolcati C, Sciuto L, Ruggeri C, Feliciangeli A. Powered wheelchairs and independence in young children with tetraplegia. *Dev Med Child Neurol* 2001;43:769–777.
16. Bremner, JG. Motor abilities as causal agents in infant cognitive development. In: Salvesberg G, ed. *The Development of Co-ordination in Infancy*. Amsterdam: Elsevier, 1993:347–377.
17. Bril B, Breniere Y. Posture and independent locomotion in early childhood: learning to walk or learning dynamic postural control? In: Salvesberg G, ed. *The Development of Co-ordination in Infancy*. Amsterdam: Elsevier, 1993:337–358.
18. Bril B, Ledebt A. Head coordination as a means to assist sensory integration in learning to walk. *Neurosci Biobehav Rev* 1998;22: 555–563.
19. Burnett CN, Johnson EW. Development of gait in childhood. II. *Dev Med Child Neurol* 1971;13:207–215.
20. Bushnell EW, Boudreau JP. Motor development and the mind: The potential role of motor abilities as a determinant of aspects of perceptual development. *Child Dev* 1993;64:1005–1021.
21. Butler C. Effects of powered mobility on self-initiated behaviors of very young children with locomotor disability. *Dev Med Child Neurol* 1986;28:325–332.
22. Byl NN, Merzenich M. Principles of neuroplasticity: implications for neurorehabilitation and learning. In: Gonzalez EG Myers SJ, Edelstein JE, Lieberman JS, Downey JA eds. *Downey and Darling's Physiological Basis of Rehabilitation Medicine*, 3rd ed. Boston: Butterworth Heinemann, 2001:609–628.
23. Campos JJ, Bertenthal B, Kermoian R. Early experience and emotional development: The emergence of wariness of heights. *Psychol Sci* 1992;3:61–64.
24. Campos JJ, Kermoian R, Zumbahlen MR. Socioemotional transformation in the family system following infant crawling onset. *New Dir Child Dev* 1992;55:25–40.
25. Chad KE, McKay HA, Zello GA, Bailey A, Faulkner A, Snyder RE. Body composition in nutritionally adequate ambulatory and non-ambulatory children with cerebral palsy and a healthy reference group. *Dev Med Child Neurol* 2000;42:334–339.
26. Chad EK, Bailey DA, McKay HA, Zello GA, Snyder RE. The effect of a weight-bearing physical activity program on bone mineral content and estimated volumetric density in children with spastic cerebral palsy. *J Pediatr* 1999;135:115–117.
27. Clark JE, Whitall J, Phillips SJ. Human interlimb coordination: the first 6 months of independent walking. *Dev Psychobiol* 1998;21:445–456.

28. Clearfield MW. The role of crawling and walking experience in infant spatial memory. *J Exp Child Psycho* 2004;89:214–241.
29. Cupp T, Oeffinger D, Tylkowski C, et al. Age-related kinetic changes in normal pediatrics. *J Pediatr Orthop* 1999;19:475–478.
30. Deitz J, Swinth Y, White O. Powered mobility and preschoolers with complex developmental delays. *Am J Occup Ther* 2002;56: 86–96.
31. De Jaeger D, Willems PA, Heglund NC. The energy cost of walking in children. *Pflugers Arch* 2001;441:538–543.
32. Diop M, Rahmani A, Calmels P, et al. Influence of speed variation and age on the intrasubject variability of ground reaction forces and spatiotemporal parameters of children's normal gait. *Ann Readapt Med Phys* 2004;47:72–80.
33. Draganski B, Baser C, Busch V, Schuierer G, Bogdahn U, May A. Changes in grey matter induced by training. *Nature* 2004;427: 311–312.
34. Farmer SE. Key factors in the development of lower limb coordination: implications for the acquisition of walking in children with cerebral palsy. *Disabil Rehabil* 2003;25:807–816.
35. Forssberg H. Neural control of human motor development. *Curr Opin Neurobiol* 1999;9:676–682.
36. Forssberg H. Ontogeny of human locomotor control. I. Infant stepping, supported locomotion and transition to independent locomotion. *Exp Brain Res* 1985;57:480–493.
37. Grasso R, Assaiante C, Prevost P, Berthoz A. Development of anticipatory orienting strategies during locomotor tasks in children. *Neurosci Biobehav Rev* 1998;22:533–539.
38. Grieve DW, Gear RJ. The relationship between length of stride, step frequency, time of swing and speed of walking for children and adults. *Ergonomics* 1966;9:379–399.
39. Herbert J, Gross J, Hayne H. The effect of age and locomotor experience on deferred imitation in human infants. *Dev Psych*. (In Press)
40. Hempel MS. Neurological development during toddling age in normal children and children at risk of developmental disorder. *Early Hum Dev* 1992;34:47–57.
41. Henderson RC. Bone density and other possible predictors of fracture risk in children and adolescents with spastic cerebral palsy. *J Bone Joint Surg Am* 1995;77:1617–1618.
42. Higgins CI, Campos JJ, Kermoian R. Effect of self-produced locomotion on infant postural compensation to optic flow. *Dev Psychol* 1996;32:836–841.
43. Hof AL, Zijlstra W. Comment on "Normalization of temporal-distance parameters in pediatric gait." *J Biomech* 1997;30:299,301–302.
44. Holands MA, Sorensen KL, Patla AE. Effects of head immobilization on the coordination and control of head and body reorientation and translation during steering. *Exp Brain Res* 2001;140:223–233.
45. Holt KG, Ratcliffe R, Jeng SF. Head stability in walking in children with cerebral palsy and in children and adults without neurological impairment. *Phys Ther* 1999;79:1153–1162.
46. Jouen F. Visual-proprioceptive control of posture in newborn infants. In: Amblard B, Berthoz A, Clarac F, eds. *Posture and Gait: Development, Adaptation and Modulation.* Elsevier Science Publishers B.V.; 1988:59–65.
47. Katoh M, Mochizuki T, Moriyama A. Changes of sagittal-plane ankle motion and ground reaction force (fore-aft shear) in normal children aged 4 to 10 years. *Dev Med Child Neurol* 1993;35:417–423.
48. Kermoian R. Locomotor experience and psychological development in infancy. In: Furumasu J, ed. *Pediatric Powered Mobility: Developmental Perspectives, Technical Issues, Clinical Approaches.* Washington, DC: RESNA Press; 1997;7–21.
49. Kermoian R. Locomotor experience facilitates psychological functioning. In: Gray D, Quatrano L, Lieberman M, eds. *Designing and Using Assistive Technology: The Human Perspective.* Baltimore, MD: Paul Brookes Publishing Company; 1997:249–266.
50. Kermoian R, Campos JJ. Locomotor experience: a facilitator of spatial cognitive development. *Child Dev* 1988;18:299–307.
51. Knudsen EI. Sensitive Periods in the Development of the Brain and Behavior. *J Cogn Neurosci* 2004;16:1412–1425.
52. Lanyon LE, Rubin CT. Static vs dynamic loads as an influence on bone remodelling. *J Biomech* 1984;17:897–905.
53. Ledebt A, Bril B. Acquisition of upper body stability during walking in toddlers. *Dev Psychobiol* 2000;36:311–324.
54. Ledebt A, Bril B, Wiener-Vacher S. Trunk and head stabiliza-

tion during the first months of independent walking. *Neuroreport* 1995;6:1737–1740.
55. Ledebt A, Wiener-Vacher S. Head co-ordination in the sagittal plane in toddlers during walking: preliminary results. *Brain Research Bulletin* 1996;40:371–373.
56. Li Y, Wang W, Crompton RH, Gunther MM. Free vertical movements and transverse forces in human walking and their role in relation to arm-swing. *J Exp Biol* 2001;204:47–58.
57. MacKelvie KJ, Khan KM, McKay HA. Is there a critical period for bone response to weight bearing exercise in children and adolescents? A systematic review. *Br J Sports Med* 2002;36:250–257.
58. Marder E, Bucher D. Central pattern generators and the control of rhythmic movements. *Curr Biology* 2001;11:R986–R996.
59. Mattiello D, Woollacott M. Posture control in children: development in typical populations and in children with cerebral palsy and down syndrome. In: Connolly KJ, Forssberg H, eds. *Neurophysiology and Neuropsychology of Motor Development: Clinics in Developmental Medicine No. 143/144.* London: Mac Keith Press; 1977;54–77.
60. Merzenich M, Recanzone M, Jenkins W, Grajski KA. Adaptive mechanisms in cortical networks underlying cortical contributions to learning and nondeclarative memory. *Cold Spring Harbor Symposia on Quantitative Biology, LV,* 1990:873–887.
61. Newell K. Change in movement and skill: learning, retention and transfer. In: Latash M, Turvey M, eds. *Dexterity and Its Development.* Mahwah: LEA; 1996:393–430.
62. Noguchi M. (Development of gait in children–characteristics of gait in children from the viewpoint of ground reaction force) *Nippon Seikeigeka Gakkai Zasshi* 1986;60:787–799.
63. O'Malley MJ. Normalization of temporal-distance parameters in pediatric gait. *J Biomech* 1996;29:619–625.
64. Ornitz EM. Normal and pathological maturation of vestibular function in the human child. In Romand R, ed. *Development of Auditory and Vestibular Systems.* New York: Academic Press; 1983: 479–535.
65. Petit MA, McKay HA, MacKelvie KJ, Heinonen A, Khan KM, Beck TJ. A randomized school-based jumping intervention confers site and maturity-specific benefits on bone structural properties in girls: hip structural analysis study. *J Bone Miner Res* 2002;17:363–372.
66. Pozzo T , Levik Y, Berthoz A. Head and trunk movements in the frontal plane during complex dynamic equilibrium tasks in humans. *Exp Brain Res* 1995;106:327–338.
67. Preis S, Klemms A, Muller K. Gait analysis by measuring ground reaction forces in children: changes to an adaptive gait pattern between the ages of one and five years. *Dev Med Child Neurol* 1997;39:228–233.
68. Rendeli C, Salvaggio E, Sciascia-Cannizzaro G, Bianchi E, Caldarelli M, Guzzetta F. Does locomotion improve the cognitive profile of children with meningomyelocele? *Child's Nerv Syst* 2002; 18:231–234.
69. Riviere J, Lecuyer R. Spatial cognition in young children with spinal muscular atrophy. *Dev Neuropsychol* 2002;21:273–283.
70. Rose J, Gamble JG, Medeiros J, Buygos A, Haskell WL. Energy cost of walking in normal children and in those with cerebral palsy: comparison of heart rate and oxygen uptake. *J Pediatr Orthop* 1989; 9:276–279.
71. Rubin CT, Lanyon LE. Regulation of bone formation by applied loads. *J Bone Joint Surg Am* 1984;66:397–402.
72. Schafer G. Infants can learn decontextualized words before their first birthday. *Child Dev* 2005;76:87–96.
73. Shaw NJ, Weite CP, Fraser WD, Rosenbloom L. Osteopenia in cerebral palsy. *Arch Phys Med Rehab* 1994;7:235–238.
74. Sienko-Thomas S, Moore, CA, Kelp-Lenane C, Norris C. Simulated gait patterns: the resulting effects on gait parameters, dynamic, electromyography, joint moments, and physiological cost index. *Gait Posture* 1996;4:100–107.
75. Simms B. The route learning ability of young people with Spina Bifida and hydrocephalus and their able-bodied peers. *Z Kinderchir* 1987;42(suppl 1):53–56.
76. Sival DA, Prechtl HF, Sonder GH, Touwen BC. The effect of intrauterine breech position on postnatal motor functions of the lower limbs. *Early Hum Dev* 1993;32:161–176.
77. Stallings VA, Cronk CE, Zemel BS, Charney EB. Body composition in children with spastic quadriplegic cerebral palsy. *J Pediatr* 1995;126:833–839.

78. Stansfield BW, Hillman SJ, Hazlewood ME, et al. Normalized speed, not age, characterizes ground reaction force patterns in 5- to 12-year-old children walking at self-selected speeds. *J Pediatr Orthop* 2001;21:395–402.

79. Stansfield BW, Hillman SJ, Hazlewood ME, et al. Sagittal joint kinematics, moments, and powers are predominantly characterized by speed of progression, not age, in normal children. *J Pediatr Orthop* 2001;21:403–411.

80. Stanton D, Wilson PN, Foreman N. Effects of early mobility on shortcut performance in a simulated maze. *Beh Brain Res* 2002;136(1):61–66.

81. Statham L, Murray MP. Early walking patterns of normal children. *Clin Orthop* 1971;70:8–24.

82. Stiles J. Neural plasticity and cognitive development. *Dev Neuropsychol* 2000;18:237–272.

83. Sutherland D, Olshen R, Biden E, et al. *The Development of Mature Walking*. Philadelphia: Lippincott; 1988.

84. Takegami Y. Wave pattern of ground reaction force of growing children. *J Pediatr Orthop* 1992;12:522–526.

85. Thelen E. Motor development: a new synthesis. *Am Psychol* 1995;50:79–94.

86. Thelan E. Treadmill-elicited stepping in seven-month-old infants. *Child Dev* 1986;57:1498–1506.

87. Thelen E, Cooke DW. Relationship between newborn stepping and later walking: a new interpretation. *Dev Med Child Neurol* 1987;29:380–393.

88. Thelen E, Fisher DM, Ridley-Johnson R. The relationship between physical growth and a newborn reflex. *Infant Behavior Dev* 1984;7:479–493.

89. Todd FN, Lamoreux LW, Skinner SR, et al. Variations in the gait of normal children. A graph applicable to the documentation of abnormalities. *J Bone Joint Surg Am* 1989;71:196–204.

90. van der Linden ML, Kerr AM, Hazlewood ME, et al. Kinematic and kinetic gait characteristics of normal children walking at a range of clinically relevant speeds. *J Pediatr Orthop* 2002;22:800–806.

91. Vaughn CL, Langerak NG, O'Malley MJ. Neuromaturation of human locomotion revealed by non-dimensional scaling. *Exp Brain Res* 2003;153:123–127.

92. Waters RL, Hislop HJ, Thomas L, et al. Energy cost of walking in normal children and teenagers. *Dev Med Child Neurol* 1983;25:184–188.

93. Wedell K, Newman CV, Reid P, Bradbury IR. An exploratory study of the relationship between size constancy and experience of mobility in cerebral palsied children. *Dev Med Child Neurol* 1972;14:615–620.

94. Weisglas-Kuperus N, Baerts W, Fetter WP, et al. Minor neurological dysfunction and quality of movement in relation to neonatal cerebral damage and subsequent development. *Dev Med Child Neurol* 1994;36:727–735.

95. Wheelwright EF, Minns RA, Law HT, et al. Temporal and spatial parameters of gait in children. I: Normal control data. *Dev Med Child Neurol* 1993;35:102–113.

96. Wiener-Vacher S, Ledebt A, Bril B. Changes in otolithic vestibulo-ocular reflex of off vertical axis rotation in infants learning to walk: preliminary results of a longitudinal study. *Ann N Y Acad Sci* 1996;781:709–712.

97. Wiener-Vacher SR, Toupet F, Narcy P. Canal and otolith vestibulo-ocular reflexes to vertical and off vertical axis rotations in children learning to walk. *Act Otolaryngol* (Stockh) 1996;116:657–665.

98. Wilmshurst S, Ward K, Adams JE, Langton CM, Mughal MZ. Mobility status and bone density in cerebral palsy. *Arch Dis Childhood* 1996;7:5,164–165.

99. Woollacott M, Assaiante C. Developmental changes in compensatory reponses to unexpected resistance of leg lift during gait initiation. *Exp Brain Res* 2002;144:385–396.

100. Woollacott M, Burtner P, Jensen J, Jasiewicz J, Roncesvalles N, Sveistrup H. Development of postural responses during standing in healthy children and children with spastic diplegia. *Neuroscience Biobehav Rev* 1998;22:583–589.

APPENDIX

The set of equations described below make it possible to determine if a child achieves an appropriate stride length given their body height and chosen walking speed. The graph shown in Figure 7-3 illustrates the mathematical relationship between stride length, cadence, and body height for normal children walking over a range of speeds. In order to relate mathematically the gait variables to height, a three-dimensional surface was fitted to experimental data from 324 children (Todd et al., 1989). Data points were plotted against three perpendicular scales representing walking speed, stride length, and body height.

Two equations define the normal reference curves in Figure 7-3, one for boys, and one for girls. Each equation depends on six constants (C1-C6), which, taken together with a child's height, enable computation of a second order curve relating stride length and walking speed. In these computations, "H" represents the child's height in centimeters, and "C1" through "C6" are constants, defined in the table below, which were derived from normal data. Two intermediate values (A and B) are calculated as follows:

For example, using the equations to calculate the predicted stride length for a 6-year-old girl, 112 cm in height, who is walking 53.3 m per minute, yields the following:

Intermediate value $A = 9.8$; intermediate value $B = 11$. Thus, her predicted stride length in cm. = 82.5 cm. If her actual measured stride length is 76.5 cm, her stride length normalized to height and walking speed is 93% of her non-impaired peers.

ACKNOWLEDGMENTS

This project was supported in part by a Distinguished Research Fellowship from the National Institute of Disability and Rehabilitation Research (NIDRR) awarded to Rosanne Kermoian. M. Elise Johanson's contribution was made possible in part by the Department of Veteran Affairs, Rehabilitation Research and Development Service, Project #B2785R.

$$Stride\ Length = A * \sqrt{Speed} + B$$

$$A = C1 * H^2 + C2 * H + C3 \qquad\qquad B = C4 * H^2 + C5 * H + C6$$

	C1	C2	C3	C4	C5	C6
BOYS	-0.0002802	0.1544256	-3.5589657	-0.0010762	0.2803360	-10.3155200
GIRLS	-0.0005145	0.1896516	-5.0245599	-0.0002684	0.2465649	-13.2757848

Chapter 8

Gait Adaptations in Adulthood: Pregnancy, Aging, and Alcoholism

Erin E. Butler, Maurice Druzin, and Edith V. Sullivan

In this chapter we describe the changes to the normal adult gait pattern that occur with pregnancy, aging, and alcoholism. We present an overview of the physiological processes enabling healthy gait and balance and how changes with pregnancy and the normal aging process contribute to changes in the normal adult gait pattern. We also identify some factors that can predict when a person will fall and provide information about practices that can reduce the risk of falling and improve gait and overall health. Finally, we discuss the changes that occur with acute alcohol use and chronic alcoholism, where the effects of alcohol disrupt normal balance and gait.

From the time gait matures in childhood (28,209), it remains stable through midlife. For example, velocity, one of the most basic parameters of gait, remains relatively unchanged between the ages of 10 to 59 years (25,156). A decline in the comfortable walking speed does not occur until after 60 years of age. Many gait variables are highly correlated with walking speed (118), suggesting that gait kinematics also remain stable until the age of 60 years. Similarly, postural equilibrium is most stable between the ages of 16 to 60 years and declines thereafter (91). Thus, there are few natural changes in gait or postural stability until later in life, other than the transient changes that occur during pregnancy.

PREGNANCY

Throughout the 280 days of human gestation, numerous physical and hormonal changes take place in a woman's body. Many of these changes, including weight gain, position of the body's center of gravity, increased joint laxity, and alterations in skeletal alignment, lead to an altered posture and gait. These changes influence postural stability and may cause musculoskeletal pain and discomfort.

Physiological Changes and Posture

The majority of women experience musculoskeletal pain during the course of pregnancy (85). On average, the total weight gain is approximately 9 to 14 kg (2,197). Most of the weight gained is due to the enlarging uterus, fetus, and breasts. The lower trunk has significantly greater rates of change than all other body segments during the second and third trimester of pregnancy (97). This weight gain leads to increased forces on the articular cartilage at the joints. As the fetus grows, the position of the mother's center of gravity moves superiorly and anteriorly (68). The developing fetal load places an increased demand on the lumbar spine and abdominal muscles (92). The changing shape and inertia of the lower trunk requires postural adjustments that can cause back pain.

Increased ligamentous laxity during pregnancy allows for greater joint motion at the pelvis (3) and the peripheral joints (32,52,188). Beginning in the tenth to twelfth week of pregnancy, the sacroiliac synchondroses and symphysis pubis begin to widen. The hormone relaxin is thought to be a major contributor to increases in joint laxity (123). The dramatic decrease in the strength of the abdominal muscles is related to excessive lengthening and overstretching of the muscles to accommodate the fetus (57,71).

A qualitative assessment of standing posture during pregnancy reveals an elevation of the head, hyperextension of the cervical spine, and extension of the knee and ankle joints (68). Similarly, a quantitative analysis of standing posture reveals a more posterior head position and an increase in lumbar lordosis and anterior pelvic tilt (65).

These alterations in joint laxity, weight, and alignment of the spine are related to decreased postural stability and the development of physical discomfort. Indeed, the most common areas of pain during pregnancy are the low-back, pelvis, hips, knees, and calves (180).

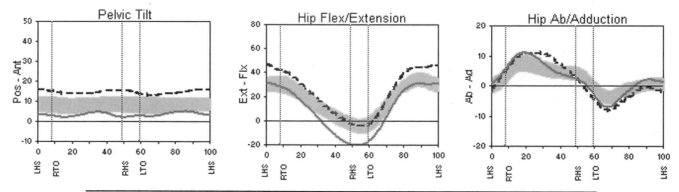

FIGURE 8-1. Comparison of pelvic and hip kinematic measures of gait during the first trimester (*solid line*) and the third trimester (*dashed line*) for one pregnant subject. Note the increased maximum anterior pelvic tilt, increased maximum hip flexion, and increased stance-phase hip adduction. Motion & Gait Analysis Laboratory, Lucile Packard Children's Hospital at Stanford.

Gait and Balance during Pregnancy

Gait during pregnancy has been described by the temporospatial characteristics of velocity, stride length, steps taken per minute (cadence), and time spent in single or double support, i.e., with one or both feet on the ground. Gait can be further analyzed in terms of joint kinematics and kinetics. However, to date, only a few studies have addressed these parameters during pregnancy.

A cinematographic analysis of two young pregnant subjects during treadmill walking revealed no differences in temporal measures or sagittal plane kinematics of the lower limbs throughout the term of pregnancy (210). The authors speculate that the gradual advancement of pregnancy allows the body time to adjust to the new loads. However, this study failed to address the impact of pregnancy on kinetics and on movement in the frontal and transverse planes. Golomer et al. (76) studied ten women between the third and eighth months of pregnancy. Although the subjects' velocity remained constant during that time, there was a trend indicating an increased cadence and decreased step length. The authors proposed that the maintenance of velocity throughout pregnancy reflects the body's ability to adapt to the change in posture and economize total energy expenditure.

A three-dimensional kinematic and kinetic gait analysis performed on 15 women between 35 and 40 weeks of pregnancy revealed statistically significant increases in maximum anterior pelvic tilt, maximum hip flexion, and stance-phase hip adduction during walking, compared to values at 1 year postpartum (64). Increases were found in the maximum hip extensor moment, maximum hip abductor moments, maximum hip power generation in the sagittal and frontal planes, the maximum ankle plantar flexor moment, and maximum ankle plantar flexion power absorption. However, these changes were determined to be secondary to substantial increases in body mass and an anterior shift of the center of gravity. There was also a sig-

nificant increase in double-support time and a decrease in single-support time. In a similar analysis performed at our laboratory, we found a trend toward increased maximum anterior pelvic tilt, increased maximum hip flexion, and increased stance-phase hip adduction between the first and third trimester of pregnancy (Figure 8-1).

Base of support during walking has been found to increase significantly in pregnant women (22). Although step width increases, pelvic width also increases; thus, the ratio of base of support to pelvic width remains constant (64). An investigation of plantar foot pressures in pregnant women at 38 weeks gestational age revealed increased loads on the lateral side of the foot and the hindfoot compared to nonpregnant controls (155). Most physiologic and morphologic changes of pregnancy persist for 4 to 6 weeks postpartum (6).

Static postural sway has been found to increase throughout pregnancy (68). Good static postural control is characterized by a small sway path, and by a small area covered by the center of foot pressure movements (217). While it might be suspected that this decreased postural stability is related to an increase in the height of the center of gravity and the development of the fetal load, much of this sway remains present at six weeks postpartum (68). The authors speculated that the decrease in postural stability may be related to laxity of the pelvic ligaments, since laxity does not readily return to pregravida conditions, unlike other mechanical factors.

Approximately 25% of all women employed during pregnancy experience a fall, a rate comparable to elderly persons aged 65 years and older (53). The leading causes of falls at work for pregnant women include slippery floors, moving at a fast pace, and carrying an object or a child. The aforementioned physiological changes and the increased levels of postural instability during pregnancy may lead to this high incidence of falls in the (employed) pregnant population.

Exercise during Pregnancy

The American College of Obstetricians and Gynecologists states, "in the absence of medical or obstetric complications, 30 minutes or more of moderate exercise a day on most, if not all, days of the week is recommended for pregnant women" (6). This recommendation is based on research which shows that women who exercise more during pregnancy have decreased lengths of hospital stays, reduced incidence of cesarean section, higher Apgar scores of newborn infants (81), and a 24% reduced risk of preeclampsia (199) than women who do not exercise during pregnancy. Additionally, regular exercise during pregnancy is related to reduced discomforts of swelling, leg cramps, fatigue, and shortness of breath (87,202). Exercise may also be beneficial in the prevention of gestational diabetes, especially in morbidly obese women (6).

Walking is one of the most beneficial forms of exercise during pregnancy, and is the preferred exercise by the majority of pregnant women (87,149,154). In a study of nearly 10,000 pregnant women, 43% of women reported walking as their leading activity, followed by swimming (12%), and aerobics (12%) (234). However, pregnant women should be aware of the decreased levels of oxygen available for aerobic exercise and modify the intensity of their workouts accordingly (6).

In summary, pregnancy results in physical and hormonal changes that affect postural balance and gait. Research to date indicates that the most prominent changes in gait are increased maximum anterior pelvic tilt, increased maximum hip flexion, and increased stance-phase hip adduction. The majority of gait and postural stability measures return to baseline after 6 weeks postpartum.

AGING

Over the last 40 years, the elderly population in the United States, age 65 years and older, has increased by 110% (220). The elderly population at age 85 and older is projected to be the fastest growing age group, doubling in size from 1995 to the year 2030, and increasing fivefold by the year 2050. This extension in lifespan is unfortunately often associated with diminished walking ability and decreased postural stability that results in frequent falls and injury. It has been documented that a large proportion (45%) of falls occur during walking (157,170,226).

Falls account for nearly half of all geriatric trauma cases (77,177), representing a leading cause of injury death in persons aged 65 to 79 years, second only to motor vehicle traffic accidents (150). For persons over 80 years, falls are the leading cause of death (150). Upwards of 90% of hip fractures are directly related to falling (146) and approximately 75% of patients who were independent ambulators prior to hip fracture become functionally dependent for walking 6 to 12 months after injury (99,135,139).

Considerable financial costs are associated with the functional dependence that occurs after falls in the elderly. Functionally dependent elderly incur $10,000 more in healthcare expenditures over 2 years than similarly aged independent persons (67). In 1995, $26. 1 billion was spent on healthcare for the 1.4 million persons making the transition from an independent to a dependent living status (128). Although less than 12% of the population is older than the age of 65 years (221), this group sustains 25% to 28% of all fatal injuries and accounts for 33% to 38% of the total US trauma care costs (43,61,148,160). Therefore, it is of general public concern to understand the impact of the aging process on falling and investigate methods to combat the risks of falling in the elderly.

Normal Age-Related Changes that Affect Gait and Balance

Changes associated with aging that negatively affect balance and gait include declining strength, muscle mass, and bone density; redistributed body mass; impaired respiratory capacity; selective atrophy of central nervous system components controlling balance and gait; and deterioration in peripheral sensory functions. Additionally, the increased use of medications in the elderly may also have a negative impact on balance and gait.

Strength, Muscle Mass and Bone Density, Respiratory Capacity. Strength, muscle mass, and bone density decline with age. The age-related change in muscle mass and function is called 'sarcopenia,' *sarx* meaning flesh and *penia* meaning loss in Greek (183). Consequences of sarcopenia include decreased strength, metabolic rate, and maximal oxygen consumption (138). Sarcopenia is multifactorial and affects mostly type II (fast-twitch) skeletal muscle fiber number (129) and cross-sectional area (8,129). Lack of regular physical activity, change in protein metabolism (i.e., a deficit between protein synthesis and degradation), alterations in the endocrine system, including decreases in growth hormone and testosterone and an increase in cortisol and cytokines, loss of neuromuscular function, altered gene expression, and cell apoptosis all underlie the age-related change in muscle mass (138). Cross-sectional and longitudinal studies have found a significant relation between muscle strength and gait velocity (9,19,59,93).

Associated with a decline in muscle mass are changes in body composition. Body fat increases while muscle mass decreases (8,89,90,198). This shift in body composition with age is often masked by relative stability in overall body weight and occurs even in physically active older adults who exercise (138). With advancing age, the mass of the upper body increases at the expense of the lower body, thereby elevating the body's center of mass (158).

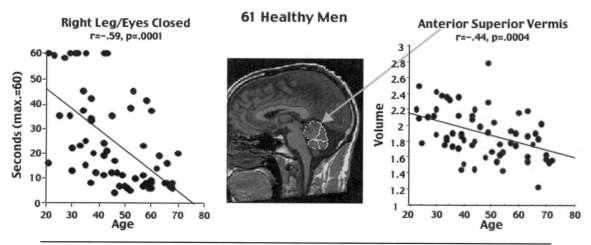

FIGURE 8-2. The data presented are based on 61 healthy men, spanning the normal adult age range and are taken from Sullivan et al. (204). *Left panel:* Number of seconds an individual was able to stand on one leg with eyes closed. Note the marked decline in ability with advancing age. Middle panel: Midsagittal slice of a high-resolution MRI, displaying manual outlining of regions of the cerebellar vermis (44). The anterior superior vermis declines in volume with age (*right panel*), and its volume is related to balance ability (204,205).

Additionally, a change in body posture as a result of skeletal changes may lead to the stooped posture observed in the elderly, causing an anterior shift in the body's center of mass and an increased demand on the posterior muscles, further stressing the balance control system (29,158). In addition, muscle strength and age have been shown to be independent predictors of loss of balance (102). Thus, with increasing age and decreasing muscle strength, loss of balance becomes more probable.

In a multisite study of over 54,000 healthy, non-smoking men and women, aged 30 to 70 years, measurements showed a loss of 0.36% per year for the musculoskeletal system and a loss of 0.84% per year for the respiratory system (193). These losses may lead to a reduced resistance to fatigue and an inability to sustain long periods of walking. Reduction in maximal energy capacity (lower VO_2 maximum) results in a proportionally higher cost of energy during walking (158). Zeleznik (233) reported a qualitative emphysematous change in lung histology and lung-thorax mechanics in the elderly. Although these changes, along with altered lung volumes, affect oxygenation and oxygen consumption levels, there is no evidence that the changes in the respiratory system with aging have a negative impact on the daily activities of older adults. Only when physiologic demands reach the limits of supply do they become evident.

Central Nervous System. Age-related changes of the central nervous system may negatively affect gait and balance. These changes include shrinkage of neuronal soma and processes of the cerebral cortex (110), especially in the frontal lobe, and similar degradation of cell structure in the vermis of the cerebellum (161,162). Although neuronal loss does not necessarily occur with aging (50),

decreases in dendritic connections and receptor sites do occur (62,108,163) and likely contribute to compromise of neurotransmitter activity, especially of the dopamine system affected in Parkinson's disease and other movement disorders (for reviews, see [78,79]). A notable exception is the substantia nigra, which loses 5% to 10% of its cells per decade (179). White matter also shows disruptive age-related degradation (110) of myelin and microtubules and axon deletion (1,145). These white matter changes may contribute to motor slowing and other features of gait that characterize normal aging, including stooped posture, shortened stride, and loss of motion fluidity.

Magnetic resonance imaging (MRI) studies have documented volume shrinkage of tissue in regional cerebral and cerebellar cortex in normal aging (23,24,41,79,98,166,172,175,204,207) that can contribute to postural instability. Degradation of basal ganglia motor and attentional systems (173), cerebellar-pontine circuitry (208), and frontal lobes (167,172) associated with aging can also exert untoward forces on gait and balance. For example, declines in the gray matter of the anterior superior vermis may underlie imbalance in static posture, measured quantitatively with the Fregley-Graybiel Walk-a-Line Test battery (66) (Figure 8-2).

A general relation has been noted between brain white matter abnormalities and falls in the elderly. Early studies using computed tomography (CT) reported correlations between the numbers of hypodensities read on CT films and impaired gait and disequilibrium (140). Later studies using MRI (98,189) noted greater frequency and extent of white matter signal hyperintensities, typically occurring in deep white matter and periventricularly, as predictive of impaired gait or high incidence of falls (16,18,31,35,211).

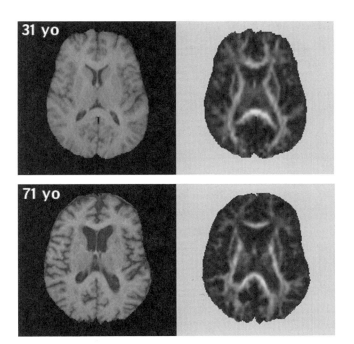

FIGURE 8-3. Left two axial images are from high-resolution MRI at the level of the lateral ventricles. Right two axial images are from diffusion tensor imaging, where the brighter the white, the higher the white matter anisotropy, a measure of fiber tract integrity. Note the expanded ventricles and sulci in the 71 year old (*bottom left*) and less intense anisotropy (*bottom right*), especially in the frontal regions of the brain. (Images reproduced from reference 168).

The volume of white matter on MRI has been shown to be significantly correlated with the development of gait and balance impairments in the elderly over a 10-year period (17). Neuropathologic correlation with antemortem MRI indicate that the white matter signals abnormalities that are associated with degradation of myelin, thinning of ventricular membrane, and increased interstitial spaces (16). Recent studies using diffusion tensor imaging, a measure of white matter microstructural fiber coherence, provide further evidence that widespread degradation of brain white matter in normal aging is predictive of declines in static balance (203) (Figure 8-3).

Peripheral Sensory and Motor Loss. In addition to age-related changes in the central nervous system, older people experience a number of peripheral sensory deficits that significantly affect their ability to maintain balance and avoid falls. The peripheral nervous system suffers age-related compromise that may affect gait and balance, including cell dysmorphology of motor neurons of the spinal cord and decreased density and number of peripheral nerve fibers (187).

Older adults typically have significantly poorer visual acuity (both high- and low-contrast), contrast sensitivity, and depth perception than younger adults (147). Consequently, healthy older persons require approximately three

times as much contrast as younger persons for the detection of objects in the environment (213). Unfortunately, while visual acuity is decreasing, there is an increased reliance on the visual system to guide locomotion in the elderly (158). When elderly and young subjects were asked to walk a straight path while wearing liquid crystal glasses that provided a view of the terrain only when they pressed a handheld switch, the elderly subjects had longer viewing durations of the terrain than the younger subjects. In addition, the elderly had a 50% success rate changing their step length when cued 1 to 2 steps before, versus an 80% success rate for the younger group. Thus, the increased reliance on vision for guidance during walking may serve to compensate for a decreased ability to alter step lengths in avoiding an unstable or dangerous surface. In short, the elderly need to pay more attention to the terrain in order to allow more time to plan required avoidance and compensation strategies.

Medications. The elderly take more medication than younger individuals do, and these prescription medications by themselves or in combination can negatively affect the neuromuscular and vestibular systems (213). Benzodiazepines, tricyclic antidepressants, neuroleptics, and psychotropic medications are the most common problem sources related to declines in gait and balance (51,131,187).

CHANGES IN GAIT WITH AGE

Temporal and Spatial Parameters. Older persons generally adopt a more conservative gait pattern than young people; that is, older persons walk more slowly, take shorter steps, and are more variable in step timing than younger people (147). Walking on an irregular surface increases the characteristics of this type of conservative gait in the elderly. The age-related decrease in overall strength means that older people need to use a greater percentage of muscle power during gait. This can lead to the use of alternative muscles for propulsive power (158) that can alter temporospatial parameters, such as stride length and velocity. As mentioned previously, there is a direct relation between muscle strength and gait velocity (9,19,59,93).

Decreased gait velocity in the elderly is a function of greater time spent in double support and decreased step length, rather than decreased cadence (25,100,156,187,227). The increase in double support times may reflect impaired motor control of the body during single support (104). Table 8-1 shows the average results for these temporospatial parameters for a typical healthy young adult, a healthy elderly adult, and an elderly adult with pathologic gait tested in our laboratory.

A study investigating the relationship between step length and joint kinetics in older subjects (average age 79 years) and younger subjects (average age 26 years)

▶ **TABLE 8-1 Comparison of Temporospatial Parameters Between Healthy and Impaired Elderly Adults and Young Adults**

Temporal-Spatial Parameters	Healthy 30-Year-Old	Healthy 75-Year-Old	Impaired 80-Year-Old
Velocity (cm/s)	140.9 ± 2.77	88.3 ± 7.47	71.7 ± 6.29
Cadence (steps/min)	110.6 ± 2.13	95.3 ± 4.21	99.7 ± 5.35
Stride Length (cm)	145.1 ± 3.06	117.8 ± 4.75	87.2 ± 6.37
Double Support (% cycle)	22.0 ± 1.70	25.3 ± 2.50	33.4 ± 7.50
Step Width (cm)	12.5 ± 1.36	13.0 ± 0.93	15.8 ± 0.88

Notice the trend toward decreased velocity and stride length, and increased double support time and step width with increasing age and pathology. Motion & Gait Analysis Laboratory, Lucile Packard Children's Hospital at Stanford.

found that older persons had a 12% shorter step length during normal walking, when corrected for leg length, than younger persons (104). Elble et al. (54) found a 17% to 20% reduction in gait velocity and stride length in an elderly group compared with young adults. Stride width variability has also been found to increase with age (26,78).

A diminished ability to maintain high levels of speed with advancing age occur even in elite athletes. Sprint performance, for example, declines with age in elite runners (120). This decline becomes most evident around 65 to 70 years of age. Master runners of both sexes (men, 40 to 88 years, women, 35 to 87 years) were recorded with high-speed cameras at the European Veterans Athletic Championships. The velocity during a 100-m sprint decreased 5% to 6% per decade in men and 5% to 7% per decade in women. Stride length showed clear reductions with increasing age, whereas cadence remained relatively unchanged. Ground contact time was significantly longer, and flight time was shorter in older age groups.

Kinematics and Kinetics. Increased joint stiffness and reduced functional range of motion with age may limit the ability of otherwise healthy muscles to generate power at the variable speeds required to navigate different terrains (158). Supporting this possibility are the observations of decreased push-off power at the ankle and a more flat-footed landing in the elderly compared with young adults (227). The joint motions most likely to be limited by musculotendinous tightness or articular disease include peak ankle dorsiflexion, peak knee extension, and peak hip extension (105). Figures 8-4 and 8-5 illustrate some of the ways in which typical young, healthy elderly, and impaired elderly persons differ in kinematic and kinetic parameters at the ankle and hip. Elderly persons may also exhibit reductions in maximum toe-floor clearance, arm swing, and rotations of the hips and knees; however, these differences may be due to reductions in velocity and stride length, rather than age alone (54).

Healthy older people exhibit increased anterior pelvic tilt, reduced peak hip extension in stance, and decreased peak ankle plantar flexion in swing, independent of speed (100,113,115). The consistent reduction in peak hip extension and compensatory increase in anterior pelvic tilt during both comfortable and fast speeds indicate the prevalence of hip flexion contractures in the elderly population (115).

Maximum gait velocity and leg power decline with advancing age and are positively correlated (121). In a group of elderly women, weaker subjects demonstrated lower concentric ankle and eccentric knee mechanical energy expenditures and higher eccentric low-back mechanical energy expenditures than stronger subjects (144). As previously noted, a decrease in overall strength requires a greater percentage of muscle activation during gait, which may lead to the use of alternative muscles for propulsive power, such as hip and low-back muscles, and also suggests a more proximal mechanism of motor control during gait with advancing age.

At self-selected walking speeds, elderly adults generate less joint torque and power in the lower extremities than young adults. Several studies have reported a decrease in ankle plantar flexor power during the late stance phase of gait in the elderly, when adjusted for speed (45). The decline in ankle plantar flexor power across the age and health status is illustrated in Figure 8-4. DeVita and Hortobagyi (45) report increases in hip extensor moment and power in healthy elderly subjects, with simultaneous reductions in ankle and knee power. Figure 8-5 illustrates the increase in hip extensor moments in stance with age, especially notable between the healthy 30-year-old and the healthy 75-year-old. Judge et al. (100) report an increase hip flexor power in older persons to compensate for reduced plantar flexor power, and McGibbon and Krebs (143) report increases in knee power absorption in late stance and hip extensor power in early stance. While not all of these studies agree in the specific aspects of change, they do suggest that neuromuscular changes that occur with aging cause changes in gait characteristics.

Changes in Static Balance with Age

Stability during walking is dependent upon normal postural control (104). Postural equilibrium is most stable between the ages of 16 to 60 years (91). Function of

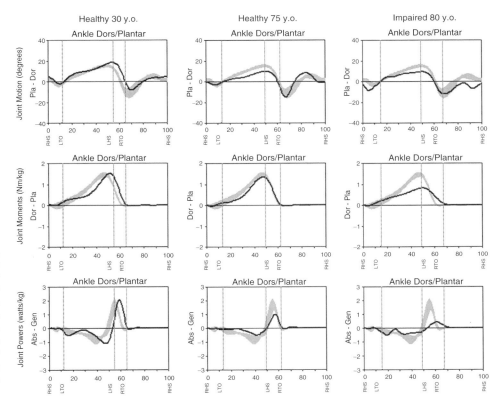

FIGURE 8-4. Sagittal plane ankle motion, moments, and power for a healthy 30-year old, a healthy 75-year old, and an 80-year old with pathological gait. Note the reduced ankle dorsiflexion and diminished ankle power generation in late stance in both of the elderly subjects. Motion & Gait Analysis Laboratory, Lucile Packard Children's Hospital at Stanford.

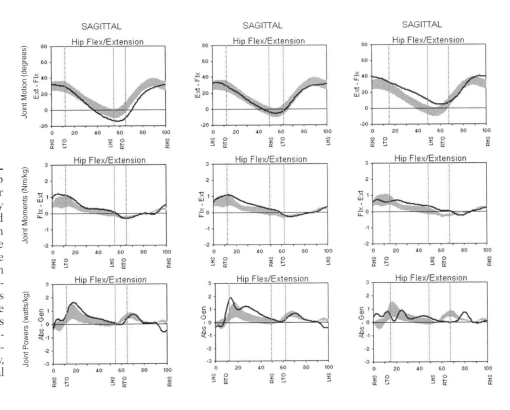

FIGURE 8-5. Sagittal plane hip motion, moments, and power for a healthy 30-year-old, a healthy 75-year old, and an 80-year old with pathologic gait. A reduction in peak hip extension and an increase in hip power during late stance can be observed, particularly in the healthy elderly subject, compared to the young subject. It has been suggested that this increase in hip power in late stance serves to compensate for diminished plantar flexor power in late stance. Motion & Gait Analysis Laboratory, Lucile Packard Children's Hospital at Stanford.

the sensory system begins to degrade after the age of 65 years, adversely affecting balance and contributing to falls. A reduction in somatosensation and vestibular function has been strongly linked to postural instability in elderly adults (133,137,165). After age 60 years, sway velocity during quiet standing increases, with the largest values found in persons older than 76 years of age (91). Advancing age correlates significantly with longer sway path lengths and greater postural sway velocity during quiet standing (12,84,194) and occurs regardless of visual conditions (eyes open, eyes open with visual feedback, and eyes closed) (13,37,56,80,119,182).

The increased reliance on the visual system to guide locomotion in the elderly also applies to postural stability. An investigation of women, aged 20 to 80 years, found an age-related increased reliance on vision for postural stability, beginning at the age of 40 years (37). Sway velocities increase with the eyes closed in all age groups, but improve with eyes open, even in the elderly (91). Indeed, reduced visual input increases the odds of a loss of balance fivefold (102).

The use of multiple sensorimotor (tactile, visual, and stance) cues can also improve postural sway (94,218). Figure 8-6 demonstrates the anterior-posterior and medial-lateral postural sway paths for a young healthy woman and an elderly healthy woman during quiet standing. Notice how the sensorimotor cues improve postural sway in both the young and elderly subjects.

The range of trunk angular sway and angular velocity in the medial-lateral and anterior-posterior planes is greater in elderly subjects (ages 65 to 75 years) than middle-aged (45 to 55 years) or young subjects (15 to 25 years) in stance and stance-related tasks, such as tandem walking (70). Increased trunk angular sway and angular velocity indicate an increase in balance instability and may be useful in detecting balance disorders in individuals prone to falling (70).

Amiridis et al. (7) measured center of pressure variations, ankle and hip electromyographic activity (tibialis anterior, medial gastrocnemius, rectus femoris, and semitendinosus) and hip and ankle kinematics in older adults (mean age 70.1 ± 4.3 years) and younger adults (20.1 ± 2.4 years). The elderly group had significantly greater and more variable center of pressure excursions than the younger adults in normal quiet standing, tandem Romberg stance (nondominant heel in front of the dominant toe, arms on the hips), and one-legged stance (standing on the dominant leg with the nonsupporting leg flexed and stabilized on the standing leg). In addition, the elderly showed an increased reliance on the hip muscles for maintaining upright balance during tandem Romberg stance and one-legged stance tasks. No significant difference was noted in the ankle muscles. This overreliance on the hip muscles has also been noted in elderly gait (100).

Physiological control mechanisms considered to contribute to static posture involve two basic component processes: a short-term and long-term component. The short-term component behaves like an open-loop control system mostly devoid of feedback, whereas the long-term component behaves like a closed-loop system with feedback based on afferent input (145,146). The open-loop component is affected little by attentional and other cognitive

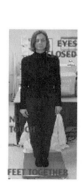

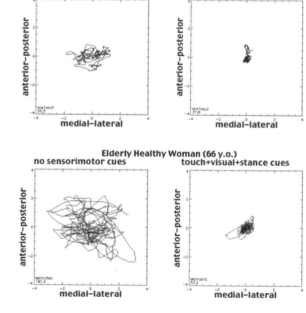

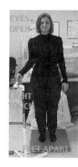

FIGURE 8-6. Postural sway for a young healthy woman and an elderly healthy woman without (*left panels*) and with (*right panels*) the aid of sensorimotor cues. The plots are stabilograms, taken from center of pressure calculations; sampling rate was 50 Hz and the resulting sway paths are averages of three 30-second trials. Note the significant reduction in sway path length for the younger (*top two plots*) and the older (*bottom two plots*) when cues are available. Without cues, the sway path of the older woman is substantially longer than that of the younger woman.

processes and is temporally brief (40,49,96). The closed-loop component can be affected by internal and external perceptual information. Several experiments demonstrated that the sway paths of young healthy adults (176), elderly adults (195), sober alcoholics (205), and individuals with fetal alcohol exposure (181) can increase under conditions of sensory challenge that influence the open-loop control component of balance.

Sway can increase while engaging in a cognitive task that influences closed–loop control, indicating that static balance is not solely under automatic control. A study quantifying cognitive demands of secondary tasks demonstrated a linear relationship between increased sway and task difficulty (159). Sway can also be affected by the nature of a secondary task. Tasks requiring articulation cause more interference to stability than do mental tasks (42) and may be related to timing factors intrinsic to speech prosody (157). The difficulty levels of the primary balance and the secondary cognitive tasks may increase independently without interacting (112,122) to permit separate assessment of each task (232). However, the presence of pathology associated with aging or neurologic conditions may introduce an interaction between tasks as a function of difficulty.

Slips and Falls

A fall is defined as "an event which results in a person coming to rest inadvertently on the ground or other lower level, and other than a consequence of the following: sustaining a violent blow, loss of consciousness, sudden onset of paralysis, as in a stroke, or an epileptic seizure" (69). For the elderly, falls may be an outcome of the deficits in gait and static balance described above.

Independent risk factors for serious falls are older age; white race; decreased bone and mineral density; low body mass index; cognitive impairment; abnormal neuromuscular findings, such as decreased reaction time or balance disturbance; poor visual acuity; previous history of falls and fall injuries; and specific chronic illnesses (216).

In a study of the biomechanics of slips and falls, kinematic and kinetic measurements of young and elderly participants were obtained on slippery and nonslippery walking surfaces. Older subjects were found to have a significantly faster horizontal heel contact velocity, shorter step length, and slower transitional acceleration of the whole body center of mass during walking than younger subjects (130). Older participants were also found to slip longer and faster and fall more often than younger participants.

Gait Predictors of Falls. A number of kinematic and kinetic gait variables distinguish elderly fallers from nonfallers. In general, the age-related effects on walking that occur in healthy nonfallers are exaggerated in elderly fallers. Fallers have a slower velocity and longer double support phase than elderly nonfallers (109), although these gait changes may be fear-related adaptations, rather than risk factors that increase the likelihood of falling. In a kinematic analysis of elderly gait, fallers had a reduced range of motion at the ankle and a delay in the maximum stance phase ankle dorsiflexion, which the authors speculate may be predictive of falls (109). An isolated and consistent reduction in hip extension during walking occurs with aging, but is exaggerated in elderly fallers compared with elderly nonfallers (113). Elderly fallers relative to nonfallers have also been shown to exhibit a substantially smaller first step at gait initiation, and the first step length variability of elderly fallers is more than twice that observed for nonfallers (142). An increased stride-to-stride variability in stride length, velocity, and double support time significantly increases the odds that an elderly person will experience future falls, regardless of fear of falling (136).

Kerrigan et al. (114) found an increase in peak external hip flexion moment in stance and reductions in the peak hip extension moment, knee flexion moment in preswing, and knee power absorption in preswing in elderly fallers compared with nonfallers, at both comfortable and fast speeds. Similarly, McGibbon et al. (144) found that the disabled elderly expend less ankle energy in late stance and more low-back energy in midstance than the healthy elderly. When controlling for walking speed, the difference in ankle mechanical energy expenditure disappeared, but midstance hip mechanical energy expenditure remained significantly higher in the disabled group. The authors suggest that increased energy transfer to the low-back and pelvis may be a strategy used to assist in advancing the swing leg. However, increased trunk energy may also compromise dynamic stability and increase the risk of falling.

Balance Predictors of Falls. Measures of balance also correlate with the number of falls a person sustains. Disequilibrium is often associated with frequent falls and concerns about falling (111).

To determine the physiological basis of age-related changes in postural control, center-of-pressure displacements and electromyographic data were collected from the tibialis anterior, soleus, vastus lateralis, and biceps femoris during quiet standing in elderly fallers, elderly nonfallers, and healthy young subjects (125). Elderly fallers demonstrated significantly greater sway in the anterior-posterior direction and greater muscle activity during quiet standing than the young subjects. Elderly nonfallers had significantly greater muscle activation and coactivation compared with younger subjects. Short-term postural sway was significantly correlated with muscle activity in each group. This study suggests that high levels of muscle activity are characteristic of age-related declines in postural stability and that such activity is correlated with short-term increases in postural sway.

Functional base of support is the anterior-posterior proportion of foot length used in maximal sustained forward and backward leaning. Base of support declines with age, and the extent of the decline may be a predictor of falls in older persons (117).

Fear of Falling. Falling begets falling. Fear of falling often leads to a reduction in activity levels and deconditioning, which leads to declines in the quality of life and physical well-being, and further increases the danger of falling (86,88,222). Indeed, fear of falling, which many older individuals express, is a liability because it can alter the magnitude of postural adjustment to maintain erect posture, resulting in overcorrection (4). Sway velocity on static and dynamic posturography is greater in elderly persons who report a fear of falling compared with those who do not (13,15).

EXERCISE TO IMPROVE GAIT AND AVOID FALLS

Although the physiological effects of aging are widely accepted as inevitable, physical activity and exercise throughout aging can diminish or even negate age's untoward effects (36). There are many benefits to exercise, including improved strength, flexibility, reaction time, gait, and postural control (192). Despite age-related decline in musculoskeletal and respiratory systems, the underlying plasticity of the muscles, autonomic nervous system, bones, and joints remains intact even in very elderly persons and is amenable to the effects of conditioning exercises (21,58–60). In one study of nine frail, institutionalized volunteers, average age 90 years, who underwent 8 weeks of high-intensity resistance training, strength increased 174% and mean tandem gait speed improved 48% (59).

Any exercise program designed for older individuals should incorporate the following four goals: increase conditioning, especially endurance; improve muscle strength, particularly of the lower extremities; minimize risk of injury; and promote enjoyment without causing excessive fatigue (124). The two main components of a good exercise program are dynamic aerobic exercise and strength training. Dynamic aerobic exercise includes walking, swimming, cycling, and jogging. In fact, brisk walking has been deemed one of the most ideal forms of exercise readily available to the elderly population (55) and has been shown to improve velocity, standing balance, speed of muscular contraction, and lead to an increase in the maximal rate of oxygen consumption and VO_2 maximum (30).

Gait velocity is directly related to muscle strength (9,19,59,93). Progressive resistive training, including hip and knee flexion/extension, ankle dorsi/plantar flexion, and hip ab/adduction exercises have been shown to significantly increase muscle strength in older persons (107,171,186,196). Strength training of the plantar flexor

muscles may also contribute to maintenance of step length in advanced age (100). A combination of resistance and balance training has been found to increase gait velocity by 13% in older persons (106), improve postural control (103,134) and reduce the incidence of falls (33,34,186). A hip flexor-stretching program for the elderly results in improvements in gait, with an increase in dynamic hip extension during both comfortable and fast walking speeds (116). The improved hip extension also leads to significant improvements in peak ankle plantar flexion and a tendency toward improved ankle power generation.

Home-based exercise programs have recently gained considerable attention for their ability to improve gait and functional performance. In one study (152), 70 community dwelling, elderly men and women completed a 6-month clinical trial. Half of the participants were given an exercise program focusing on strength and balance training and encouraged to increase overall physical activity; the other half of the participants were given 6 months of nutrition education. The exercise group was asked to perform body weight exercises, lower body strength training with ankle weights, upper body strength training with dumbbells, and balance training exercises 3 times per week. Exercises were demonstrated by an exercise physiologist and explained in a detailed booklet outlining the program. At the end of the six months, the exercise group saw a significant improvement in functional performance and balance and coordination, compared to the group who only received nutrition education. The authors concluded that a home-based, multidimensional exercise program in community-dwelling elders is feasible and can be effective in improving functional performance, despite limited supervision.

Additionally, Tai Chi has been shown to improve balance in the elderly (101,219,230). Tai Chi was originally developed as a martial art form but has been used by elderly Chinese people as an exercise form for the past 300 years (231). Tai Chi focuses on slow sequential movements, providing a smooth, continuous and low intensity activity. After only 4 weeks of intensive Tai Chi training, community-dwelling elderly subjects (mean age 69 years) significantly improved their ability to use somatosensory, visual, and vestibular information to control body sway during quiet standing, and an improved ability to voluntarily weight shift to various spatial positions within their base of support, compared to the control group (219). Furthermore, the improved balance performance at week 4 of the elderly subjects was comparable to that of experienced Tai Chi practitioners. One investigator points out that with Tai Chi training there is a counterintuitive reduction in anticipatory postural adjustments of standing posture while stability of standing is improved (63). These findings suggest that practicing Tai Chi may lead to a greater use of the elasticity of the peripheral structures involving muscles, ligaments, and tendons and a decrease in the participation of the central neutral structures in postural equilibrium, thereby improving postural stability.

Elderly adults who participate in sports and a high level of total physical activity, walking, or household activity experience a smaller decline in mobility over time than older adults who are inactive. In a 3-year prospective study of over 2,000 men and women aged 55 to 85 years, two mobility tests (timed 6 meter walk and repeated chair stands) were performed at baseline and again 3 years later. Continued physical activity was associated with the smaller decline in mobility (225). Older persons who exercise regularly perform better on tests of strength, flexibility, reaction time, walking, and balance maneuvers than older persons who do not exercise on a regular basis (20,132). Similarly, older adults who participate in 20 to 30 minutes of moderate-intensity exercise on most days of the week (1,000 kcal per week) have better physical function, e.g., endurance, lower extremity strength, gait speed, and balance, than older persons who are active throughout the day but do not exercise, or who are inactive (27).

Even if exercise has not been a lifelong habit, research shows that adults who participate in sports and physical activities in old age have better postural ability than adults who only exercised at an early age. In a study of 65 adults over the age of 60 years, those subjects who only started participating in sports and physical activities after age 60 had postural performances close to that of the subjects who had always exercised, and had significantly better balance than those subjects who only exercised at an early age or never exercised (164).

ALCOHOL AND ALCOHOLISM

Falling is one of the leading causes of morbidity and mortality in otherwise healthy individuals and its liability is exacerbated with alcohol (214,215). In an investigation of ground-level falls, ethanol was present in nearly 50% of all cases tested (83). Acute alcohol ingestion reduces the function of the vestibular system and leads to balance and gait disturbances. The acute effects of alcohol use include positional nystagmus and gaze nystagmus (127), reductions in the gain of the vestibulo-ocular reflex (169,190,212), and increases in body sway during static and dynamic posturography (75,127,153). A comparison of the sway pattern of subjects after acute alcohol ingestion closely resembles that of patients with chronic lesions of the cerebellar anterior lobe, i.e., the spinocerebellum (48,153).

The incidence of alcohol abuse and dependence is high, estimated at upwards of 15% of the US population and 30% to 35% of patients treated at university medical centers, making it a significant public health concern, although it is often overlooked in clinical interview (10). Thus, acknowl-

edgment of alcoholism, its potential effects on postural stability, its mechanisms of action, and strategies for mitigating imbalance should be pursued. In a recent survey of alcoholic men and women who volunteered for research studies, proportionately more alcoholics (60%) than controls (30%), regardless of sex, reported a history of at least one fall in the past year (184). Contributing special liability to falling is alcoholism and alcoholism's interaction with aging (47,72,204,223). The chronic effects of alcohol intoxication on balance and gait can linger in alcoholics who have withdrawn from alcoholism and remain sober (224).

Gait ataxia in alcoholics has traditionally been attributed to damage to the anterior superior vermis of the cerebellum, as determined with postmortem study (11,82,224). More recently, *in vivo* neuroimaging studies confirm these speculations and have reported significant correlations between alcoholism-related ataxia and low regional glucose metabolism quantified with positron emission tomography (73) and anterior superior vermian shrinkage quantified with MRI (204).

Balance platform studies of recovering alcoholics provide evidence for enduring instability measurable with static (46,126,223) or dynamic posturography, that is, stance during platform perturbation (126). Although degree of impaired postural control has been related to the amount of alcohol drunk in the 6 months prior to examination (228,229), persistent deficits in balance diminish with protracted sobriety in recovering alcoholics but do not necessarily fully resolve (185,206). Although peripheral neuropathy, which can be a concomitant of chronic alcoholism, may exacerbate imbalance, neuropathy does not necessarily account for imbalance (191). Another likely factor mitigating against full recovery is the presence of cerebellar pathology, noted in chronic alcoholics and also in children with prenatal alcohol exposure (200). Lesions in this vermian region characteristically result in postural tremor (~3 Hz) (74,151), which is prominent in the anterior-posterior direction (141,223) and detectable with spectral analysis of sway velocity (14).

A study from our laboratory (205) assessed sway during quiet standing in alcoholic men who had been sober for several months and examined whether postural instability, measured in terms of sway path length and direction, could be ameliorated by sensorimotor visual, tactual, or stance cues, which are known to exert stabilizing forces in normal, healthy adults (95). The alcoholics were significantly less stable than the controls when maintaining erect posture in the absence of visual, tactile, or stance cues. Although longer sobriety was predictive of shorter sway paths, residual imbalance without stabilizing cues was still measurable months after cessation of drinking. In the presence of cues, however, the sway paths of the alcoholics were indistinguishable from those of the controls, indicating

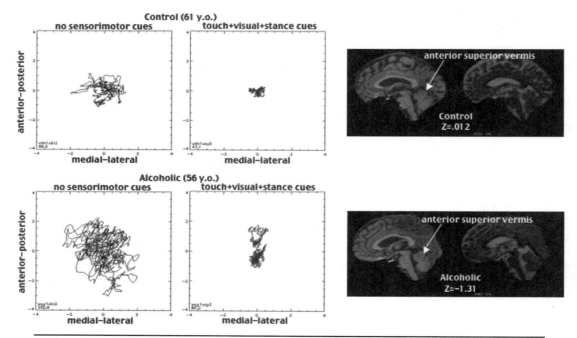

FIGURE 8-7. *Left panels:* Force plate stabilograms collected with and without sensorimotor cues in a 61-year-old control man (*top*) and a 56-year-old alcoholic man (*bottom*). The MRI images on the right are midsagittal MRI (proton density weighted on the left and T2-weighted on the right), showing a volume deficit in the anterior superior vermis of the alcoholic relative to the control (205).

that the alcoholics had functionally adequate sensorimotor integration skills despite the likely cerebellar basis for imbalance (Figure 8-7). The frequency characteristics of sway velocity in the 2 to 7 Hz frequencies was also greater in alcoholics than controls, but postural tremor at all of these frequencies was ameliorated with sensorimotor cues. These results provide support for a cerebellar vermian basis of alcoholism-related postural instability and indicate that alcoholics can successfully engage in sensorimotor integration to override CNS-related deficits in static balance (205).

Stabilization that availed with sensorimotor cues has implications for rehabilitation strategies for individuals recovering from chronic alcoholism and probably also for nonalcoholic patients with similar postural instability. The progressive improvement in balance and decrease in sway with increasing numbers of cues suggests that that when external cues are present, impaired individuals can adapt mechanisms to compensate for underlying cerebellar insult and such cues may even reduce fear of falling.

ACKNOWLEDGMENTS

The authors thank Margaret J. Rosenbloom, M.A. for help in manuscript editing and preparation, Adolf Pfefferbaum, M.D. for the balance platform and MRI figures, and Jessica Rose, Ph.D. for the gait analysis studies. Partial support for this project was obtained from the National Institute on Aging (AG17919) and the National Institute on Alcohol Abuse and Alcoholism (AA10723) granted to E.V.S.

REFERENCES

1. Aboitiz F, Rodriguez E, Olivares R, Zaidel E. Age-related changes in fibre composition of the human corpus callosum: sex differences. *Neuroreport* 1996;7:1761–1764.
2. Abrams B, Parker JD. Maternal weight gain in women with good pregnancy outcome. *Obstet Gynecol* 1990;76:1–7.
3. Abramson D, Roberts SB, Wilson P. Relaxation of the pelvic joints in pregnancy. *Surg Gynecol Obstet* 1934;58:595–613.
4. Adkin AL, Frank JS, Carpenter MG, Peysar GW. Fear of falling modifies anticipatory postural control. *Exp Brain Res* 2002;143:160–170.
5. Ahmad S, Rohrbaugh JW, Anokhin AP, Sirevaag EJ, Goebel JA. Effects of lifetime ethanol consumption on postural control: a computerized dynamic posturography study. *J Vestibul Res* 2002;12:53–64.
6. American College of Obstetricians and Gynecologists. Exercise during pregnancy and the postpartum period. *Clin Obstet Gynecol* 2003;46:496–499.
7. Amiridis IG, Hatzitaki V, Arabatzi F. Age-induced modifications of static postural control in humans. *Neurosci Lett* 2003;350:137–140.
8. Aniansson A, Hedberg M, Henning GB, Grimby G. Muscle morphology, enzymatic activity, and muscle strength in elderly men: a follow-up study. *Muscle Nerve* 1986;9:585–591.
9. Aniansson A, Rundgren A, Sperling L. Evaluation of functional capacity in activities of daily living in 70-year-old men and women. *Scand J Rehab Med* 1980;12:145–154.
10. Arciniegas DB, Beresford TP. *Neuropsychiatry: An Introductory Approach*. Cambridge: Cambridge University Press; 2001.
11. Baker K, Harding A, Halliday G, Kril J, Harper C. Neuronal loss in functional zones of the cerebellum of chronic alcoholics with and without Wernicke's encephalopathy. *Neuroscience* 1999;91:429–438.

12. Baloh RW, Corona S, Jacobson KM, Enrietto JA, Bell T. A prospective study of posturography in normal older people. *J Am Geriatr Soc* 1998;46:438–443.

13. Baloh RW, Fife TD, Zwerling L, et al. Comparison of static and dynamic posturography in young and older normal people. *J Am Geriatr Soc* 1994;42:405–412.

14. Baloh RW, Jacobson KM, Beykirch K, Honrubia V. Static and dynamic posturography in patients with vestibular and cerebellar lesions. *Arch Neurol* 1998;55:649–654.

15. Baloh RW, Spain S, Socotch TM, Jacobson KM, Bell T. Posturography and balance problems in older people. *J Am Geriatr Soc* 1995;43:638–644.

16. Baloh RW, Vinters HV. White matter lesions and disequilibrium in older people: 2. clinicopathologic correlation. *Arch Neurol* 1995;52:975–981.

17. Baloh RW, Ying SH, Jacobson KM. A longitudinal study of gait and balance dysfunction in normal older people. *Arch Neurol* 2003;60:835–839.

18. Baloh RW, Yue Q, Socotch TM, Jacobson KM. White matter lesions and disequilibrium in older people: 1. case-control comparison. *Arch Neurol* 1995;52:970–974.

19. Bassey EJ, Bendall MJ, Pearson M. Muscle strength in the triceps surae and objectively measured customary walking activity in men and women over 65 years of age. *Clin Sci (Lond)* 1988;74:85–89.

20. Baylor AM, Spirduso WW. Systematic aerobic exercise and components of reaction time in older women. *J Gerontol* 1988;43:P121–126.

21. Beere PA, Russell SD, Morey MC, Kitzman DW, Higginbotham MB. Aerobic exercise training can reverse age-related peripheral circulatory changes in healthy older men. *Circulation* 1999;100:1085–1094.

22. Bird AR, Menz HB, Hyde CC. The effect of pregnancy on footprint parameters. A prospective investigation. *J Am Podiatr Med Assoc* 1999;89:405–409.

23. Blatter DD, Bigler ED, Gale SD, et al. Quantitative volumetric analysis of brain MRI: Normative database spanning five decades of life. *Am J Neuroradiol* 1995;16:241–245.

24. Blatter DD, Bigler ED, Gale SD, et al. Quantitative volumetric analysis of brain MR: normative database spanning 5 decades of life. *Am J Neuroradiol* 1995;16:241–251.

25. Bohannon RW. Comfortable and maximum walking speed of adults aged 20–79 years: reference values and determinants. *Age Ageing* 1997;26:15–19.

26. Brach JS, Berthold R, Craik R, VanSwearingen JM, Newman AB. Gait variability in community-dwelling older adults. *J Am Geriatr Soc* 2001;49:1646–1650.

27. Brach JS, Simonsick EM, Kritchevsky S, Yaffe K, Newman AB. The association between physical function and lifestyle activity and exercise in the health, aging and body composition study. *J Am Geriatr Soc* 2004;52:502–509.

28. Bril B, Breniere Y. Postural requirements and progression velocity in young walkers. *J Motor Behav* 1992;24:105–116.

29. Brocklehurst JC, Robertson D, James-Groom P. Skeletal deformities in the elderly and their effect on postural sway. *J Am Geriatr Soc* 1982;30:534–538.

30. Brown M, Holloszy JO. Effects of walking, jogging and cycling on strength, flexibility, speed and balance in 60- to 72-year olds. *Aging* 1993;5:427–434.

31. Cahn DA, Malloy PF, Salloway S, et al. Subcortical hyperintensities on MRI and activities of daily living in geriatric depression. *J Neuropsychiatry Clin Neurosci* 1996;8:404–411.

32. Calguneri M, Bird HA, Wright V. Changes in joint laxity occurring during pregnancy. *Ann Rheum Dis* 1982;41:126–128.

33. Campbell AJ, Robertson MC, Gardner MM, Norton RN, Buchner DM. Falls prevention over 2 years: a randomized controlled trial in women 80 years and older. *Age Ageing* 1999;28:513–518.

34. Campbell AJ, Robertson MC, Gardner MM, Norton RN, Tilyard MW, Buchner DM. Randomised controlled trial of a general practice programme of home based exercise to prevent falls in elderly women. *Br Med J* 1997;315:1065–1069.

35. Carmelli D, Kelly-Hayes M, Wolf PA, et al. The contribution of genetic influences to measures of lower-extremity function in older male twins. *J Gerontol A Biol Sci Med Sci* 2000;55:B49–53.

36. Chakravarthy MV, Joyner MJ, Booth FW. An obligation for primary care physicians to prescribe physical activity to sedentary patients to reduce the risk of chronic health conditions. *Mayo Clin Proc* 2002;77:165–173.

37. Choy NL, Brauer S, Nitz J. Changes in postural stability in women aged 20 to 80 years. *J Gerontol A Biol Sci Med Sci* 2003;58:525–530.

38. Collins JJ, De Luca CJ, Burrows A, Lipsitz LA. Age-related changes in open-loop and closed-loop postural control mechanisms. *Exp Brain Res* 1995;104:480–492.

39. Collins JJ, De Luca CJ. Open-loop and closed-loop control of posture: A random-walk analysis of center-of-pressure trajectories. *Exp Brain Res* 1993;95:308–318.

40. Collins JJ, De Luca CJ. The effects of visual input on open-loop and closed-loop postural control mechanisms. *Exp Brain Res* 1995;103:151–163.

41. Courchesne E, Chisum HJ, Townsend J, et al. Normal brain development and aging: quantitative analysis at in vivo MR imaging in healthy volunteers. *Radiology* 2000;216:672–682.

42. Dault MC, Yardley L, Frank JS. Does articulation contribute to modifications of postural control during dual-task paradigms? *Cogn Brain Res* 2003;16:434–440.

43. DeMaria EJ, Merriam MA, Casanova LA, Gann DS, Kenney PR. Do DRG payments adequately reimburse the costs of trauma care in geriatric patients? *J Trauma* 1988;28:1244–1249.

44. Deshmukh A, Desmond JE, Sullivan EV, et al. Quantification of cerebellar structures with MRI. *Psychiatr Res Neuroimaging* 1997;75:159–172.

45. DeVita P, Hortobagyi T. Age causes a redistribution of joint torques and powers during gait. *J Appl Physiol* 2000;88:1804–1811.

46. Diener H-C, Dichgans J, Bacher M, Guschlbauer B. Characteristic alteration of long-loop "reflexes" in patients with Friedreich's disease and late atrophy of the cerebellar anterior lobe. *J Neurol, Neurosurg, Psychiatry* 1984;47:679-685.

47. Diener H-C, Dichgans J, Bacher M, Guschlbauer. Improvement in ataxia in alcoholic cerebellar atrophy through alcohol abstinence. *J Neurol* 1984;231:258–262.

48. Diener HC, Dichgans J, Bacher M, Hulser J, Liebich H. Mechanisms of postural ataxia after intake of alcohol. *Z Rechtsmed* 1983;90:159–165.

49. Diener HC, Dichgans J, Guschlbauer B, Bacher M, Langenbach P. Disturbances of motor preparation in basal ganglia and cerebellar disorders. In: Allun JHH, Hulliger M, eds. *Progress in Brain Research, Vol 80, Afferent Control of Posture and Locomotion*. Amsterdam: Elsevier Scientific Publishers B.V.; 1989:481–488.

50. Dlugos CA, Pentney RJ. Morphometric evidence that the total number of synapses on Purkinje neurons of old F344 rats is reduced after long-term ethanol treatment and restored to control levels after recovery. *Alcohol Alcohol* 1997;32:161–172.

51. Dominguez RO, Bronstein AM. Assessment of unexplained falls and gait unsteadiness: the impact of age. *Otolaryngol Clin North Am* 2000;33:637–657.

52. Dumas GA, Reid JG. Laxity of knee cruciate ligaments during pregnancy. *J Orthop Sports Phys Ther* 1997;26:2–6.

53. Dunning K, LeMasters G, Levin L, Bhattacharya A, Alterman T, Lordo K. Falls in workers during pregnancy: risk factors, job hazards, and high risk occupations. *Am J Ind Med* 2003;44:664–672.

54. Elble RJ, Thomas SS, Higgins C, Colliver J. Stride-dependent changes in gait of older people. *J Neurol* 1991;238:1–5.

55. Elward K, Larson EB. Benefits of exercise for older adults. A review of existing evidence and current recommendations for the general population. *Clin Geriatr Med* 1992;8:35–50.

56. Era P, Heikkinen E, Gause-Nilsson I, Schroll M. Postural balance in elderly people: changes over a five-year follow-up and its predictive value for survival. *Aging Clin Exp Res* 2002;14:37–46.

57. Fast A, Weiss L, Ducommun EJ, Medina E, Butler JG. Low-back pain in pregnancy. Abdominal muscles, sit-up performance, and back pain. *Spine* 1990;15:28–30.

58. Fiatarone MA, Evans WJ. The etiology and reversibility of muscle dysfunction in the aged. *J Gerontol* 1993;48:77–83.

59. Fiatarone MA, Marks EC, Ryan ND, Meredith CN, Lipsitz LA, Evans WJ. High-intensity strength training in nonagenarians. Effects on skeletal muscle. *JAMA* 1990;263:3029–3034.
60. Fiatarone MA, O'Neill EF, Ryan ND, et al. Exercise training and nutritional supplementation for physical frailty in very elderly people. *N Engl J Med* 1994;330:1769–1775.
61. Finelli FC, Jonsson J, Champion HR, Morelli S, Fouty WJ. A case control study for major trauma in geriatric patients. *J Trauma* 1989; 29:541–548.
62. Flood DG. Critical issues in the analysis of dendritic extent in aging humans, primates, and rodents. *Neurobiol Aging* 1993;14:649–654.
63. Forrest WR. Anticipatory postural adjustment and T'ai Chi Ch'uan. *Biomed Sci Instrum* 1997;33:65–70.
64. Foti T, Davids JR, Bagley A. A biomechanical analysis of gait during pregnancy. *J Bone Joint Surg Am* 2000;82:625–632.
65. Franklin ME, Conner-Kerr T. An analysis of posture and back pain in the first and third trimesters of pregnancy. *J Orthop Sports Phys Ther* 1998;28:133–138.
66. Fregly AR, Graybiel A, Smith MS. Walk on floor eyes closed (WOFEC): A new addition to an ataxia test battery. *Aerosp Med* 1972;43:395–399.
67. Fried TR, Bradley EH, Williams CS, Tinetti ME. Functional disability and health care expenditures for older persons. *Arch Intern Med* 2001;161:2602–2607.
68. Fries EC, Hellebrandt FA. The influence of pregnancy on the location of the center of gravity, postural stability, and body alignment. *Am J Obstetr Gynecol* 1943;46:374–380.
69. Gibson MJ. The prevention of falls in later life. *Dan Med Bull* 1987; 34(suppl 4):1–24.
70. Gill J, Allum JH, Carpenter MG, et al. Trunk sway measures of postural stability during clinical balance tests: effects of age. *J Gerontol A Biol Sci Med Sci* 2001;56:M438–447.
71. Gilleard WL, Brown JM. Structure and function of the abdominal muscles in primigravid subjects during pregnancy and the immediate postbirth period. *Phys Ther* 1996;76:750–762.
72. Gilman S, Adams K, Koeppe RA, et al. Cerebellar and frontal hypometabolism in alcoholic cerebellar degeneration studied with positron emission tomography. *Ann Neurol* 1990;28:775–785.
73. Gilman S, Adams K, Koeppe RA, et al. Cerebellar and frontal hypometabolism in alcoholic cerebellar degeneration studied with Positron Emission Tomography. *Ann Neurol* 1990;28:775–785.
74. Gilman S, Bloedel JR, Lechtenberg R. *Disorders of the Cerebellum.* Philadelphia: F.A. Davis Co; 1981.
75. Goebel JA, Dunham DN, Rohrbaugh JW, Fischel D, Stewart PA. Dose-related effects of alcohol on dynamic posturography and oculomotor measures. *Acta Otolaryngol Suppl* 1995;520 Pt 1:212–215.
76. Golomer E, Ducher D, Arfi GS, Sud R. [Simple locomotion and during load carrying in pregnant women]. *J Gynecol Obstet Biol Reprod (Paris)* 1991;20:406–412.
77. Gomberg BF, Gruen GS, Smith WR, Spott M. Outcomes in acute orthopaedic trauma: a review of 130,506 patients by age. *Injury* 1999;30:431–437.
78. Grabiner PC, Biswas ST, Grabiner MD. Age-related changes in spatial and temporal gait variables. *Arch Phys Med Rehabil* 2001;82:31–35.
79. Gur RC, Gunning-Dixon FM, Turetsky BI, Bilker WB, Gur RE. Brain region and sex differences in age association with brain volume: a quantitative MRI study of healthy young adults. *Am J Geriatr Psychiatr* 2002;10:72–780.
80. Hageman PA, Leibowitz JM, Blanke D. Age and gender effects on postural control measures. *Arch Phys Med Rehabil* 1995;76:961–965.
81. Hall DC, Kaufmann DA. Effects of aerobic and strength conditioning on pregnancy outcomes. *Am J Obstet Gynecol* 1987;157:1199–1203.
82. Harper CG, Kril JJ. Neuropathological changes in alcoholics. In: Hunt WA, Nixon SJ eds. *Alcohol Induced Brain Damage: NIAAA Research Monograph No 22.* Rockville, MD: National Institute of Health; 1993:39–69.
83. Hartshorne NJ, Harruff RC, Alvord EC, Jr. Fatal head injuries in ground-level falls. *Am J Forensic Med Pathol* 1997;18:258–264.
84. Hasselkus BR, Shambes GM. Aging and postural sway in women. *J Gerontol* 1975;30:661–667.
85. Heckman JD, Sassard R. Musculoskeletal considerations in pregnancy. *J Bone Joint Surg Am* 1994;76:1720–1730.
86. Hindmarsh JJ, Estes EH, Jr. Falls in older persons. Causes and interventions. *Arch Intern Med* 1989;149:2217–2222.
87. Horns PN, Ratcliffe LP, Leggett JC, Swanson MS. Pregnancy outcomes among active and sedentary primiparous women. *J Obstet Gynecol Neonatal Nurs* 1996;25:49–54.
88. Howland J, Lachman ME, Peterson EW, Cote J, Kasten L, Jette A. Covariates of fear of falling and associated activity curtailment. *Gerontologist* 1998;38:549–555.
89. Hughes VA, Frontera WR, Roubenoff R, Evans WJ, Singh MA. Longitudinal changes in body composition in older men and women: role of body weight change and physical activity. *Am J Clin Nutr* 2002;76:473–481.
90. Hughes VA, Frontera WR, Wood M, et al. Longitudinal muscle strength changes in older adults: influence of muscle mass, physical activity, and health. *J Gerontol A Biol Sci Med Sci* 2001;56:B209–217.
91. Hytonen M, Pyykko I, Aalto H, Starck J. Postural control and age. *Acta Otolaryngol* 1993;113:119–122.
92. Ireland ML, Ott SM. The effects of pregnancy on the musculoskeletal system. *Clin Orthop* 2000; 169–179.
93. Ito H, Nagasaki H, Maruyama H, Hashizume K, Nakamura R. [Age related changes in the walking cycle during fastest walking in healthy male subjects]. *Nippon Ronen Igakkai Zasshi* 1989;26:347–352.
94. Jeka JJ, Lackner JR. Fingertip contact influences human postural control. *Exp Brain Res* 1994;100:495–502.
95. Jeka JJ, Lackner JR. Fingertip contact influences human postural control. *Exp Brain Res* 1994;100:495–502.
96. Jeka JJ, Schoner G, Dikjstra T, Ribeiro P, Lackner JR. Coupling of fingertip somatosensory information to head and body sway. *Exp Brain Res* 1997;113:475–483.
97. Jensen RK, Doucet S, Treitz T. Changes in segment mass and mass distribution during pregnancy. *J Biomech* 1996;29:251–256.
98. Jernigan TL, Archibald SL, Berhow MT, Sowell ER, Foster DS, Hesselink JR. Cerebral structure on MRI .1. Localization of age-related changes. *Biol Psychiatry* 1991;29:55–67.
99. Jette AM, Harris BA, Cleary PD, Campion EW. Functional recovery after hip fracture. *Arch Phys Med Rehabil* 1987;68:735–740.
100. Judge JO, Davis RB, 3rd, Ounpuu S. Step length reductions in advanced age: the role of ankle and hip kinetics. *J Gerontol A Biol Sci Med Sci* 1996;51:M303–312.
101. Judge JO, Kenny AM, Kraemer WJ. Exercise in older adults. *Conn Med* 2003;67:461–464.
102. Judge JO, King MB, Whipple R, Clive J, Wolfson LI. Dynamic balance in older persons: effects of reduced visual and proprioceptive input. *J Gerontol A Biol Sci Med Sci* 1995;50:M263–270.
103. Judge JO, Lindsey C, Underwood M, Winsemius D. Balance improvements in older women: effects of exercise training. *Phys Ther* 1993;73:254–262; discussion 263–255.
104. Judge JO, Ounpuu S, Davis RB, 3rd. Effects of age on the biomechanics and physiology of gait. *Clinical Geriatric Medicine* 1996;12:659–678.
105. Judge JO, Ounpuu S, Davis RB, 3rd. Effects of age on the biomechanics and physiology of gait. *Clin Geriatr Med* 1996;12:659–678.
106. Judge JO, Underwood M, Gennosa T. Exercise to improve gait velocity in older persons. *Arch Phys Med Rehabil* 1993;74:400–406.
107. Judge JO, Whipple RH, Wolfson LI. Effects of resistive and balance exercises on isokinetic strength in older persons. *J Am Geriatr Soc* 1994;42:937–946.
108. Kaasinen V, Aalto S, K NA, Hietala J, Sonninen P, Rinne JO. Extrastriatal dopamine D(2) receptors in Parkinson's disease: a longitudinal study. *J Neural Transm* 2003;110:591–601.
109. Kemoun G, Thoumie P, Boisson D, Guieu JD. Ankle dorsiflexion delay can predict falls in the elderly. *J Rehabil Med* 2002;34:278–283.
110. Kemper TL. Neuroanatomical and neuropathological changes during aging and dementia. In: Albert ML, Knoefel JE, eds. *Clin Neurol Aging* New York: Oxford University Press; 1994:3–67.
111. Kerber KA, Enrietto JA, Jacobson KM, Baloh RW. Disequilibrium in older people: a prospective study. *Neurology* 1998;51:574–580.

112. Kerr B. Processing demands during mental operations. *Mem Cognit* 1973;1:401–412.

113. Kerrigan DC, Lee LW, Collins JJ, Riley PO, Lipsitz LA. Reduced hip extension during walking: healthy elderly and fallers versus young adults. *Arch Phys Med Rehabil* 2001;82:26–30.

114. Kerrigan DC, Lee LW, Nieto TJ, Markman JD, Collins JJ, Riley PO. Kinetic alterations independent of walking speed in elderly fallers. *Arch Phys Med Rehabil* 2000;81:730–735.

115. Kerrigan DC, Todd MK, Della Croce U, Lipsitz LA, Collins JJ. Biomechanical gait alterations independent of speed in the healthy elderly: evidence for specific limiting impairments. *Arch Phys Med Rehabil* 1998;79:317–322.

116. Kerrigan DC, Xenopoulos-Oddsson A, Sullivan MJ, Lelas JJ, Riley PO. Effect of a hip flexor-stretching program on gait in the elderly. *Arch Phys Med Rehabil* 2003;84:1–6.

117. King MB, Judge JO, Wolfson L. Functional base of support decreases with age. *J Gerontol* 1994;49:M258–263.

118. Kirtley C, Whittle MW, Jefferson RJ. Influence of walking speed on gait parameters. *J Biomed Eng* 1985;4:282–288.

119. Kollegger H, Baumgartner C, Wober C, Oder W, Deecke L. Spontaneous body sway as a function of sex, age, and vision: posturographic study in 30 healthy adults. *Eur Neurol* 1992;32:253–259.

120. Korhonen MT, Mero A, Suominen H. Age-related differences in 100-m sprint performance in male and female master runners. *Med Sci Sports Exerc* 2003;35:1419–1428.

121. Kozakai R, Tsuzuku S, Yabe K, Ando F, Niino N, Shimokata H. Age-related changes in gait velocity and leg extension power in middle-aged and elderly people. *J Epidemiol* 2000;10:S77–81.

122. Lajoie Y, Teasdale N, Bard C, Fleury M. Attentional demands for static and dynamic equilibrium. *Exp Brain Res* 1993;97:139–144.

123. Laros Jr RK. Physiology of normal pregnancy. In: Willson JR, Carrington ER, eds. *Obstetrics and Gynecology.* St. Louis, MO: Mosby Year Book; 1991:242.

124. Larson EB, Bruce RA. Exercise. In: Cassell CK, Leipqiz RM, Cohen HJ, Larson EB, Meier DE, Capello C, eds. *Geriatric Medicine: An Evidence-Based Approach.* New York: Springer-Verlag; 2003: 1023–1029.

125. Laughton CA, Slavin M, Katdare K, et al. Aging, muscle activity, and balance control: physiologic changes associated with balance impairment. *Gait Posture* 2003;18:101–108.

126. Ledin T, Odkvist L. Abstinent chronic alcoholics investigated by dynamic posturography, ocular smooth pursuit and visual suppression. *Acta Otolaryngol* 1991;111:646–655.

127. Ledin T, Odkvist LM. Effect of alcohol measured by dynamic posturography. *Acta Otolaryngol Suppl* 1991;481:576–581.

128. Levit KR, Olin GL, Letsch SW. Americans' health insurance coverage, 1980–91. *Health Care Financ Rev* 1992;14:31–57.

129. Lexell J, Taylor CC, Sjostrom M. What is the cause of the ageing atrophy? Total number, size and proportion of different fiber types studied in whole vastus lateralis muscle from 15- to 83-year-old men. *J Neurol Sci* 1988;84:275–294.

130. Lockhart TE, Woldstad JC, Smith JL. Effects of age-related gait changes on the biomechanics of slips and falls. *Ergonomics* 2003;46:1136–1160.

131. Lord SR, Anstey KJ, Williams P, Ward JA. Psychoactive medication use, sensori-motor function and falls in older women. *Br J Clin Pharmacol* 1995;39:227–234.

132. Lord SR, Caplan GA, Ward JA. Balance, reaction time, and muscle strength in exercising and nonexercising older women: a pilot study. *Arch Phys Med Rehabil* 1993;74:837–839.

133. Lord SR, Clark RD, Webster IW. Physiological factors associated with falls in an elderly population. *J Am Geriatr Soc* 1991;39:1194–1200.

134. Lord SR, Ward JA, Williams P. Exercise effect on dynamic stability in older women: a randomized controlled trial. *Arch Phys Med Rehabil* 1996;77:232–236.

135. Magaziner J, Simonsick EM, Kashner TM, Hebel JR, Kenzora JE. Predictors of functional recovery one year following hospital discharge for hip fracture: a prospective study. *J Gerontol* 1990;45:M101–107.

136. Maki BE. Gait changes in older adults: predictors of falls or indicators of fear. *J Am Geriatr Soc* 1997;45:313–320.

137. Manchester D, Woollacott M, Zederbauer-Hylton N, Marin O. Visual, vestibular and somatosensory contributions to balance control in the older adult. *J Gerontol* 1989;44:M118–127.

138. Marcell TJ. Sarcopenia: causes, consequences, and preventions. *J Gerontol A Biol Sci Med Sci* 2003;58:M911–916.

139. Marottoli RA, Berkman LF, Cooney LM, Jr. Decline in physical function following hip fracture. *J Am Geriatr Soc* 1992;40:861–866.

140. Masdeu JC, Wolfson L, Lantos G, et al. Brain white matter changes in the elderly prone to falling. *Arch Neurol* 1989;46:1292–1296.

141. Mauritz KH, Dichgans J, Hufschmidt A. Quantitative analysis of stance in late cortical cerebellar atrophy of the anterior lobe and other forms of cerebellar ataxia. *Brain* 1979;102:461–482.

142. Mbourou GA, Lajoie Y, Teasdale N. Step length variability at gait initiation in elderly fallers and non-fallers, and young adults. *Gerontology* 2003;49:21–26.

143. McGibbon CA, Krebs DE. Discriminating age and disability effects in locomotion: neuromuscular adaptations in musculoskeletal pathology. *J Appl Physiol* 2004;96:149–160.

144. McGibbon CA, Puniello MS, Krebs DE. Mechanical energy transfer during gait in relation to strength impairment and pathology in elderly women. *Clin Biomech (Bristol, Avon)* 2001;16:324–333.

145. Meier-Ruge W, Ulrich J, Bruhlmann M, Meier E. Age-related white matter atrophy in the human brain. *Ann N Y Acad Sci* 1992;673:260–269.

146. Melton LJ. Epidemiology of Fractures. In: Riggs BL, Melton LK, eds. *Osteoporosis: Etiology, Diagnosis, and Management.* New York: Raven Press; 1988:111–131.

147. Menz HB, Lord SR, Fitzpatrick RC. Age-related differences in walking stability. *Age Ageing* 2003;32:137–142.

148. Morris JA, Jr., MacKenzie EJ, Damiano AM, Bass SM. Mortality in trauma patients: the interaction between host factors and severity. *J Trauma* 1990;30:1476–1482.

149. Mottola MF, Campbell MK. Activity patterns during pregnancy. *Can J Appl Physiol* 2003;28:642–653.

150. National Center for Injury Prevention and Control. 10 Leading Causes of Injury Deaths, United States. http://wwwcdcgov/ncipc/ 2004.

151. Neiman J, Lang AE, Fornazzari L, Carlen PL. Movement disorders in alcoholism: a review. *Neurology* 1990;40:741–746.

152. Nelson ME, Layne JE, Bernstein MJ, et al. The effects of multidimensional home-based exercise on functional performance in elderly people. *J Gerontol A Biol Sci Med Sci* 2004;59:154–160.

153. Nieschalk M, Ortmann C, West A, Schmal F, Stoll W, Fechner G. Effects of alcohol on body-sway patterns in human subjects. *Int J Legal Med* 1999;112:253–260.

154. Ning Y, Williams MA, Dempsey JC, Sorensen TK, Frederick IO, Luthy DA. Correlates of recreational physical activity in early pregnancy. *J Matern Fetal Neonatal Med* 2003;13:385–393.

155. Nyska M, Sofer D, Porat A, Howard CB, Levi A, Meizner I. Planter foot pressures in pregnant women. *Isr J Med Sci* 1997;33:139–146.

156. Oberg T, Karsznia A, Oberg K. Basic gait parameters: reference data for normal subjects, 10–79 years of age. *J Rehabil Res Dev* 1993;30:210–223.

157. Overstall PW, Exton-Smith AN, Imms FJ, Johnson AL. Falls in the elderly related to postural imbalance. *Br Med J* 1977;1:261–264.

158. Patla AE. A framework for understanding mobility problems in the elderly. In: Craik RL, Oatis CA, eds. *Gait Analysis: Theory and Application.* St. Louis, MO: Mosby-Year Book Inc; 1995:436–449.

159. Pellecchia GL. Postural sway increases with attentional demands of concurrent cognitive task. *Gait Posture* 2003;18:29–34.

160. Pellicane JV, Byrne K, DeMaria EJ. Preventable complications and death from multiple organ failure among geriatric trauma victims. *J Trauma* 1992;33:440–444.

161. Pentney R, Quackenbush LJ, O'Neill M. Length changes in dendritic networks of cerebellar Purkinje cells of old rats after chronic ethanol treatment. *Alc Clin Exp Research* 1989;13:413–419.

162. Pentney RJ, Dlugos CA. Cerebellar Purkinje neurons with altered terminal dendritic segments are present in all lobules of the cerebellar vermis of ageing, ethanol-treated F344 rats. *Alcohol Alcohol* 2000;35:35–43.

163. Pentney RJ. Remodeling of neuronal dendritic networks with aging and alcohol. *Alcohol Alcohol* 1991;(suppl 1):393–397.

164. Perrin PP, Gauchard GC, Perrot C, Jeandel C. Effects of physical and sporting activities on balance control in elderly people. *Br J Sports Med* 1999;33:121–126.

165. Peterka RJ, Black FO. Age-related changes in human posture control: sensory organization tests. *J Vestib Res* 1990;1:73–85.

166. Pfefferbaum A, Mathalon DH, Sullivan EV, Rawles JM, Zipursky RB, Lim KO. A quantitative magnetic resonance imaging study of changes in brain morphology from infancy to late adulthood. *Arch Neurol* 1994;51:874–887.

167. Pfefferbaum A, Sullivan EV, Rosenbloom MJ, Mathalon DH, Lim KO. A controlled study of cortical gray matter and ventricular changes in alcoholic men over a five year interval. *Arch Gen Psychiatry* 1998;55:905–912.

168. Pfefferbaum A, Sullivan EV. Diffusion MR imaging in psychiatry and ageing. In: Gillard J, Waldman A, Barker P eds. *Physiological Magnetic Resonance in Clinical Neuroscience.* Cambridge: Cambridge University Press; 2005, pp. 558–578.

169. Post RB, Lott LA, Beede JI, Maddock RJ. The effect of alcohol on the vestibulo-ocular reflex and apparent concomitant motion. *J Vestib Res* 1994;4:181–187.

170. Prudham D, Evans JG. Factors associated with falls in the elderly: a community study. *Age Ageing* 1981;10:141–146.

171. Pyka G, Lindenberger E, Charette S, Marcus R. Muscle strength and fiber adaptations to a year-long resistance training program in elderly men and women. *J Gerontol* 1994;49:M22–27.

172. Raz N, Gunning FM, Head D, et al. Selective aging of the human cerebral cortex observed in vivo: Differential vulnerability of the prefrontal gray matter. *Cereb Cortex* 1997;7:268–282.

173. Raz N, Rodrigue KM, Kennedy KM, Head D, Gunning-Dixon F, Acker JD. Differential aging of the human striatum: longitudinal evidence. *Am J Neuroradiol* 2003;24:1849–1856.

174. Reeves S, Bench C, Howard R. Ageing and the nigrostriatal dopaminergic system. *Int J Geriatr Psychiatry* 2002;17:359–370.

175. Resnick SM, Goldszal AF, Davatzikos C, et al. One-year changes in MRI brain volumes in older adults. *Cereb Cortex* 2000;10:464–472.

176. Riley MA, Clark S. Recurrence analysis of human postural sway during the sensory organization test. *Neurosci Lett* 2003;342:45–48.

177. Riley R. Accidental falls and injuries among seniors. *Health Rep* 1992;4:341–354.

178. Rinne JO, Lonnberg P, Marjamaki P. Age-dependent decline in human brain dopamine-D1 and dopamine-D2 receptors. *Brain Res* 1990;508:349–352.

179. Rinne JO, Rummukainen J, Paljarvi L, Sako E, Molsa P, Rinne UK. Neuronal Loss in the Substantia Nigra in Patients with Alzheimer's Disease and Parkinson's Disease in Relation to Extrapyramidal Symptoms and Dementia. *Alzheimer's Disease and Related Disorders* 1989;317:325–332.

180. Ritchie JR. Orthopedic considerations during pregnancy. *Clin Obstet Gynecol* 2003;46:456–466.

181. Roebuck RM, Simmons RW, Mattson SN, Riley EP. Prenatal exposure to alcohol affects the ability to maintain postural balance. *Alc Clin Exp Res* 1998;22:252–258.

182. Rogind H, Lykkegaard JJ, Bliddal H, Danneskiold-Samsoe B. Postural sway in normal subjects aged 20–70 years. *Clin Physiol Funct Imaging* 2003;23:171–176.

183. Rosenberg IH. Sarcopenia: origins and clinical relevance. *J Nutr* 1997;127:990S–991S.

184. Rosenbloom MJ, O'Reilly A, Sassoon SA, Sullivan EV, Pfefferbaum A. Persistent cognitive deficits in community treated alcoholic men and women volunteering for research: Limited contribution from psychiatric comorbidity. *J Stud Alcohol* 2005;66:254–265.

185. Rosenbloom MJ, Pfefferbaum A, Sullivan EV. Recovery of short-term memory and psychomotor speed but not postural stability with long-term sobriety in alcoholic women. *Neuropsychology* 2004;18:589–597.

186. Rubenstein LZ, Josephson KR, Trueblood PR, et al. Effects of a group exercise program on strength, mobility, and falls among fall-prone elderly men. *J Gerontol A Biol Sci Med Sci* 2000;55:M317–321.

187. Rubino FA. Gait disorders. *Neurologist* 2002;8:254–262.

188. Schauberger CW, Rooney BL, Goldsmith L, Shenton D, Silva PD, Schaper A. Peripheral joint laxity increases in pregnancy but does not correlate with serum relaxin levels. *Am J Obstet Gynecol* 1996;174:667–671.

189. Scheltens P, Barkhof F, Leys D, Wolters EC, Ravid R, Kamphorst W. Histopathologic correlates of white matter changes on MRI in Alzheimer's disease and normal aging. *Neurology* 1995;45:883–888.

190. Schmal F, Thiede O, Stoll W. Effect of ethanol on visual-vestibular interactions during vertical linear body acceleration. *Alcohol Clin Exp Res* 2003;27:1520–1526.

191. Scholz E, Diener H, Dichgans J, Langohr H, Schied W, Schupmann A. Incidence of peripheral neuropathy and cerebellar ataxia in chronic alcoholics. *J Neurol* 1986;233:212–217.

192. Seguin R, Nelson ME. The benefits of strength training for older adults. *Am J Prev Med* 2003;25:141–149.

193. Sehl ME, Yates FE. Kinetics of human aging: I. Rates of senescence between ages 30 and 70 years in healthy people. *J Gerontol A Biol Sci Med Sci* 2001;56:B198–208.

194. Sheldon JH. The effect of age on the control of sway. *Gerontol Clin (Basel)* 1963;5:129–138.

195. Shumway-Cook A, Woollacott M, Kerns KA, Baldwin M. The effects of two types of cognitive tasks on postural stability in older adults with and without a history of falls. *J Gerontol* 1997;52:M232–240.

196. Skelton DA, Young A, Greig CA, Malbut KE. Effects of resistance training on strength, power, and selected functional abilities of women aged 75 and older. *J Am Geriatr Soc* 1995;43:1081–1087.

197. Soltani H, Fraser RB. A longitudinal study of maternal anthropometric changes in normal weight, overweight and obese women during pregnancy and postpartum. *Br J Nutr* 2000;84:95–101.

198. Song MY, Ruts E, Kim J, Janumala I, Heymsfield S, Gallagher D. Sarcopenia and increased adipose tissue infiltration of muscle in elderly African American women. *Am J Clin Nutr* 2004;79:874–880.

199. Sorensen TK, Williams MA, Lee IM, Dashow EE, Thompson ML, Luthy DA. Recreational physical activity during pregnancy and risk of preeclampsia. *Hypertension* 2003;41:1273–1280.

200. Sowell ER, Jernigan TL, Mattson SN, Riley EP, Sobel DF, Jones KL. Abnormal development of the cerebellar vermis in children prenatally exposed to alcohol: size reduction in lobules I–V. *Alc Clin Exp Res* 1996;20:31–34.

201. Spencer RM, Zelaznik HN, Diedrichsen J, Ivry RB. Disrupted timing of discontinuous but not continuous movements by cerebellar lesions. *Science* 2003;300:1437–1439.

202. Sternfeld B, Quesenberry CP, Jr., Eskenazi B, Newman LA. Exercise during pregnancy and pregnancy outcome. *Med Sci Sports Exerc* 1995;27:634–640.

203. Sullivan EV, Adalsteinsson E, Hedehus M, et al. Equivalent disruption of regional white matter microstructure in aging healthy men and women. *Neuroreport* 2001;12:99.

204. Sullivan EV, Deshmukh A, Desmond JE, Lim KO, Pfefferbaum A. Cerebellar volume decline in normal aging, alcoholism, and Korsakoff's syndrome: Relation to ataxia. *Neuropsychology* 2000; 14:341–352.

205. Sullivan EV, Rose J, Pfefferbaum A. Effect of vision, touch, and stance on cerebellar vermian-related sway and tremor: A quantitative MRI and physiological study. *Cereb Cortex* 2005;in press.

206. Sullivan EV, Rosenbloom MJ, Lim KO, Pfefferbaum A. Longitudinal changes in cognition, gait, and balance in abstinent and relapsed alcoholic men: Relationships to changes in brain structure. *Neuropsychology* 2000;14:178–188.

207. Sullivan EV, Rosenbloom MJ, Serventi KL, Pfefferbaum A. Effects of age and sex on volumes of the thalamus, pons, and cortex. *Neurobiol Aging* 2004;25:185–192.

208. Sullivan EV. Compromised pontocerebellar and cerebellothalamo-cortical systems: speculations on their contributions to cognitive and motor impairment in nonamnesic alcoholism. *Alc Clin Exp Research* 2003;27:1409–1419.

209. Sutherland DH, Olshen RA, Biden EN, Wyatt MP. *The Development of Mature Walking. Clinics in Developmental Medicine No. 104–105.* London: MacKeith Press; 1988.

210. Taves C, Charteris J, Wall JC. The kinematics of treadmill walking during pregnancy. *Physiotherapy Canada* 1982;34:321–324.

211. Tell GS, Lefkowitz DS, Diehr P, Elster AD. Relationship between

balance and abnormalities in cerebral magnetic resonance imaging in older adults. *Arch Neurol* 1998;55:73–79.

212. Tianwu H, Watanabe Y, Asai M, Shimizu K, Takada S, Mizukoshi K. Effects of alcohol ingestion on vestibular function in postural control. *Acta Otolaryngol Suppl* 1995;519:127–131.
213. Tideiksaar R. *Falling in Old Age*. New York: Springer Publishing Company, Inc; 1997.
214. Tinetti M, Doucette J, Claus E. The contribution of predisposing and situational risk factors to serious fall injuries. *J Am Geriatr Soc* 1995;43:1207–1213.
215. Tinetti M, Williams C. The effect of falls and fall injuries on functioning in community-dwelling older persons. *J Gerontol* 1998;53A: M112–M119.
216. Tinetti ME, Doucette JT, Claus EB. The contribution of predisposing and situational risk factors to serious fall injuries. *J Am Geriatr Soc* 1995;43:1207–1213.
217. Toupet M, Gagey PM, Heuschen S. Vestibular patients and aging subjects lose use of visual input and expend more energy in static postural control. In: Vellas BJ, Toupet M, Rubenstein L, et al, eds. *Balance and Gait Disorders in the Elderly*. Paris: Elsevier; 1992: 183–198.
218. Tremblay F, Mireault AC, Dessureault L, Manning H, Sveistrup H. Postural stabilization from fingertip contact: I. Variations in sway attenuation, perceived stability and contact forces with aging. *Exp Brain Res* 2004;157:275–285.
219. Tsang WW, Hui-Chan CW. Effect of 4- and 8-wk intensive Tai Chi Training on balance control in the elderly. *Med Sci Sports Exerc* 2004; 36:648–657.
220. U.S. Census Bureau. Aging in the United States: Past, Present, and Future. *http://wwwcensusgov/ipc/prod/97agewcpdf* 2004.
221. U.S. Census Bureau. Census 2000 PHC-T-9. Population by Age, Sex, Race, and Hispanic or Latino Origin for the United States: 2000. *http://wwwcensusgov/population/cen2000/phc-t9/tab01pdf* 2000.
222. Vellas BJ, Wayne SJ, Romero LJ, Baumgartner RN, Garry PJ. Fear of falling and restriction of mobility in elderly fallers. *Age Ageing* 1997;26:189–193.
223. Victor M, Adam RD, Mancell EL. A restricted form of cerebellar de-

generation occurring in alcoholic patients. *Arch Neurol* 1959;1:577–688.
224. Victor M, Adams RD, Collins GH. *The Wernicke-Korsakoff Syndrome and Related Neurologic Disorders Due to Alcoholism and Malnutrition*, 2nd ed. Philadelphia: F.A. Davis Co; 1989.
225. Visser M, Pluijm SM, Stel VS, Bosscher RJ, Deeg DJ. Physical activity as a determinant of change in mobility performance: the Longitudinal Aging Study Amsterdam. *J Am Geriatr Soc* 2002;50:1774–1781.
226. Wild D, Nayak US, Isaacs B. Description, classification and prevention of falls in old people at home. *Rheumatol Rehabil* 1981;20:153–159.
227. Winter DA, Patla AE, Frank JS, Walt SE. Biomechanical walking pattern changes in the fit and healthy elderly. *Phys Ther* 1990;70:340–347.
228. Wober C, Wober-Bingol C, Karwautz A, Nimmerrichte RA, Deecke L, Lesch OM. Postural control and lifetime alcohol consumption in alcohol-dependent patients. *Acta Neurol Scand* 1999;99: 48–53.
229. Wober C, Wober-Bingol C, Karwautz A, Nimmerrichter A, Walter H, Deecke L. Ataxia of stance in different types of alcohol dependence-a posturographic study. *Alcohol* 1998;33:393–402.
230. Wolf SL, Barnhart HX, Kutner NG, McNeely E, Coogler C, Xu T. Reducing frailty and falls in older persons: an investigation of Tai Chi and computerized balance training. Atlanta FICSIT Group. Frailty and Injuries: Cooperative Studies of Intervention Techniques. *J Am Geriatr Soc* 1996;44:489–497.
231. Wolf SL, Coogler C, Xu T. Exploring the basis for Tai Chi Chuan as a therapeutic exercise approach. *Arch Phys Med Rehabil* 1997;78: 886–892.
232. Woollacott M, Shumway-Cook A. Attention and the control of posture and gait: a review of an emerging area of research. *Gait Posture* 2002;16:1–14.
233. Zeleznik J. Normative aging of the respiratory system. *Clin Geriatr Med* 2003;19:1–18.
234. Zhang J, Savitz DA. Exercise during pregnancy among US women. *Ann Epidemiol* 1996;6:53–59.

Chapter 9

Walking for Health

William L. Haskell and Leslie Torburn

Evolutionary theory and data have demonstrated that humans carrying genetic alleles favoring such motor skills as stamina, endurance, strength, speed, and agility at relevant genes were more likely to experience better reproductive fitness than their counterparts who were not so endowed (7). Good mobility was critical for survival, and walking became an increasingly important feature of daily life in the evolving human. Without other means of transportation, people who could walk considerable distances during a day or on consecutive days were more likely to survive. This increase in physical activity activated gene expression that further enhanced their motor fitness or capacity (29). For more than 99.5% of the last 100,000 years, modern *Homo sapiens* have primarily relied on walking for moving about and muscular work to perform most daily chores. It is only within the past 200 years that man has been able to reduce systematically his required daily physical activity and especially walking through a variety of technological developments. Thus, modern man has inherited a body exquisitely designed for a wide range of physical activities, and it functions best when activities, such as walking, are a significant part of daily life.

Throughout much of recorded western history, physicians, philosophers, educators, and scientists have promoted the idea that being physically active contributes to improved health, better physical functioning, and increased longevity. Taking frequent walks or similar activity to help prevent or treat various chronic diseases and promote "successful aging" has been a frequent recommendation by a number of early major thought leaders *("Before supper take a little walk, after supper do the same"* – Erasmus [1514] or *"Of all exercises walking is the best"* – Thomas Jefferson [1791]).

While these personal observations or clinical impressions were valuable in promoting a healthier lifestyle, it was not until the mid-1900s that data collected and analyzed scientifically were published describing some of the health benefits of walking and other moderate or vigorous intensity activities. The fact that walking and similar activities need to be included in the lives of many children as well as adults is highlighted by the recent rapid

increase in obesity and type II diabetes mellitus in many technologically advanced cultures (46). The present increase in obesity, type II diabetes, and cardiovascular disease indicate that walking and other physical activity needs to be included in the daily life of both children and adults. One way to reverse this decline and effectively combat this "hypokinetic state" is to increase substantially the amount of brisk or vigorous walking performed by a large segment of the sedentary population. This chapter primarily will review the evidence that supports the health and performance benefits of walking, how much walking the population currently performs, and some issues surrounding attempts to improve health through increased walking.

> *"I find in the domestic duck that bones of the wing weigh less and the bones of the leg more, in proportion to the whole skeleton, than do the same bones in the wild-duck; and I presume this change may be safely attributed to the domestic duck flying much less and walking more, than its wild parent" Charles Darwin – 1859 (9)*

WALKING IN THE USA

Data from Surveys

Based on various physical activity surveys of representative samples of the United States adult population conducted over the past 30 years, walking is the most frequently reported physical activity. Most surveys have only assessed the walking performed during leisure time or for transportation and have not included walking involved during occupational work or household chores. Data collected in 2000 using the Behavioral Risk Factor Surveillance System by the Centers for Disease Control and Prevention indicated that about 30% of men and 47% of women reported walking as a leisure-time physical activity (47). Both men and women who reported walking for leisure time walked an average of 2.87 times per week, with an average duration of 34.4 minutes for men and 29.9 minutes for women. The prevalence for walking during leisure time was highest for men and women age 45 to 54 years

(53.5%) and lowest for those age 18 to 24 years (38.1%), whereas 52% of college graduates reported walking for leisure time but only 35.6% of participants reporting less than a high school education reported such walking. Non-Hispanics reported the highest rate of walking (49.4%), while Hispanic men and women reported the lowest prevalence (39.9%). These data are quite similar to the results of a random sample survey of 1,818 United States men and women collected during 1999 to 2000, where 34% of the population were identified as regular walkers (5 times per week for ≥30 minutes), 45.6% as occasional walkers (<5 times per week or <30 minutes per session) and 20.7% as never walkers (13).

Walking Based on Data from Pedometers

Pedometers and motion sensors (usually accelerometers) have been used to evaluate the physical activity habits, especially walking, of various groups of individuals. Accelerometers have been used to study habitual physical activity or changes in activity and have been preferred over pedometers because they can be used to evaluate a variety of different types of activity, not just ambulation, and they have greater accuracy in determining an overall activity profile (27). However, the substantially greater costs and logistical challenges when using accelerometers as compared to pedometers to collect data over extended periods of time in a large number of participants has made pedometers a popular instrument for recording walking. Systematic evaluations of pedometers have demonstrated that a number of well-made pedometers can provide accurate data on the amount of walking performed by most adults (45). Pedometers may be less accurate in children and older adults who have limited mobility and an altered (shuffle) gait.

The results of several studies have been reported where pedometers were used to assess the amount of walking performed throughout the day in representative samples of the adult population. These data indicate that for adults the number of steps per day typically ranges between 2,500 and 15,000, with very sedentary people achieving less than 4,000 steps per day. Sedentary people being in the range of 4,000 to 6,000, moderately active in the range of 6,000 to 9,000, active (achieving public health recommendations for physical activity) 9,000 to 12,000, and the very active at more than 12,000 steps per day (51). Pedometer data collected over a seven-day period on a representative sample of adults living in South Carolina indicated that the average number of steps taken per day was 5,931 (sd ± 3,634) with men recording 7,192 ± 3,596 and women 5,210 ± 3,518 steps per day (52). Adults at the age of 35 to 44 years accumulated more steps per day than either younger or older adults did, with those 65+ years recording only 3,766 ± 2,805 steps per day. The number of steps

per day was strongly associated with degree of adiposity: normal weight (BMI <25) = 7,029, overweight (BMI 25–29.9) = 5,813, and obese (BMI ≥30) = 4,618 steps per day.

The idea that a good walking goal for promoting health is 10,000 steps per day was introduced in Japan in the 1960s (17). This 10,000-step level as a physical activity goal for adults was exported to many countries in the late 1990s. Since then, a number of investigators have evaluated how this amount of walking relates to current public health recommendations, such as the CDC/ACSM public health guidelines for physical activity that recommends at least 30 minutes of moderate intensity activity on most, preferably all, days of the week (41). The results of these evaluations generally indicate that when most adults regularly achieve 10,000 steps per day, they meet the current recommendations for physical activity. For example, in healthy adults who reported at least 30 minutes of moderate intensity activity per day on a seven-day physical activity recall, 73% recorded at least 10,000 steps per day on a pedometer (58). Practitioners have rapidly adopted the idea of a 10,000-step goal for the promotion of physical activity in a variety of clinical and community settings. However, little systematically collected data have been published on how successful this approach is in maintaining an increase in daily walking as compared to other approaches.

WALKING AND MAINTAINING GOOD HEALTH THROUGHOUT THE LIFESPAN

Over the past 50 years, scientific data have continued to accumulate supporting the association between increased habitual moderate intensity physical activity, including brisk walking, with a significantly lower prevalence of various chronic diseases, greater physical independence in the elderly and a better overall health status and quality of life among many adults. Men and women who include bouts of brisk walking on most days have lower occurrences of fatal and nonfatal heart attack and stroke, hypertension, type II diabetes mellitus, site-specific cancers (especially of the colon and breast), osteoporosis, and depression. Frequent walking by older persons helps to maintain and/or increase cardiorespiratory and muscle endurance, as well as muscle strength, balance and gait speed, all important factors for retaining the capacity to perform a wide range of tasks of daily living and maintain independent living.

Cardiovascular Disease

Men and women who accumulate 120 minutes or more per week of brisk walking during most weeks generally have lower rates of cardiovascular disease (CVD) and clinical events caused primarily by the atherothrombotic process. The initial support for this relationship using modern scientific methods was published by Morris and colleagues in 1953 (34). They reported an inverse association between on-the-job activity and future CVD clinical events in two occupations, double-decker bus conductors and postal carriers as compared to their sedentary counterparts, bus drivers, and civil service workers who sat at desks most of the day. The rate of first clinical episodes of coronary artery disease (CAD) in the conductors was about 30% lower than in the drivers. While actual walking time or distance was not measured, the major activity of the bus conductors was walking up and down the stairs collecting fares on the double-decker buses and all of the postal carriers completed most of their routes by walking.

Over the past 50 years, since this initial report by Morris and colleagues, there have been a number of well-designed, prospective observational studies that have linked increased amounts of walking with lower CVD risk for men and women. In most cases the walking intensity has been defined as "usual pace" or "brisk" and the amount in minutes per day or hours per week. In the data analysis of several of these reports, the amount of walking has been separated from other activities, especially more vigorous activities. This approach allows for a more refined analysis of the association between walking amount and clinical CVD events independent of other physical activity. A summary of the results of such a study is presented in Figures 9-1 and 9-2. These data are from the Observational Study of the Women's Health Initiative (30). Participants were 73,743 healthy women (without cardiovascular disease or cancer) 50 to 79 years of age at study entry who were evaluated in 42 clinics and represented a broad spectrum of the US population. At a baseline visit, a variety of health and lifestyle measurements were recorded, including a detailed assessment of recreational physical activities classified as mild, moderate, or vigorous intensity. Questions were asked regarding the frequency of walks performed outside the home for a duration of ≥10 minutes without stopping, the average duration of each walk, and the walking pace. Using energy expenditure data provided in the Physical Activity Compendium (2), the estimated amount of energy expended while walking was calculated as MET-hours per week. The average length of follow-up was 3.7 years with 232,971 person-years of exposure and 1,551 CVD events.

In Figure 9-1 the relation between amount of energy spent per week walking and development of CVD during follow-up is provided for women ages 50 to 59, 60 to 69, and 70 to 79 years. Women were categorized into quintiles according to MET-hours per week while walking with the values for low to high quintiles being 0, 0.1 to 2.5, 2.6 to 5.0, 5.1 to 10.0, >10.0 MET-hours per week. There was a highly significant association ($p < 0.001$) between higher amounts of walking and decreased risk of having a CVD clinical event over the next two to six years. The relationship was similar for women in all three age groups, with a somewhat less strong association in the oldest women. The association between pace of walking and CVD clinical events was also analyzed in this study. Women were categorized by usual self-reported walking pace into five categories: 1) rarely or never walk, 2) <2 mph, 3) 2 to 3 mph, 4) 3 to 4 mph, and 5) >4 mph. As can be seen in Figure 9-2, there was a highly significant trend (p for trend = 0.002) with women who report walking faster having less CVD during follow-up. The overall favorable association between walking and better cardiovascular health was seen in women representing different ages, ethnicities, and body size as determined by body mass index.

A number of other studies reporting on the relation of routine walking amount and risk of CVD are quite consistent with the overall results of the Women's Health Initiative. For example, results from the US Nurses Health Study demonstrated that the incidence of CHD among 72,488

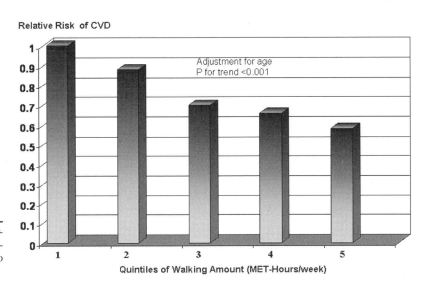

FIGURE 9-1. Age-adjusted relative risks for cardiovascular disease according to quintile of walking amount (MET–hours/week) in women age 50 to 79 years (Women's Health Initiative Study).

Relative Risk for CVD

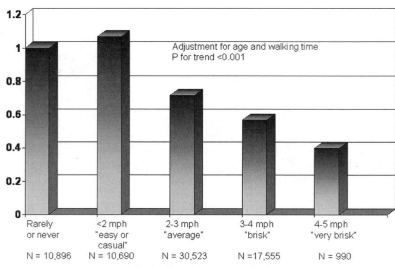

FIGURE 9-2. Age and walking amount adjusted relative risks for cardiovascular disease according to average speed of walking in women age 50 to 79 years (Women's Health Initiative Study).

women age 40 to 65 years during 8 years of follow-up was much lower in women who accumulated ≥ 10 MET-hours per week while walking than those who accumulated ≤ 0.5 MET-hours per week (R^2 adjusted for age $= 0.46$, $p < 0.001$) (31). The authors concluded from the results of this study "brisk walking and vigorous exercise are associated with substantial and similar reductions in the incidence of coronary heart disease among women." In the Honolulu Heart Program, men age 71 to 93 years who reported walking at least 1.5 miles per day had nearly 50% lower CHD incidence over a 2- to 4-year follow-up period compared to men reporting walking less than 0.25 miles per day (age adjusted, $p = 0.002$) (16). Also, in a random sample of generally healthy men and women enrollees in a health maintenance organization age ≥ 65 years, walking more than 4 hours per week was associated with a significantly lower rate of hospitalizations due to CVD compared to their contemporaries who reported walking <1 hour per week ($R^2 = 0.69$, $p < 0.01$) (24). Total mortality rate was lower in those who walked more than 4 hours per week, especially in women ($R^2 = 0.45$, $p < 0.01$).

Stroke

A lower stroke rate in more physically active or physically fit persons compared to the least active or fit in the study population has been reported in a number of studies. In a meta-analysis of data available in 2002, Lee and colleagues concluded that moderate and high amounts of physical activity are associated with a reduced risk of total, ischemic, and hemorrhagic strokes in men and women (26). This report points to the need for more data on physical activity amount and intensity and stroke incidence, especially for hemorrhagic stroke. However,

in most of these studies, the design of the physical activity assessments did not allow for just an analysis of walking independent of other activity. In the Nurses Health Study involving 72,488 women aged 40 to 65 years, where walking was analyzed independent of other activities, women reporting walking ≥ 3.3 miles per week versus those walking <0.2 miles per week experienced a significantly lower incidence of stroke ($R^2 = 0.66$, $p < 0.01$) during an average follow-up period of eight years (19).

Peripheral Arterial Disease

In patients with peripheral arterial disease (PAD), stenosis of the arteries in the legs reduces blood flow causing hypoxia to the contracting muscles during exercise, especially during walking. This condition, frequently referred to as intermittent claudication, is caused by the atherothrombotic process that develops most frequently in the intermediate-size arteries of the lower legs. When the reduced capacity for blood flow in such arteries cannot meet the increased demands for flow caused by exercise, tissue ischemia and local muscle pain occurs. As the exercise continues in duration and/or intensity, the ischemia increases until the patient stops the exercise due to leg pain. Major risk factors for developing PAD include cigarette smoking, diabetes mellitus, hypertension, hypercholesterolemia, a diet high in animal fats and low in plant products, and a sedentary lifestyle (8). Limited observational data support the idea that frequent walking helps to prevent the development of PAD in older men and women, but compared to the data linking walking to the reduced risk of CHD, the data on walking and PAD prevention is still quite sparse (38).

In patients with PAD, frequent walking is considered to be one of the cornerstones of therapy. In conjunction with pharmacologic treatment and possibly surgery, frequent walking is prescribed to maintain physical functioning and independence. In a systematic review of the effects of exercise training in patients with PAD, Gardner and Poehlman concluded that exercise, especially walking, was effective in reducing the clinical symptoms and increasing walking performance (15). The claudication pain end point used during exercise rehabilitation (i.e., intermittent exercise to near-maximal pain) was the most important program component for producing improvements in distance walked, as it explained 55% and 40% of the variance in the increases in the distances to onset and to maximal claudication pain, respectively. Exercise programs that had patients walk to near-maximal claudication pain (high pain end point) demonstrated greater improvements in claudication symptoms than programs that had patients stop walking at the onset of claudication pain (low pain end point). These data support the notion that greater amounts of ischemia induced within the claudicating musculature may produce greater improvements in pain symptoms, possibly due to greater hemodynamic and metabolic adaptations.

Physiological Changes Contributing to Less CVD

A number of biological measures causally linked to the development of CVD and/or the precipitation of clinical events are known to be altered favorably with moderately intense physical activity. These include the decrease in arterial blood pressure, alterations in the lipoprotein profile, especially the reduction in triglyceride and the increase in high-density cholesterol concentrations, enhancement of insulin-mediated glucose uptake (glucose tolerance), less of a tendency for red blood cell clotting and/or increased

fibrinolysis, a decrease in myocardial oxygen demand at rest and work along with an increase in aerobic capacity (maximal oxygen uptake), and an increase in endothelium-mediated coronary artery vasodilatation capacity and angiogenesis. While not all of the changes have been shown to be produced specifically by an increase in walking, most appear to improve to some degree by moderately intense physical training. For example, substantial data exist that increased walking will help prevent the development of hypertension and reduce arterial blood pressure. In a study of 6,017 generally healthy Japanese men age 35 to 60 years who had a baseline blood pressure <140/90 mm Hg, it was observed that men who walked more had a lower rate of developing hypertension than men who walked little (50). During 59,574 person-years of follow-up, the multivariate relative risk for developing hypertension was 29% lower (*p* for trend = 0.002) for men who reported walking >20 minutes to work each day compared to men reporting a walk to work of ≤10 minutes per day. In this population, for every 26 men who walked more than 20 minutes to work daily, one case of hypertension was prevented.

In people who are quite inactive and have a low aerobic capacity, brisk walking puts a sufficient stress (overload) on a number of the body's tissues or systems to produce an increase in their efficiency or capacity (42). That increased exercise intensity, within the normal range of walking, produces step-wise increases in cardiorespiratory function (aerobic capacity) in inactive women was effectively demonstrated by Duncan and colleagues (10). Displayed in Figure 9-3 are changes in maximal oxygen uptake measured during walking on a treadmill and HDL-cholesterol concentrations for 102 sedentary, healthy premenopausal women randomly assigned to control (no change in physical activity), "strollers" who walked at 3 mph, "walkers" who walked at 4.0 mph, and "brisk walkers" who walked at 5.0 mph. All the women assigned to walking walked 3 miles per day, five times per week for 24 weeks. All

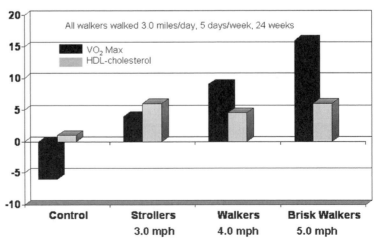

FIGURE 9-3. Percent changes after 24 weeks in maximal oxygen uptake (VO₂ max) and high-density lipoprotein cholesterol (HDL-C) in response to walking at different speeds but the same distance.

three exercise groups achieved a significant increase in maximal oxygen uptake, but those who walked faster (but still just 3 miles per day) had greater increases than the women who walked slower. These data support the idea that by increasing walking speed while holding the walking distance constant, a person can gain a greater increase in cardiorespiratory capacity. However, this does not appear to be true for changes in HDL-cholesterol as all three exercise groups had significant but similar increases in HDL-cholesterol concentration over the 24 weeks. Thus, for HDL-cholesterol, it appears here and in other studies the total amount of walking performed is more important than the speed of walking or intensity of the exercise. For a number of health related measures, such as blood lipids, insulin-mediated glucose uptake and obesity prevention, the total amount of exercise performed is more important than performing it at a very high intensity (22,48).

Type II Diabetes

Since the 1980s there has been a steady and rapid increase in the prevalence of type II diabetes in the populations of most technologically developed countries. In addition to the increase in prevalence, the age of onset of type II diabetes has continued to decrease with an increasing number of cases being reported in boys and girls in their teens (11). This increase in prevalence and earlier age of onset is beginning to cause major havoc with health care costs due to the long-term and expensive care to deal not only with the medical management of the diabetes but also the treatment of the blindness, leg amputations, end state renal disease, and coronary heart disease caused by the diabetes. While there is genetic variation among individuals in their susceptibility to type II diabetes, a major cause of this disease is a chronic exposure to inactivity, overeating, positive energy balance and the resulting obesity (21). The process of type II diabetes is initiated when there is an increase in the resistance to insulin-mediated glucose uptake (insulin resistance) and the pancreas has to produce more and more insulin in order to move glucose from the blood into tissues. Eventually, the pancreas is not able to produce sufficient insulin to overcome this resistance and blood sugar rises to a level where diabetes is diagnosed.

The major tissue involved in this "insulin resistance" is the skeletal muscle. Substantial experimental data collected in animals and humans have demonstrated that frequent muscle contractions, such as occur while walking, play a critical role in maintaining or increasing insulin sensitivity or decreasing insulin resistance in the skeletal muscle (43). These increases in insulin-mediated glucose uptake produced by exercise can significantly reduce blood glucose levels following an oral glucose challenge (glucose tolerance test) (23). The amount of insulin needed to produce this improved glucose uptake is significantly reduced. Rather than being mainly an "exercise training"

effect where an improvement in insulin sensitivity is detected only after weeks or months of increased exercise, the improvement is seen after only a few sessions of moderate intensity walking (acute response). Rogers and colleagues reported that after only seven sessions of brisk walking and cycling (50 to 60 minutes per session on seven consecutive days) by 10 men with poor glucose tolerance, they had a significant reduction in both glucose and insulin concentrations over three hours following an oral glucose load of 100 g (Figure 9-4) (44).

Men and women who are habitually more physically active, including more walking, are significantly less likely to develop type II diabetes in the future than less active persons. In the Nurses Health Study, women in the upper quintile of reported walking had a relative risk for developing type II diabetes over an 8-year follow-up period of 0.58 ($p = 0.001$ for trend) and 0.74 when adjusted for BMI ($p = 0.01$ for trend) compared to women in the lowest quintile of walking. A faster pace of walking was

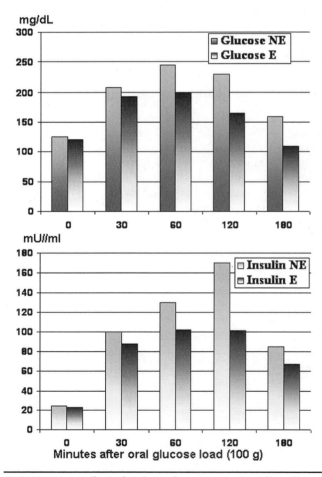

FIGURE 9-4. Effect of 7 days of exercise (primarily walking) on plasma glucose and insulin response to a 100 gram glucose tolerance test (OGTT) in 10 men with abnormal glucose tolerance. OGTT was performed 18 hours after last exercise bout. NE = non-exercise control group; E = exercise group.

independently associated with a lower risk of type II diabetes (18). British men age 40 to 59 years who reported moderate intensity activity (including a lot of walking) had a relative risk of 0.42 (p <0.001 for trend across activity levels) for developing type II diabetes during eight years of follow-up compared to men considered inactive (56). The results of these prospective observational studies showing a reduced risk of developing type II diabetes in more active men are supported by experimental studies where inactive persons at high risk of developing type II diabetes are randomized to an exercise group or a sedentary control group. Data from the Da Qing IGT and Diabetes Study in China support the idea that an increase in physical activity by men and women with elevated blood glucose levels significantly reduces the rate of development of type II diabetes as compared to an inactive control group (39). Over a 6-year period of intervention, there were 15.7 new cases per 100 person years in the control and 8.3 new cases per 100 person years in the exercise group, (46% decrease, p <0.001). The exercise program for patients included a mixture of mild to vigorous activities, with slow to fast speed walking being one of the major forms of exercise. The exercise benefits occurred in subjects who were either lean or overweight at baseline.

Walking and the Obesity Epidemic

The relation between physical activity and obesity in the general public is complex because body-weight gain or loss depends on the energy intake from food as well as the energy expenditure through physical activity. When one looks at the extreme ends of the physical activity continuum in a population, those at the low end generally have a higher prevalence of being overweight (BMI = 25.0 to 29.9) or obese (BMI ≥30) than those at the high end. However, in the broad and relatively homogenous middle range of energy expenditure in the adult population, the reported level of physical activity amount usually does not correlate well with measures of adiposity. This is particularly true more recently as "daily required physical activity" has decreased for a greater and greater proportion of the population because of technological advances. People now have a reduced need to move in the home and on the job. Furthermore, economic policies and incentives favor sitting at a desk for long hours, as the work environment constrains a person's opportunities for daily activity (25).

Bassett and colleagues documented that high levels of daily physical activity, especially substantial walking, are associated with a healthy body weight in Old Order Amish men and women (4). These Old Order Amish living in Ontario, Canada, refrain from driving automobiles, using electrical appliances, and employing other modern conveniences, and manual labor farming was the primary occupation. The amount of physical activity performed daily by 98 men and women was assessed using standard question-

naires, pedometers, and a log for seven consecutive days. The average number of steps per day for men was 18,425 and 14,196 for women and the men reported walking 12.0 hours per week and the women 5.7 hours per week. None of Amish men and only 9% of the women were obese (BMI ≥30), while 25% of the Amish men and 26% of the women were overweight or obese (BMI >25). By contrast, in the general population, the majority of adults do not walk more than 2 to 3 hours per week, accumulate less than 5,000 steps per day, and approximately 56% have BMI >25 and 20% are obese (BMI ≥30) (33).

The contribution of increased walking to weight loss in overweight adults has been investigated repeatedly over the past 30 years with mixed results. Programs that have included an increase in walking ≥12 miles per week for more than 12 weeks frequently have reported significant weight loss, while programs that included less exercise typically have not. Pollock and colleagues (42) had sedentary middle-aged men walk 40 minutes per session, 4 days per week for 20 weeks, with walking distance averaging 12 to 13 miles per week over the last 12 weeks. Compared with sedentary controls, these men lost an average of 1.3 kg body weight (p <0.05) and reduced their percentage of body fat 1.1% (p <0.01). In a 12-month weight loss study involving 201 premenopausal, overweight sedentary women, Jakicic and colleagues demonstrated that the magnitude of weight loss was related to the amount of exercise performed (20). As displayed in Figure 9-5, women who walked <150 minutes per week had about a 6% weight loss at 6 and 12 months, while those women who walked >200 minutes per week had a 12% to 14% weight loss during the same period. In some studies where an increase in physical activity is provided during structured sessions, no or little weight loss was observed because participants reduced activity performed during other times of the day.

Osteoporosis, Osteoarthritis, and Bone Health

Most current recommendations for improving general bone health, especially for increasing or maintaining bone mineral density and preventing fractures related to osteoporosis include the frequent performance of moderate or vigorous intensity weight-bearing physical activity, including walking. Osteoporosis is a disease characterized by decreased bone mass and leading to increased bone fragility and susceptibility to fracture. Compression and bending forces placed on the skeleton during muscle contractions and the action of gravity during exercise stimulate bone formation and strength. Generally, vigorous intensity or high-impact exercise produces the greatest stimulus for increased bone strength, but most weight-bearing activities provide benefit. Walking briskly (see section on power walking) as well as up and down hills or stairs provides sufficient stress on the bones of the hip, legs,

% Weight Change

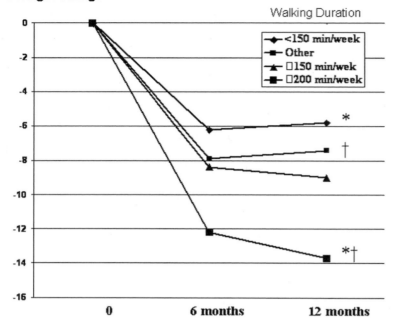

FIGURE 9-5. Percent changes in body weight based on exercise duration (walking on treadmill in home) in 196 premenopausal women participating in a comprehensive weight loss program. Group assignment based on average amount of exercise at 6 and 12 months. Groups that have the same symbol (astrisk or dagger) are significantly different from one another.

and feet to stimulate increased bone growth in children and young adults and decrease the rate of bone density loss in postmenopausal women and older men (55). As with many of the health benefits of walking, other good health habits such as not smoking and adequate calcium intake are important in maximizing bone health.

In addition to evidence that frequent exercise helps to maintain bone strength, it has been shown that leisure-time physical activity, including walking, reduces the risk of hip fractures in postmenopausal women (14). A total of 61,200 generally healthy women aged 40 to 77 years were followed for a period of 12 years during which time incidence of hip fracture was assessed. After controlling for age, body mass index, use of postmenopausal hormones, smoking, and dietary intake, the most active women had a 55% lower incidence of hip fracture than the least active women ($R^2 = 0.45$, 95% CI $= 0.32$–0.63). Among women who did no other exercise, walking at least 4 hours per week was associated with 41% lower risk of hip fracture ($R^2 = 0.59$, 95% CI $= 0.37$–0.94) compared to women who walked <1 hour per week.

Osteoarthritis is a chronic degenerative joint disease characterized primarily by progressive loss of articular cartilage, which leads to the narrowing of the joint space, pain, restriction in motion, crepitus, and deformity. Chronic, repetitive muscular loading of the joint, especially during occupational work and vigorous athletic training and competition can lead to an increase in the risk of osteoarthritis (40,54). However, joints tolerate slowly applied loads much better than sudden impact or torsional loading. There is no good evidence that increased walking or

similar activities prevent the development of osteoarthritis, but there are data from observational and experimental studies showing that moderate-intensity resistance and aerobic exercise, including walking, can help reduce joint pain and swelling and increase functional capacity in patients with osteoarthritis (53). Ettinger and colleagues conducted an 18-month randomized clinical trial comparing walking or resistance exercise to participation in a health education class in 365 men and women age ≥60 years with osteoarthritis of the knee (12). The walking and resistance exercise sessions lasted 60 minutes and were performed three times per week. Overall compliance with the exercise sessions was 68% in the walking group and 70% in the resistance-training group. When compared with participants in the health education class (exercise controls) patients in both exercise groups showed significant improvements in self-reported pain and disability scores, six-minute walk time, stair climb test, and time to lift and carry 10 pounds. These data support the use of supervised walking in the comprehensive medical management of osteoarthritis.

Cancer

Over the past two decades data have continued to accumulate supporting an inverse relationship between level of habitual physical activity and overall cancer incidence as well as selected site-specific cancers, especially of the colon and breast. For many other cancers there are inadequate data to determine if a significant relationship exists, but favorable trends have been reported for lung and some reproductive organ cancers. However, due to the complex nature of the etiology of most cancers, including the long delay between risk exposure and the clinical display of the tumor, the relatively low-prevalence of most site-specific cancers in the general population and our lack of understanding about biological mechanisms by which exercise might protect against a cancer, it has not yet been possible to establish a causal link between physical activity and cancer morbidity or mortality. There is no consistent evidence that an increase in physical activity, including walking, decreases a person's risk of acquiring cancer. In the numerous observational studies that have investigated either occupational or leisure-time physical activity and cancer risk, it appears that moderate intensity activities (4–5 METS or higher) are more strongly associated with lower cancer risk than activities that require less than 4 METS (49). Thus, for walking to meet these criteria for cancer prevention, walking briskly ($\geq$4 mph), walking up stairs or hills or hiking with a pack all should be considered.

Recently, some cancer treatment centers have been providing supervised aerobic and resistance exercise training programs for patients following surgery, radiation, or chemotherapy for their cancer. These programs are designed to improve physical performance and independence, increase lean body mass and reduce adiposity, and enhance health-related quality of life. The effects of a home-based walking program on fatigue, physical functioning, and emotional distress were evaluated in 46 women during a 6-week program of radiation therapy for breast cancer (32). Women randomly assigned to the walking program experienced significantly greater improvements in physical functioning, fatigue, emotional distress, and sleeping compared to women assigned to usual care.

Cognitive Function and Dementia

Moderate intensity exercise when performed on a regular basis appears to have favorable influences on a variety of mental and psychological functions. It has been reported that frequent walking contributes to a higher level of cognitive function and to lower occurrence of dementia in older women and men. Among 18,766 women aged 70 to 81 years who reported no vigorous physical activity, those women in the upper two quartiles of walking duration (1.5 to 2.8 hours per week and >2.8 hours per week) had significantly higher cognitive scores on all measures as compared to women in the lowest quartile of walking (<38 minutes per week) (59). The average speed of walking was estimated at 21 to 30 minutes per mile or 2 to 3 mph. The relationship of walking to the development of cognitive impairment was studied in 5,925 community-dwelling women aged $\geq$65 years without baseline cognitive impairment or physical limitations who were followed for 6 to 8 years (60). Cognitive decline occurred in 17%, 18%, 22%

and 24% of those women in the highest to lowest quartiles of blocks walked (p <0.001 for trend). After adjustment for age, educational level, comorbid conditions, smoking status, estrogen use, and functional limitations, women in the highest quartile of walking remained 34% less likely than women in the lowest quartile to develop cognitive decline. Walking has been reported to protect against cognitive decline in older men as well as women (3).

Distance walked per day was assessed by questionnaire in 2,257 physically capable men aged 71 to 93 years as part of the Honolulu-Asia Aging Study (1). During the course of a 6- to 8-year follow-up, men who walked the least (<0.25 miles per day) had a 1.8-fold excess risk of developing dementia compared to those who walked more than 2 miles per day (17.8 versus 10.3/1,000 person-years). Somewhat similar results have been reported from the Canadian Study of Health and Aging in which a nationwide population-based sample of 4,615 men and women aged $\geq$65 years free of dementia at baseline were evaluated 5 years later (28). One of the stronger predictors of developing Alzheimer disease was baseline level of physical activity. Subjects reporting regular physical activity (a substantial amount being walking) had a 41% lower risk of developing Alzheimer disease compared to persons reporting no regular physical activity. A biological basis for such an effect is not known but could be related to less vascular disease and a lower rate of multi-infarct dementia in the more physically active older persons.

POWER WALKING FOR FITNESS AND HEALTH

In order to achieve the beneficial effects of exercise, adults must participate in moderate-intensity physical activity on most days of the week, for at least 30 minutes (41). In terms of energy expenditure, moderate-intensity activity is defined as 3 to 6 METS (work metabolic rate/resting metabolic rate). Brisk walking at a pace of 4 mph meets this criterion for most adults (2). The actual energy expenditure for an individual will vary depending on walking speed, surface (smooth or uneven, soft or hard, etc.), and gradient (horizontal, up, down) (2). Personal factors such as mechanical efficiency (e.g., inefficient gait due to hip or leg deformity) may also affect energy expenditure in some individuals.

Comfortable walking speed is typically about 3 mph, or 80.5 m/min (36,57). To achieve brisk walking speed of 4 mph (107 m/min), or a vigorous exercise pace of 5 mph (134 m/min), the mechanics of walking must be altered from that of regular comfortable walking. Murray et al. studied walking at slow, free, and fast speeds. When comparing free walking (85 m/min) to fast walking (115 m/min), they found fast walking resulted in an increased arc of hip motion due to increased

▶ **TABLE 9-1 Velocity, Stride Length, and Cadence of Free Versus Power Walking**

Subject	Walking Pace	Velocity (m/min)	Cadence (steps/min)	Stride Length (cm)
Subject 1	Free	91.9	123	150.0
Subject 1	Power	148.8	146	200.0
Subject 2	Free	91.5	126	145.7
Subject 2	Power	139.1	169	165.6

flexion in terminal swing and increased extension in terminal stance; increased knee flexion in early stance; increased shoulder and elbow arc of motion; and an increase in the vertical excursion of the head. Fast walking also resulted in increased stride length and increased cadence (36). Race walkers use different joint motions than that observed for fast walking, and have an increased stride

length and cadence beyond that of normal controls during fast walking (35).

Many people participate in walking for fitness and health. Brisk walking (4 mph, or 107 m/min) is sufficient to achieve the physiological benefits of exercise (37). However, to achieve a higher level of fitness than that afforded by moderate intensity of brisk walking, people may choose

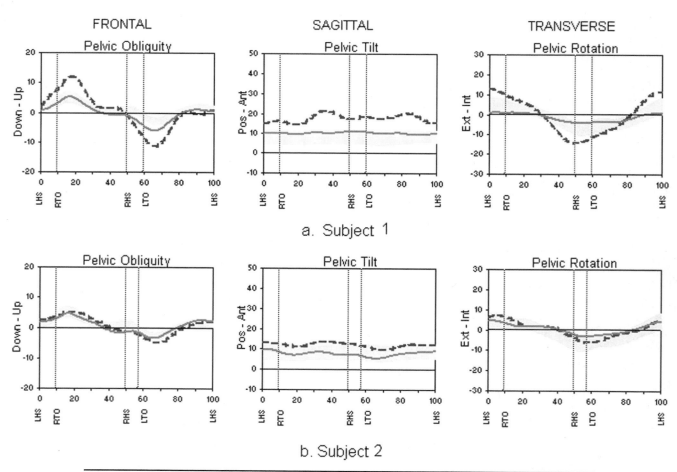

FIGURE 9-6. Pelvic kinematics for **(a)** Subject 1 and **(b)** Subject 2. *Solid line* is free walking; *dashed line* is power walking; *light gray lines* represent normal comfortable speed walking ± 2 standard deviations. LHS = left heel strike; RTO = right toe off; RHS = right heel strike; LTO = left toe off. X-axis is percent of gait cycle. Y-axis is degrees of motion. LHS to LTO represents stance phase. LTO to LHS represents swing phase. LHS to RTO is loading response (initial double limb support) and RHS to LTO is preswing (terminal double limb support).

to participate in vigorous exercise (greater than 6 METS) (41). Fitness, or power, walking (5.0 mph, 134 m/min, or greater) meets the criteria of vigorous exercise (2).

There is a paucity of information in the literature describing the kinematic and kinetic data looking specifically at the recreational power walker. We studied two women (Subjects 1 and 2) who participate in power walking as part of their regular fitness routine. Both achieved walking speeds sufficient to generate an exercise effect as described in the literature (2,41). Both subjects had a free walking pace faster than that reported by Murray et al. of 85.0 m/min, as shown in Table 9-1 (36).

An increased speed, or velocity, of walking, can be obtained by increased cadence and/or increased stride length. During power walking, Subject 1 increased her velocity by 62% over free walking primarily with an increased stride length (33% increase) and a small increase (19%) in cadence. Subject 2 achieved a 52% increase in velocity primarily through an increase in her cadence (34%) with only a slight increase (14%) in stride length (Table 9-1).

Kinematics

During power walking, both subjects had the elbows flexed from 75 to 100 degrees and had an increased arc of shoulder motion during reciprocal arm swing. During free walking, the elbows have an arc of motion from about 20 to

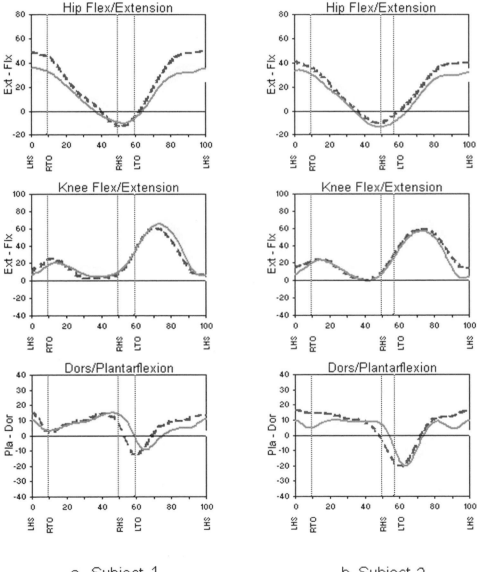

FIGURE 9-7. Hip, knee, and ankle kinematics for **(a)** Subject 1 and **(b)** Subject 2. *Solid line* is free walking; *dashed line* is power walking; *light gray lines* represent normal comfortable speed walking ±2 standard deviations. LHS = left heel strike; RTO = right toe off; RHS = right heel strike; LTO = left toe off. X-axis is percent of gait cycle. Y-axis is degrees of motion. LHS to LTO represents stance phase. LTO to LHS represents swing phase. LHS to RTO is loading response (initial double limb support) and RHS to LTO is preswing (terminal double limb support).

a. Subject 1   b. Subject 2

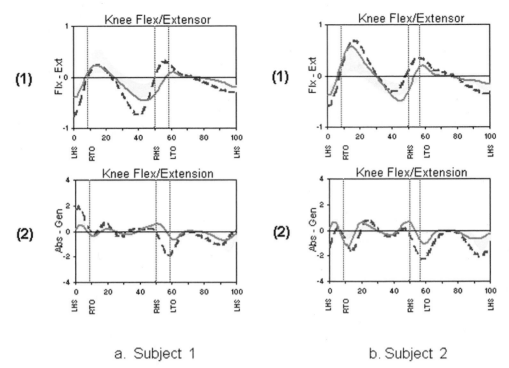

a. Subject 1   b. Subject 2

FIGURE 9-8. Knee kinetics (1) and power (2) for **(a)** Subject 1 and **(b)** Subject 2. *Solid line* is free walking; *dashed line* is power walking; *light gray lines* represent normal comfortable speed walking ± 2 standard deviations. LHS = left heel strike; RTO = right toe off; RHS = right heel strike; LTO = left toe off. X-axis is percent of gait cycle. (1) Kinetics: Y-axis is the joint moment (Nm/kg). (2) Power: Y-axis is in Watts/kg, expressed as positive for power generation, or negative for power absorption. LHS to LTO represents stance phase. LTO to LHS represents swing phase. LHS to RTO is loading response (initial double limb support) and RHS to LTO is preswing (terminal double limb support).

40 degrees of flexion. Subject 1, who used primarily an increased stride length to achieve power walking velocity, had an increase in pelvic motion in all three planes (Figure 9-6a), and increased hip flexion at initial contact, with less change in sagittal plane ankle motion than Subject 2 (Figure 9-7a). Subject 1 also demonstrated a significant increase in trunk rotation that accompanied the increase in pelvic rotation (Figure 9-6a): for the left limb at initial contact, the pelvis rotated to the left while the trunk rotated to the right and in terminal stance, the pelvis rotated to the right while the trunk rotated to the left. When using cadence as the primary means of achieving an increased velocity for power walking, Subject 2's trunk and lower extremity motion only varied by an increased anterior pelvic tilt and increased ankle dorsiflexion in swing and early stance (Figures 9-6b and 9-7b). Her peak ankle dorsiflexion position occurred at initial contact with a gradual progression toward plantar flexion during stance (Figure 9-7b).

The kinematic data from these two subjects demonstrate two different strategies used to achieve increased speed of walking. Both subjects had increased elbow flexion and increased shoulder range of motion during power walking. However, when increased cadence was chosen as the primary mode to achieve faster walking speed, there were minimal changes in the kinematics. When faster walking speed was achieved by increasing the stride length, there were significant changes in the kinematics of the trunk and pelvis. If one has mechanical pathology in the lumbar spine that may be aggravated by increased trunk and pelvis rotation, it may be best to use increased cadence, rather than increased stride length, to achieve walking speeds of vigorous exercise.

Kinetics

In loading response, both subjects had similar increases in knee flexor and hip extensor moments. In late stance (preswing) there were similar increases in knee extensor and hip flexor moments for both women (Figures 9-8 and 9-9). At the ankle, there was an increased generation of power in late stance during power walking compared to comfortable speed walking (Figure 9-10).

These two subjects demonstrated power walking at speeds adequate to generate a vigorous exercise effect. Their techniques of increasing walking speed were different in that one used primarily an increased cadence and one used primarily an increase in stride length. The resulting joint kinematics, kinetics, and power varied depending on the chosen technique. However, there were similarities in some of these variables as well. As participation in power walking grows, especially in the older population, it is important to continue to expand our understanding of the mechanics of high speed walking through research to promote safe techniques.

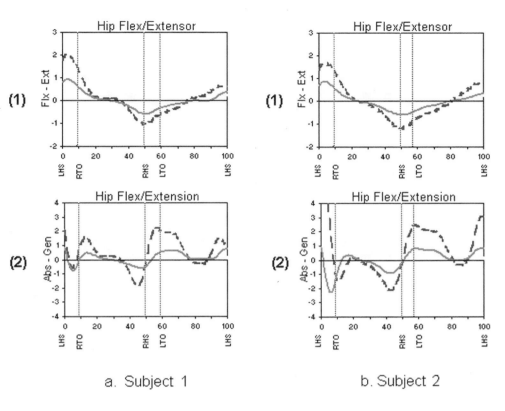

FIGURE 9-9. Hip kinetics (1) and power (2) for **(a)** Subject 1 and **(b)** Subject 2. *Solid line* is free walking; *dashed line* is power walking; *light gray lines* represent normal comfortable speed walking ± 2 standard deviations. LHS = left heel strike; RTO = right toe off; RHS = right heel strike; LTO = left toe off. X-axis is percent of gait cycle. (1) Kinetics: Y-axis is the joint moment (Nm/kg). (2) Power: Y-axis is in Watts/kg, expressed as positive for power generation, or negative for power absorption. LHS to LTO represents stance phase. LTO to LHS represents swing phase. LHS to RTO is loading response (initial double limb support) and RHS to LTO is preswing (terminal double limb support).

a. Subject 1   b. Subject 2

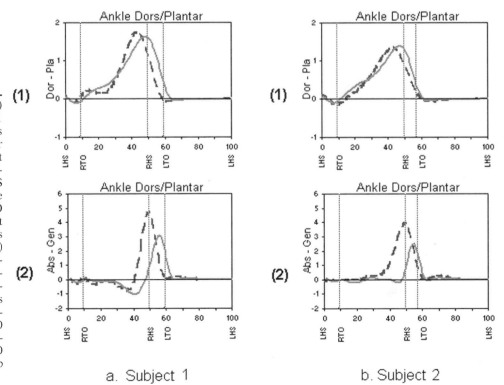

FIGURE 9-10. Ankle kinetics (1) and power (2) for **(a)** Subject 1 and **(b)** Subject 2. *Solid line* is free walking; *dashed line* is power walking; *light gray lines* represent normal comfortable speed walking ± 2 standard deviations. LHS = left heel strike; RTO = right toe off; RHS = right heel strike; LTO = left toe off. X-axis is percent of gait cycle. (1) Kinetics: Y-axis is the joint moment (Nm/kg). (2) Power: Y-axis is in Watts/kg, expressed as positive for power generation, or negative for power absorption. LHS to LTO represents stance phase. LTO to LHS represents swing phase. LHS to RTO is loading response (initial double limb support) and RHS to LTO is preswing (terminal double limb support).

a. Subject 1   b. Subject 2

Conclusion

That frequent walking has the potential to provide a number of significant health benefits throughout a person's lifespan has been scientifically documented over the past 50 years. These benefits include the reduction in the incidence of coronary heart disease, hypertension, stroke, obesity, type II diabetes, osteoporosis, and several site-specific cancers. Walking is also effective in the treatment or rehabilitation process for many of these and other disorders, including osteoarthritis. In older persons, walking contributes to enhanced physical and cognitive functioning and a lower incidence of dementia. Many of the studies report significant health benefits from brisk walking (3+ mph) for two or more hours per week, with greater benefits resulting from faster walking or longer durations. There are numerous reasons for promoting walking to improve the health of the population over a number of other activities. Compared to jogging or running, walking produces substantially fewer musculoskeletal injuries (5) and by building walking into each person's lifestyle the public health goals for physical activity can be achieved (6). Walking also provides an environmental friendly form of transportation and can be done alone or as a socially oriented group hike or trek. Most people possess the skill and ability to walk daily and special equipment requirements, other than good walking shoes and possibly a walking stick, are minimal.

REFERENCES

1. Abbott RD, White LR, Ross GW, Masaki KH, Curb JD, Petrovitch H. Walking and dementia in physically capable men. *JAMA* 2004;292:1447–1453.
2. Ainsworth BE, Haskell WL, Whitt MC, et al. Compendium of physical activities: an update of activity codes and MET intensities. *Med Sci Sports Exerc* 2000;32:S498–S516.
3. Albert MS, Jones K, Savage CR, et al. Predictors of cognitive change in older persons. MacArthur Studies of Successful Aging. *Psychol Aging* 1995;10:578–589.
4. Bassett DR, Schneider PL, Hunington GE. Physical activity in an Old Order Amish community. *Med Sci Ex Sports* 2004;36:79–85.
5. Colbert LH, Hootman JM, Macera CA. Physical activity-related injuries in walkers and runners in the Aerobics Center Longitudinal Study. *Clin J Sports Med* 2000;10:259–263.
6. Coleman KJ, Raynor HR, Mueller DM, Cerny FJ, Dorn JM, Epstein LH. Providing sedentary adults with choices for meeting their walking goals. *Prevent Med* 1999;28:510–519.
7. Cordain L, Gotshall RW, Eaton SB, Eaton SB 3rd. Physical activity, energy expenditure, and fitness: an evolutionary perspective. *Int J Sports Med* 1998;19:328–335.
8. Criqui MH. Peripheral arterial disease—epidemiological aspects. *Vasc Med* 2001;6:S3–S7.
9. Darwin C. *The Origin of Species by Means of Natural Selection, or the Preservation of Favored Races in the Struggle for Life*. Watts and Co., London; 1859:546.
10. Duncan JJ, Gordon NF, Scott CB. Women walking for health and fitness: how much is enough? *JAMA* 1991;266:295–299.
11. Engelgau MM, Gelss LS, Saaddine JB, et al. The evolving diabetes burden in the United States. *Ann Intern Med* 2004;140:945–950.
12. Ettinger WH, Burns R, Messier SP, et al. A randomized trial comparing aerobic exercise and resistance exercise with a health education program in older adults with knee osteoarthritis: The Fitness Arthritis and Seniors Trial (FAST). *JAMA* 1997;277:25–31.
13. Eyler AA, Brownson RC, Bacak SJ, Housemann RA. The epidemiology of walking for physical activity in the United States. *Med Sci Sports Ex* 2003:35:1529–1536.
14. Feskanic D, Willett W, Colditz G. Walking and leisure-time physical activity and risk of hip fracture in postmenopausal women. *JAMA* 2002;288:2300–2306.
15. Gardner AW, Poehlman ET. Exercise rehabilitation programs for the treatment of claudication pain: a meta-analysis. *JAMA* 1995;274:975–980.
16. Hakim AA, Curb D, Petrovich H, et al. Effects of walking on coronary heart disease in elderly men: The Honolulu Heart Program. *Circulation* 1999;100:9–13.
17. Hatano Y. Use of the pedometer for promoting daily walking activity. *Jap C Health Physical Ed Rec* 1993;29:4–8.
18. Hu FB, Sigal RJ, Rich-Edwards JW, et al. Walking compared with vigorous physical activity and risk of type 2 diabetes in women. *JAMA* 1999;282:1433–1439.
19. Hu FB, Stampfer MJ, Colditz GA, et al. Physical activity and risk of stroke in women. *JAMA* 2000;283:2961–2967.
20. Jakicic JM, Marcus BH, Gallagher KJ, Napolitano M, Lang W. Effect of exercise duration and intensity on weight loss in overweight sedentary women: a randomized trial. *JAMA* 2003;290:1323–1330.
21. Koh-Banerjee P, Wang Y, Hu FB, Spiegelman D, Willett WC, Rimm EB. Changes in body weight and body fat distribution as risk factors for clinical diabetes in US men. *Am J Epidemiol* 2004;159:1150–1159.
22. Kraus WE, Houmard JA, Duscha BD, et al. Effects of the amount and intensity of exercise on plasma lipoproteins. *N Engl J Med* 2002;347:1483–1492.
23. Krotkiewski M, Lonnroth P, Mandroukas K, et al. The effects of physical training on insulin secretion and effectiveness and on glucose metabolism in obesity and Type-2 (noninsulin dependent) diabetes mellitus. *Diabetologia* 1985;28:881–890.
24. LaCroix AZ, Levielle SG, Hecht JA, Grothaus LC, Wagner EH. Does walking decrease the risk of cardiovascular disease hospitalizations and death in older adults? *J Am Geriatr Soc* 1996;44:113–120.
25. Lakdawalla D, Philipson T. The growth of obesity and technological change: a theoretical and empirical examination. NBER Working Paper No 8946. *National Bureau of Economic Research*, Cambridge, MA; 2002.
26. Lee CD, Folsom AR, Blair SN. Physical activity and stroke risk: A meta-analysis. *Stroke* 2003;34:2475–2482.
27. Leenders NYJM, Sherman WM, Nagaraja HN, Kien CL. Evaluation of methods to assess physical activity in free-living conditions. *Med Sci Sports Ex* 2001;33:1233–1240.
28. Lindsay J, Laurin D, Verreault R, Helliwell B, Hill GB, McDowell I. Risk factors for Alzheimer's disease: a prospective analysis from the Canadian Study of Health and Aging. *Am J Epidemiol* 2002;156:445–453.
29. Malina RM. Darwinian fitness, physical fitness and physical activity. In: Mascie-Taylor CGN, Lasker GW, eds. *Applications of Biological Anthropology*. Cambridge: Cambridge University Press; 1991:143–184.
30. Manson JE, Greenland P, LaCroix AZ, et al. Walking compared to vigorous exercise for the prevention of cardiovascular events in women. *N Engl J Med* 2002;347:716–725.
31. Manson JE, Hu FB, Rich-Edwards JW, et al. A prospective study of walking as compared with vigorous exercise in the prevention of coronary heart disease in women. *N Engl J Med* 1999;341:650–658.
32. Mock V, Dow KH, Mears CJ, et al. Effects of exercise on fatigue, physical functioning, and emotional distress during radiation therapy for breast cancer. *Oncol Nurs Forum* 1997;24:991–2000.
33. Mokdad AH, Bowman B, Ford E, Vinicor F, Marks JS, Koplan JP. The continuing epidemic of obesity and diabetes in the United States. *JAMA* 2001;286:1195–1200.
34. Morris JN, Heady JA, Raffle PAB, et al. Coronary heart disease and physical activity of work. *Lancet* 1953;6795:1053–1057.
35. Murray MP, Guten GN, Mollinger LA, Gardner GM. Kinematic and electromyography patterns of Olympic race walkers. *Am J Sport Med* 1983;11:68–74.

36. Murray MP, Mollinger LA, Gardner GM, Sepic SB. Kinematic and EMG patterns during slow, free, and fast walking. *J Orthop Res* 1984; 2:272–280.
37. Murtagh EM, Boreham CAG, Murphy MH. Speed and exercise intensity of recreational walkers. *Prevent Med* 2002;35:397–400.
38. Newman AB. Peripheral arterial disease: insights from population studies of older adults. *J Am Geriatr Soc* 2000;48:1157–1162.
39. Pan X-R, Lei G-W, Hu Y-H, et al. Effects of diet and exercise in preventing NIDDM in people with impaired glucose tolerance. The Da Quing IGT and Diabetes Study. *Diabetes Care* 1997;20:537–544.
40. Panush RS, Inzinna JD. Recreational activities and degenerative joint disease. *Sports Med* 1994;17:1–5.
41. Pate RR, Pratt M, Blair SN, Haskell WL, et al. Physical activity and public health: a recommendation from the Centers for Disease Control and Prevention and the American College of Sports Medicine. *JAMA* 1995;273:402–407.
42. Pollock ML, Miller HS, Janeway R, Linnerud AC, Robertson B, Valentino R. Effects of walking on body composition and cardiovascular function in middle-aged men. *J Appl Physiol* 1971;30:126–130.
43. Rodnick KJ, Haskell WL, Swislocki ALM, Foley JE, Reaven GM. Improved insulin action in muscle, liver and adipose tissue in physically trained humans. *Am J Physiol* 1987;253:E489–E495.
44. Rogers MA, Yamamoto C, King DS, Hagberg JM, Ehansi AA, Holloszy JO. Improvement in glucose tolerance after one-week of exercise in patients with mild NIDDM. *Diabetes Care* 1988;11:613–618.
45. Schneider PL, Crouter SE, Lukajic O, Bassett JR. Accuracy and reliability of 10 pedometers for measuring steps over a 400-meter walk. *Med Sci Sports Ex* 2003;35:1779–1784.
46. Seidell JC. Obesity, insulin resistance and diabetes—a worldwide epidemic. *BMJ* 2000;83:S5–S8.
47. Simpson ME, Serdula M, Galuska DA, et al. Walking trends among US adults: the Behavioral Risk Factor Surveillance System, 1987–2000. *Am J Prev Med* 2003;25:95–100.
48. Slentz CA, Duscha BD, Johnson JL, et al. Effects of the amount of exercise on body weight, body composition, and measures of central obesity. *Arch Intern Med* 2004;164:31–39.
49. Thune I, Furberg A-S. Physical activity and cancer risk: dose response and cancer, all sites and site-specific. *Med Sci Sports Exerc* 2001;33:S530–S550.
50. Tomoshige H, Tsumura K, Suematsu C, Okada K, Fujii S, Endo G. Walking to work and the risk of hypertension in men: The Osaka Health Survey. *Ann Intern Med* 1999;130:21–26.
51. Tudor-Locke C, Bassett DR. How many steps/day are enough: preliminary pedometer indices for public health. *Sports Med* 2004;34:1–5.
52. Tudor-Locke C, Ham SA, Macera C, Ainsworth BE, Kirtland KA, Kinsey CD. Descriptive epidemiology of pedometer-determined physical activity. *Med Sci Sports Ex* 2004;36:1567–1573.
53. Van Barr ME, Assendelft WJJ, Dekker J, Oostendorp RAB, Bulsma JWJ. Effectiveness of exercise therapy in patients with osteoarthritis of the hip or knee. A systematic review of randomized clinical trials. *Arthritis Review* 1999;42:1361–1369.
54. Vingard E, Alfredsson L, Goldie I, Hogstedt C. Occupation and osteoarthrosis of the hip and knee: a registry-based cohort study. *Int J Epidemiol* 1991;20:1025–1031.
55. Vuori I. Dose-response of physical activity and low back pain, osteoarthritis and osteoporosis. *Med Sci Sports Ex* 2001;33:S551–S586.
56. Wannamethee SG, Shaper AG, Alberti GMM. Physical activity and metabolic factors, and the incidence of coronary heart disease and type 2 diabetes. *Arch Intern Med* 2000;160:2108–2116.
57. Waters RL, Lunsford BR, Perry J, Byrd R. Energy-speed relationship of walking: standard tables. *J Orthop Res* 1988;6:215–222.
58. Welk GJ, Differding JA, Thompson RW, et al. The utility of the Digi-walker step counter to assess daily physical activity patterns. *Med Sci Sports Ex* 2000;32:S481–S488.
59. Weuve J, Kang JH, Manson JE, Breteler MM, Ware JH, Grodstein F. Physical activity, including walking, and cognitive function in older women. *JAMA* 2004; 292:1454–1461.
60. Yaffe K, Barnes D, Nevitt M, Lui L-Y, Covinsky K. A prospective study of physical activity and cognitive decline in elderly women. *Arch Intern Med* 2001;161:1703–1708.

Chapter 10

Gait Analysis: Clinical Decision Making

Janet M. Adams and Jacquelin Perry

THE DEVELOPMENT OF GAIT ANALYSIS

Clinical use of gait analysis began as an observational skill when physicians, therapists, and prosthetists defined normal and abnormal limb motion and common deviations displayed by patients. Because the hip, knee, and ankle move at different rates and through asynchronous arcs, a systematic approach was devised corresponding to the pattern of limb motion. Critical events (i.e., heel strike) were selected to differentiate intervals and define phases. Clinicians from the Pathokinesiology and Physical Therapy Departments at Rancho Los Amigos National Rehabilitation Center developed generic terminology for both normal and abnormal gait. The functional subdivisions of the gait cycle were expanded to eight phases, each differentiating a major kinematic event. A "Full Body: Observational Gait Analysis Form" was developed which identified 35 commonly observed gait deviations and their phasic occurrence (15). Using this form as a guide, clinicians established a protocol for analysis that included observing the patient walk, identifying excessive or inadequate motion, and when it occurs in the gait cycle. Reliability and validity of this tool has been affirmed by two separate studies (4,7). The observational analysis is correlated with clinical assessments of strength, range of motion (ROM), spasticity, motor control, and sensation to determine the probable cause(s) of the deviation and its contribution to functional deficits.

Combined with an observational analysis, instrumented analysis provides a more precise and quantitative means of identifying deviations and probable cause. Orthopedists, treating children and adults with upper motor neuron lesions increasingly rely on instrumented analysis for presurgical decision making (6,14,17,22,24,25).

FUNCTIONAL PERSPECTIVE

Walking requires antigravity muscular support, joint mobility to allow smooth progression, and adequate motor control for the transition of body weight from one limb to another. Disruption of normal function by disease, trauma, degeneration, fatigue, or pain produces functional limitations. Potential for normal function varies with the severity of the primary impairment and the ability to utilize residual function for substitute action. Compensatory strategies depend on residual muscle strength, motor control, joint mobility, and sensory capabilities. Intervention depends on the ability of the clinician to identify and treat the impairment contributing to the functional loss, not the more conspicuous compensatory action.

Gait Cycle Organization & Interpretation

A stride is a complete cycle of limb motion that is divided into two periods: stance and swing. Stance, the period of foot-floor contact, is subdivided into 5 phases: initial contact, loading response, mid-stance, terminal stance, and preswing. Stance comprises 62% of the gait cycle (GC). The remaining 38% of the gait cycle constitutes the swing period, initiated as the foot leaves the support surface. It is equally divided into three phases: initial swing, mid-swing, and terminal swing.

Sequential combinations of these phases accomplish three tasks: weight acceptance, single limb support, and limb advancement. Initial contact and loading response constitute the period of *weight acceptance* (0% to 12% GC), an interval of double limb support when both feet are in contact with the floor for the transfer of body weight from one limb to the other. Mid-stance (13% to 30% gait cycle) and terminal stance (31% to 49% gait cycle) are involved in the task of *single limb support* when the weight of the body is fully supported by the stance limb. The task of *swing limb advancement* is initiated during preswing. Preswing is the period of terminal double limb support when weight is again transferred to the contralateral limb. *Swing limb advancement* includes preswing (50% to 62% GC), initial swing (63% to 74% GC), midswing (75% to 87% GC), and terminal swing (88% to 100% GC) (17,18).

165

Task 1: Weight Acceptance

The purpose of the two phases involved in weight acceptance is to protect the joints from impact injury and preserve progression. The critical functions are establishing a heel rocker and shock absorption.

Phase 1: Initial contact is a brief event that initiates stance phase. Foot position and contact point determine the availability of the *heel*, or first, rocker. Heel contact creates a moment that initiates plantar flexion and subtalar eversion resisted by eccentric action of the pretibial (anterior tibialis [AT], extensor digitorum longus [EDL], extensor hallucis longus [EHL]) muscles and posterior tibialis (17,21,23).

Abnormal foot contact patterns may be caused by pretibial muscle weakness, inadequate knee extension or plantar flexion contractures. The normal event of heel strike may be replaced by a low or abbreviated heel strike, foot-flat, or forefoot contact. All three reduce the pivotal action that the heel rocker provides, resulting in decreased momentum, reduced stride length, and decreased velocity (17).

Phase 2. Loading response is characterized by an increase in knee flexion as weight is transferred onto the limb. The eccentric action of the quadriceps limits knee flexion to 15 degrees. The knee flexes to provide shock absorption to protect proximal joints. Deviations may be either excessive or absent knee motion. Weak quadriceps (<4/5 in manual muscle testing [MMT]) result in the avoidance of knee flexion; the patient compensates by positioning body weight anterior to the knee joint axis creating an extensor moment, thereby eliminating the demand for quadriceps action. Plantar flexion contractures, spasticity, or premature activation of the gastrocnemius may prevent knee flexion during loading (13,14,20). This phase also requires peak hip extensor and abductor muscle action to increase weight-bearing stability of the limbs and pelvis (9).

Task 2: Single Limb Support

Contralateral toe-off places weight exclusively on the stance limb, defining the third and fourth phases of the gait cycle, mid and terminal stance. During this task, the body advances over a stationary foot while maintaining limb stability. Critical functions include stabilization of the hip in the sagittal and coronal planes to prevent excessive pelvic & trunk motion, as well as unrestrained ankle dorsiflexion to allow progression over a stationary foot. The second (ankle) and third (forefoot) rockers preserve momentum. The rate of tibial advancement is restrained by eccentric action of the plantar flexors (17,21,23). The critical factors include adequate strength of the plantar flexors and mobility of the ankle, knee, and hip.

Phase 3: Mid-stance is a period of flat foot support and relies on the pivotal mobility of the *ankle*, or second, rocker to preserve momentum and advance the limb over a stationary foot. Controlled ankle dorsiflexion is critical to progression. The larger soleus muscle is the predominant decelerating force, eccentrically contracting along with the gastrocnemius and perimalleolar (posterior tibialis [PT], flexor digitorum longus [FDL], flexor hallucis longus [FHL], peroneus longus [PL], and peroneus brevis [PB]) muscles (17,21,23). By the end of mid-stance, the ankle achieves 5 degrees of dorsiflexion and the center of pressure is moving toward the forefoot while the hip and knee are passively extending.

Errors in motor control that cause premature, excessive or spastic plantar flexor muscle action and contractures frequently produce premature lifting of the heel, relocating the pivotal axis to the forefoot to preserve momentum (14). When patients lack momentum to progress onto the forefoot, knee hyperextension or genu recurvatum results.

Plantar flexor weakness (<4/5) causes unrestrained dorsiflexion. The tibia accelerates forward, inducing knee flexion that increases the demand on the quadriceps. Even when the quadriceps are graded *good* or *normal* in strength (4 or 5), they no longer have a stable base over which to exert force and full knee extension cannot occur. The dorsiflexion moment increases and knee flexion persists, requiring continuous quadriceps action. Once maximum available dorsiflexion range is reached, the heel lifts off the support surface (premature heel rise). Forefoot contact results but is coupled with excess dorsiflexion and knee flexion. This pattern is often mistakenly referred to as equinus since the heel is lifted, however the ankle is dorsiflexed instead of plantar flexed.

Just as primary ankle impairments cause knee deviations, knee impairments produce changes in ankle kinematics that alter the foot contact pattern. For example, when a patient presents with a knee flexion contracture and strong calf muscles, momentum will be preserved by voluntarily plantar flexing, assuming a forefoot contact pattern. This increases the relative length of the involved limb and enables progression over a stationary foot. Similarly, hip flexion contractures induce secondary knee flexion, requiring modification of the ankle position and foot-floor contact pattern to preserve momentum.

Phase 4: Terminal stance progression relies on hip extension mobility and controlled dorsiflexion to progress the body over a stationary foot. The forefoot becomes the axis about which the weight-bearing limb pivots; it is called the *forefoot*, or third, rocker. Heel rise occurs, reducing the base of support to the metatarsal heads. Eccentric action of the soleus and gastrocnemius peak at 45% GC and 40% GC, respectively, coupled with posterior tibialis and peroneals activation which stabilizes the subtalar and transverse tarsal joints for forefoot weight bearing (17,21,23). The ankle dorsiflexes 10 degrees while the center of pressure advances over the contour of the metatarsal heads.

Inadequate plantar flexion strength allows unrestrained tibial advancement resulting in a flexed knee during stance and a possible loss of heel rise. If quadriceps strength is inadequate to support a flexed knee (<4/5), knee extension persists. Excessive plantar flexion from contracture, spasticity or disordered motor control accentuates the extensor moment causing hyperextension at the knee. The center of pressure cannot progress to the forefoot, which requires premature contralateral initial contact and leads to a reduced step length.

Task 3: Swing Limb Advancement

This task includes the final phase of stance (preswing) and all three swing phases. The initial requirement is rapid transformation of a "rigid" extended limb into a flexible mobile segment. The critical events are limb advancement and foot clearance.

Phase 5: Pre-swing is the final phase of stance (50% to 62% gait cycle). Contralateral foot contact initiates double limb support phase. The rapid transfer of weight abruptly unloads the stance limb and two events occur: 20 degrees of plantar flexion and 40 degrees of knee flexion. The energy for this action is the result of the abrupt release, in terminal stance, of the soleus and gastrocnemius eccentric action (12). At 54% of the gait cycle, there is a prominent spike of plantar flexor power that generates the dynamic elastic response characterized as "push-off" (17,21,23). The adductor longus contributes to the arc of hip flexion for limb advancement.

Spasticity of the vasti or rectus femoris may obstruct knee flexion requiring compensation at the hip and/or pelvis to achieve foot clearance (8,20). Reduced knee flexion may also result from joint effusion, pain, or the secondary effect of reduced velocity.

Phases 6, 7 & 8: Initial, Mid & Terminal Swing During initial swing the hip flexes 20 degrees, the knee flexes another 20 degrees (total arc of 60°), and the ankle begins dorsiflexing to accomplish foot clearance. Momentum from hip flexion is the primary determinant of knee flexion during this interval. Mid-swing continues the task of limb advancement and foot clearance. Hip flexion (25°) and ankle dorsiflexion to neutral are the critical events while advancing the tibia past its vertical alignment. Terminal swing completes limb advancement with full knee extension, while keeping the hip at 25 degrees of flexion and the ankle dorsiflexed to neutral. Hip flexion is terminated by the hamstring muscles while momentum and quadriceps action extend the knee to neutral. In preparation for initial contact, the gluteus maximus and adductor magnus activate (9).

The major deviation during swing is toe drag. Limb clearance is impaired if there is limited hip flexion, knee flexion, or dorsiflexion. The primary cause may be inadequate knee flexion in pre-swing. Weak dorsiflexors (manual muscle test [MMT] <3/5) causes "foot drop" requiring increased hip and knee flexion to achieve foot clearance (steppage gait). Weak contralateral abductors, spastic quadriceps, or weak dorsiflexors all produce a relative lengthening of the swing limb requiring compensatory action for clearance. In terminal swing, step length may be compromised by inadequate knee extension, tight or spastic hamstrings or disordered motor control obstructing knee extension with hip flexion.

Temporal Gait Characteristics

Walking speed for 20 to 60 year old adults at the normal self selected pace averages 80 m per minute (men 82 m per minute and women 78 m per minute) +/− 10 m per minute (1 SD) (26). At this speed, the duration of stance is 62% of the gait cycle and swing is 38%. Double limb support averages 24% GC with the remaining 38% as single limb support. Wide variability in stride characteristics exists within the normal population depending on speed, age, gender, and geographic location (2,5,11,26).

Stance as a percentage of the gait cycle increases as walking speed becomes slower (5). Among persons with a disability, a correlation between severity and self-selected velocity has been identified. Normal 20 to 60 year old individuals walking at slow speeds average 43 m per minute; consequently, disabled individuals with slower velocities must exert maximal efforts to accompany peers (26).

CLINICAL TESTING TO IDENTIFY PRIMARY IMPAIRMENTS

Strength Assessment

For patients with musculoskeletal pathology, the standard manual muscle testing (MMT) procedures are appropriate as they have the ability to isolate movement of one joint from that of adjacent joints. Clinical interpretation of the MMT grades 0 to 5 represent absent to normal strength; however, it often overestimates the patient's capabilities. Correlation of MMT grades and torque measurements of individuals with polio and age-matched controls defined a grade 4/5 ("good") was equivalent to 40% of true normal strength, grade 3/5 ("fair") was 20% of normal and grade 2/5 ("poor") was 10% of normal (1). Thus, a grade 4/5 (good) actually represents a significant loss of strength (as much as 60%) despite the ability of the examiner to offer substantial resistance. The weakness may introduce subtle deviations as a result of muscle fatigue that do not appear during the standard gait analysis (6–10 m of walking) but limit community mobility.

Mobility Assessment

Contractures restrict passive soft tissue mobility, requiring postural adaptations to preserve progression. "Rigid" and "elastic" or "yielding" contractures should be differentiated as they have different functional implications. Elastic contractures yield under the force of body weight but resist full range during a manual stretch using minimal force (2 fingers) (17). In contrast, rigid contractures do not stretch significantly regardless of the force exerted by body weight. This differentiation is especially critical at the ankle. Yielding contractures can be a valuable supplement for weak plantar flexors, acting as an internal orthosis, providing tibial stability in the absence of sufficient muscle strength. In contrast, rigid contractures are usually obstructive and require serial casting or surgical lengthening. Differentiation between the two types of contractures, especially at the ankle, is critical for deciding on an optimal intervention strategy.

The Significance of Pathology: Musculoskeletal versus Neuromuscular

An essential first step in the clinical application of gait analysis is identification of the patient's medical diagnosis as a means of classifying the primary impairments. Impairments affecting gait primarily fall into two broad practice patterns, neuromuscular and musculoskeletal. Patients with neuromuscular impairments primarily have disordered motor control resulting from upper motor neuron lesions (3). This significantly limits their ability to substitute for impaired function. Musculoskeletal impairments limit functional performance caused by pathological alteration in the peripheral structures. These patients generally have excellent substitutive capability.

Primary Impairments in Patients with Musculoskeletal Pathology

Patients with gait abnormalities often exhibit asymmetry with one limb more affected than the other. If the impairment is moderate, that limb will be the focus of disability. If, however, the impairment is severe the "strong" limb may be the symptomatic site of overuse. Thus, at least a preliminary assessment of both limbs should precede instrumented gait analysis. Even a MMT grade 2/5 can be beneficial for functional tasks despite the absence of antigravity capabilities. The initial gait modification is a reduced gait velocity.

WEAK DORSIFLEXORS: Strength requirements of the dorsiflexors (AT, EDL and EHL) vary throughout the gait cycle. When graded <3/5, drop foot is most evident in midswing. Compensatory hip and knee flexion provide foot clearance (steppage gait). The heel (first) rocker at initial contact and loading is eliminated resulting in forefoot or flatfoot contact. As only foot weight need be supported, a posterior leaf-spring dorsiflexion assist orthosis is sufficient to support the foot during swing and to preserve the heel rocker. In contrast, grade 3/5 strength (20% of normal) is suffi-cient during midswing to lift the foot against gravity for foot clearance. Thus, the patient will exhibit their most conspicuous gait deviation during loading where a grade of 4/5 is needed to eccentrically control the rate of plantar flexion following heel contact. A fair grade (3/5) introduces a "foot-slap" (the foot was sufficiently dorsiflexed in swing for heel contact but experiences uncontrolled rapid plantar flexion during loading). An alternate strategy is initial contact with a "low" or "abbreviated" heel contact (the angle to the floor ≤5°). This effectively eliminates the heel rocker, reducing the knee flexion moment during loading. A severe foot drop, 30 degrees to 50 degrees during swing, requires conspicuous lifting of the limb in swing for clearance. As the limb is lowered for stance, initial contact is made with the forefoot and the limb rapidly drops to create foot-flat. Paralysis of anterior tibialis with 4 or 5 grades of the extensor digitorum longus provides sufficient strength for foot clearance in swing; however, the medial rays of the foot drop resulting in dorsiflexion with eversion.

WEAK CALF MUSCLES: The soleus and gastrocnemius account for 91% of the force required to eccentrically control the dorsiflexing ankle during mid and terminal stance. The perimalleolar group (FDL, FHL, PT, PL, PB) provides the remaining 9% as they control the subtalar and metatarsal joints (17,21,23). The severity of gastrocsoleus muscle weakness is evident in the timing of heel rise and knee kinematics. Grade 3/5 or "fair" (20% of normal) plantar flexion strength is required to accomplish one heel rise but it is not adequate to restrain the tibia's forward translation, resulting in knee instability (10). Calf strength graded 3+/5 is sufficient to restrain the tibia in mid-stance but heel rise is delayed. Grade 4/5 will provide single stance heel rise for short distances, while unlimited community ambulation requires a 5/5.

Uncontrolled advancement of tibia during mid and terminal stance causes excessive knee flexion. This increases the demand on the quadriceps at a time when they are normally inactive. Quadriceps demand can be reduced by maintaining the center of pressure close to the calcaneus. Knee flexion can therefore be avoided by reducing the ankle dorsiflexion moment. Tibial control may be restored by an articulated ankle foot orthosis (AFO) with a dorsiflexion stop. The orthosis should allow free plantar flexion to protect the quadriceps from an exaggerated heel rocker during loading which would increase the flexor moment at the knee. If plantar flexion is blocked the patient must have sufficient quadriceps strength to meet the demand.

WEAK QUADRICEPS. The normal pattern and rate of walking requires quadriceps with grade 4+ to 5 strength. Grade 4/5 (good) is the minimum strength required to resist the knee flexion moment created by the heel rocker. Patients with quadriceps graded less than *good* (<4/5) avoid knee flexion during loading but have an otherwise normal gait as long as the hip extensors and plantar flexors are at least a grade 4/5. In patients graded <3/5, knee stability may be maintained by increased activity of the hip extensors to control the femur and premature activation of the ankle plantar flexors to retract the tibia. At initial contact, slight (10°) plantar flexion avoids the heel rocker reaction as the limb is loaded. The knee extends to its passive limit of at least 5° hyperextension for stability in the absence of an orthotic restricting recurvatum. If the hip extensor or calf muscles are less than 3/5 and knee hyperextension range is inadequate, a knee-ankle foot orthosis (KAFO) is optimal. A locked knee joint is customary but a freely mobile, posteriorly off-set orthotic joint is indicated for patients with severe recurvatum (>20°). The off-set joint is designed to enhance the extensor moment and limit recurvatum while providing flexion for swing limb clearance.

WEAK HIP EXTENSORS; Four muscles are involved in hip extension; gluteus maximus and adductor magnus are the primary extensors, and the larger hamstring muscles (semimembranosus and biceps femoris, long head) serve as a supplementary force. When the extensors are <3/5, a backward trunk lean preserves the standing posture by positioning the line of gravity posterior to the hip joint axis. Patients immediately assume this posture after initial contact. Quadriceps demand is correspondingly increased by the alignment of the ground reaction force vector posterior to the knee axis. The hamstrings may accentuate this demand. In many patients, the posterior lean is coupled with excessive lordosis, as a hip flexion contracture is common.

WEAK HIP ABDUCTORS: Four muscles contribute to hip abduction: gluteus medius and minimus, upper gluteus maximus and tensor fasciae latae (9). Lateral trunk lean over the stance limb is the sign of inadequate hip abductor strength (<4/5). The abductors counter the large adductor moment created by lifting the contralateral limb for swing. Weakness deprives the patient of the force needed to hold the pelvis level. Compensation is initiated in loading by shifting the trunk toward the stance limb to reduce the opposing adduction moment. With complete abductor paralysis, the trunk's center of mass will lie directly over the hip joint center to neutralize the abductor demand.

Primary Impairments in Patients with Neuromuscular Dysfunction

Upper motor neuron lesions resulting from cerebrovascular accidents, cerebral palsy, or traumatic brain injuries or trauma can lead to disruptions in neural control mechanisms interfering with the patients' ability to walk (3). Impairments may include spasticity, impaired or inadequate motor control, the emergence of primitive locomotor patterns, muscle weakness, restricted joint mobility, impaired balance and sensation, and may include cognitive deficits. Muscle weakness may result from loss of selective control, dependence on primitive control patterns, or lack of normal somatosensory input. Joint mobility may be restricted by antagonistic muscle activation and spasticity, as well as contracture. Cognitive and somatosensory deficits further limit the patients substitutive capabilities. Significant functional loss is common; patients typically exhibit varying degrees of impaired or inadequate selective control with difficulty modifying the rate, direction, duration, and intensity of muscle activity. Within each disability, there is a significant range of deficits, from mild to severe. All but the smallest lesions result in poor substitutive actions since the capacity to voluntarily modify the motions or postures of the paretic limb is dependent on selective motor control. Substitutive mechanisms are further limited when proprioception is impaired. The feedback needed to define limb position and balance to guide the compensatory action may be limited or absent. This limits the repertoire of movement strategies available to effectively compensate.

GAIT ANALYSIS: CLINICAL DECISION MAKING CASE STUDIES

The following case studies illustrate the use of instrumented gait analysis in clinical decision making. Recommendations include surgical decisions (by a medical doctor [MD]), as well as exercise prescription and orthotic prescription (by a physical therapist [PT])

CASE 1

Diagnosis (Dx)-Anterior Compartment Syndrome with Drop Foot

This 17-year old male was diagnosed with anterior compartment syndrome (left) following open reduction internal fixation of a tibial fracture 9 months ago at the site of a benign tumor excised 3 months previously.

Chief Complaint: Difficulty clearing the foot during swing resulting in loss of balance and fear of tripping limiting community ambulation, participation in sports, and recreational activities.

Clinical Examination:

PROM: Dorsiflexion with knee flexed: 10 degrees
              Dorsiflexion with knee extended: −5 degrees

Strength tests	MMT	Torque	Strength tests	MMT	Torque
Anterior Tibialis	2+		Gastrocnemius	2	
EDL	3+		Soleus	2	
EHL	1		PT, FHL, PL, PB	4	
Dorsiflexion		10.2% N	Plantar flexors		22.4% N

Palpation: Anterior tibialis muscle contraction palpable without tendon tension

Gait Instrumentation: 3-D motion, stride characteristics, and kinesiologic electromyography (EMG) during self selected paced walking.

Results

Foot Floor Contact: Low heel strike at initial contact (Fig. 10-1). Loading: Foot flat at 3% GC. Normal heel off in terminal stance.

			% Normal
Stride:	Velocity:	56.9 m/min	70
	Stride Length:	1.135 m	75
	Cadence:	100.3 steps/min	93
	Single limb support:	left	82

Motion:

Ankle: Initial Contact (IC) in 10 degrees of plantar flexion (PF). Terminal Stance: 5 degrees of dorsiflexion (DF) in terminal stance (yielding contracture reduces with body weight).
    Swing Phase: 10 degrees of PF throughout swing phase (Figs. 10-2 and 10-3)

Knee: IC in 5 degrees of flexion increasing to 10 degrees in loading, achieving neutral in terminal stance.

Hip: IC in 15 degrees of flexion, followed by immediate extension to neutral, reaching 10 degrees of extension in terminal stance.

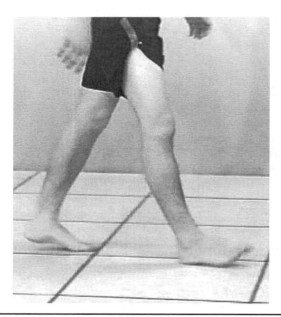

FIGURE 10-1. Initial contact in 9 degrees of plantar flexion with a "low" heel strike minimizing the flexion moment at the knee. Case 1: Drop Foot.

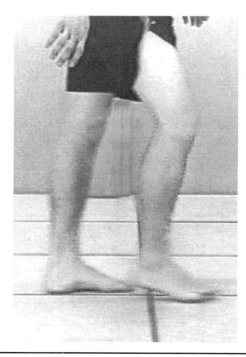

FIGURE 10-2. Mid-swing ankle dorsiflexion is inadequate; note the slight compensatory increase in hip and knee flexion with minimal clearance.

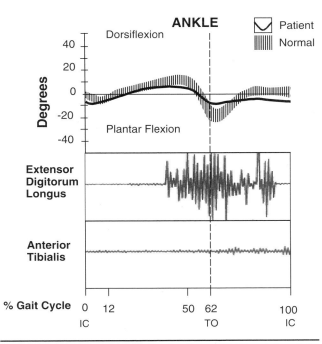

FIGURE 10-3. No functionally significant EMG activity of the anterior tibialis with 38% MVC of the EDL. Despite limitations in dorsiflexion PROM the ankle reaches 5 degrees of DF in terminal stance (yielding contracture), yet remains plantar flexed throughout swing.

EMG: (Fig. 10-3)

Anterior Tibialis:	No functionally significant EMG activity
EDL:	38% maximum voluntary contraction (MVC) with premature onset & cessation
Soleus:	41% MVC, normal phasing
Gastrocnemius:	41% MVC, normal phasing

Interpretation:
Despite moderate anterior tibialis EMG activity during manual muscle testing (2+) and torque testing (10% normal), there was no functionally significant anterior tibialis EMG activity during walking. Failure to lift foot may be a result of tendon entrapment in the operative scar or partial denervation. In contrast, the EDL demonstrated 38% MVC throughout swing with a grade of 3+, but lacked the leverage to effectively dorsiflex the foot to neutral for foot clearance.

Recommendations:
- Surgical:
  - Transfer the EDL to the dorsum of the foot with the tendon removed from the retinaculum to improve its dorsiflexion leverage. Selective lengthening of the gastrocnemius only to 10 degrees of dorsiflexion with knee extended. The soleus should be left intact to preserve plantar flexion strength.
- Physical Therapy
  - Strengthen the AT, EDL & EHL to counter disuse atrophy, Functional electrical stimulation to partially denervated muscles
  - Strengthen the plantar flexors, quadriceps & hip extensors
  - Gait & balance training
- Orthotic
  - Articulated AFO with DF-stop and a DF-assist until EDL recovers adequate strength to dorsiflex foot. Post surgically, if active dorsiflexion to neutral is not achieved (>6 mos) a posterior leaf spring is recommended.

CASE 2

Dx-Post Polio Syndrome with Excess Dorsiflexion in Stance Caused by Inadequate Plantar Flexor Strength

This 49-year-old woman was diagnosed with post polio syndrome 6 months ago.

Chief Complaint: Pain, weakness and fatigue in the right lower extremity limiting community mobility. Complaints of knee collapse in late stance inducing fear of falling with reports of instability on uneven terrain limiting community ambulation and recreation.

Clinical Examination:

PROM:		
	DF (knee extended)	−5°
	Subtalar eversion	3°
	Knee hyperextension	5°
	Straight Leg Raise (SLR)	70°

Strength Tests	MMT	Torque (% N)
Plantar flexion	2	6
Knee extension	3−	21
Hip Abductors	4+	8
Hip Extensors	4+	28

Gait Instrumentation: 3-D motion, stride characteristics, and kinesiologic EMG performed during self selected paced walking.

Results

Foot Floor Contact: IC with the heel, premature contact of 5th metatarsal (5% GC), heel off delayed until double limb support (preswing).

Stride:

		% Normal
Velocity:	30.3 m/min	39
Stride Length:	0.639 m	48
Cadence:	94.7 steps/min	80
Single limb support:	Right	48.3

Motion:

Ankle: IC in 10 degrees of plantar flexion (Fig. 10-4), reversing to 20 degrees of dorsiflexion by terminal stance (Fig. 10-5), Swing phase plantar flexion 20-5 degrees.

Knee: Hyperextension of 5 degrees at initial contact (Fig. 10-4) with increasing flexion of 15 degrees in terminal stance.

Hip: IC in 5 degrees of flexion and 30 degrees of medial rotation continuing throughout stance.

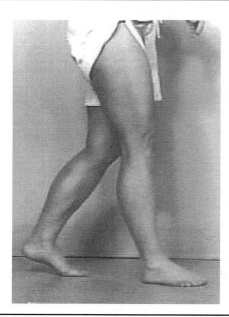

FIGURE 10-4. Loading response: avoidance of knee flexion during loading response caused by weakness and fatigue in the quadriceps (torque testing 21% N) leading to tibial instability. Case 2: Post Polio Syndrome.

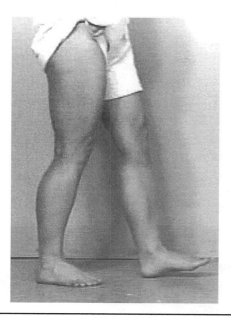

FIGURE 10-5. Terminal stance: excess dorsiflexion caused by weak calf muscles (torque testing 6% N), lack of heel rise and persistent knee flexion increasing quadriceps demand.

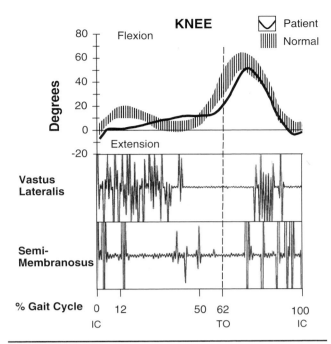

FIGURE 10-6. Knee hyperextension (5°) in loading with persistent knee flexion throughout stance. Sparse high amplitude EMG in the vastus lateralis indicative of large motor units (reinnervation) with decreased activation in terminal stance contributing to knee collapse.

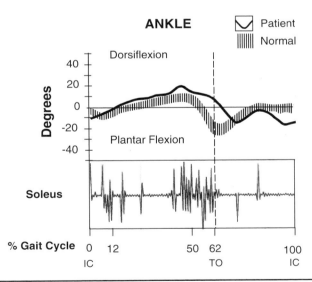

FIGURE 10-7. Ankle progressively dorsiflexes from initial contact in 10 degree of plantar flexion to 20 degrees of dorsiflexion in terminal stance and a delay reversal to plantar flexion in late preswing. In mid-swing the ankle briefly dorsiflexed to neutral but drops into plantar flexion in terminal swing.

EMG: All recordings sparse with high amplitude activity (Figs. 10-6 and 10-7)

Soleus:	(16% MVC) slightly prolonged
Vastus Lateralis:	(26% MVC) premature and prolonged
Semimembranosus:	(64% MVC) premature and prolonged
Biceps Femoris:	(8% MVC) out of phase, active in terminal stance
Gluteus Maximus:	(8% MVC) low amplitude (premature and prolonged)

Interpretation:
Sparse EMG activity indicates a reduced number of motor units available for activation. High amplitude EMG is characteristic of recovery through motor unit enlargement as a result of reinnervation by sprouting. A mild yielding PF contracture assists with tibial control in stance, however dorsiflexion is excessive (20°) increasing the quadriceps demand at the knee. With 21% N quadriceps strength and 6% N plantar flexion strength, knee instability is likely. Small arcs of joint motion and slow velocity indicate voluntary protection of the few remaining large motor units. Motor unit enlargement indicates more muscle fibers are activated simultaneously which may contribute to overuse and fatigue.

Recommendations:
- No surgical recommendations
- Physical Therapy

  Client education and guidance in modification of functional activities to avoid overuse and fatigue. (J Perry recommendations for patients diagnosed with Post-Polio) (16,19)
  - Avoid activities causing fatigue that persists more than 10 minutes
  - Interrupt active day by two rest periods
  - Stop an activity before pain develops
  - No resistive exercise causing muscle or joint pain
  - Balance training
  - Gait training with SPC (single point cane) to protect and unload overused muscles
- Orthotics
  - Articulated AFO (lightweight) modified as follows:

A dorsiflexion stop at 5 degrees to assist and protect a weak calf and reduce the flexor moment at the knee throughout stance. Allow free plantar flexion to protect the weak quads during IC and loading by attenuating the effect of the heel rocker at initial contact. The goal is to prevent fatigue and overuse of quadriceps and hip extensors.

CASE 3

Dx-Post CVA with Equinovarus Foot

This 36-year-old male had a 2-year history of right hemiparesis following a CVA

Chief Complaint: Pain in the forefoot and toes during weight bearing. Difficulty with foot clearance and impaired balance with the use of a quad cane limiting household and community ambulation.

Clinical Examination:

PROM: DF (knee flexed) $-10°$
       DF (knee extended) $-30°$

Strength Testing (in Synergy-no selective control)
Anterior Tibialis	Weak
Posterior Tibialis	Weak
Soleus & Gastrocnemius	Weak

Spasticity

Muscle	EMG response
AT	Absent
Gastrocnemius	Prolonged (>5 sec of clonus)
Soleus	Prolonged (>5 sec of clonus)
FDL & FHL	Prolonged (>5 sec of clonus)
PL	Prolonged (>5 sec) sparse EMG
PB	Normal response

Gait Instrumentation: 3-D motion, stride characteristics, and kinesiologic EMG performed during self-selected paced walking.

Results

Foot Floor Contact: IC with 5th metatarsal (MT) only, absent 1st MT or heel contact throughout stance (Fig. 10-8).

Stride: Velocity 13% N, Stride Length 25% N, Cadence 53% N, Single limb support 14% N

Motion:

Ankle: IC in 20 degrees of PF reducing to 12 degrees of PF in terminal stance (Fig. 10-9). Inversion 25 degrees.

Knee: IC: 12 degrees of flexion decreasing to 5 degrees in mid-stance with a peak of 30 degrees in initial swing (Fig. 10-11).

Hip: IC: flexed 25 degrees, reducing to 15 degrees in mid-stance increasing to 30 degrees in initial swing.

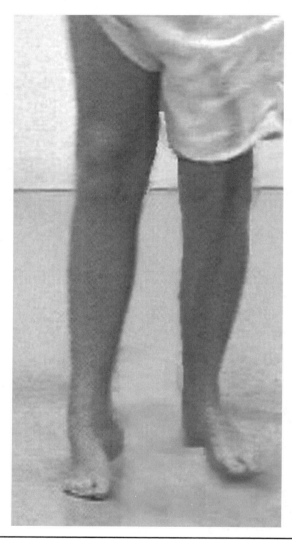

FIGURE 10-8. Mid-stance with equinovarus foot position without heel, 1st MT or toe contact. Case 3: CVA with equinovarus.

EMG: Figures 10-12 and 10-13
  Anterior Tibialis: Sparse activity throughout initial & mid-swing
  Soleus, Gastrocnemius, FHL & FDL: all exhibit premature onset in terminal swing that continues into terminal stance.
  Posterior Tibialis: delayed onset with sparse & curtailed intensity
  Peroneus Longus: no activity throughout stance
  Peroneus Brevis: sparse throughout stance

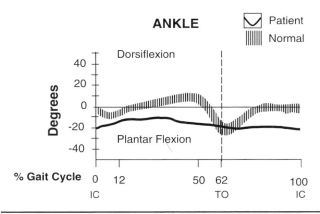

FIGURE 10-9. Ankle Motion: Initial contact in 20° of plantar flexion reducing to 12 degrees of PF in terminal stance dropping to 20° throughout swing.

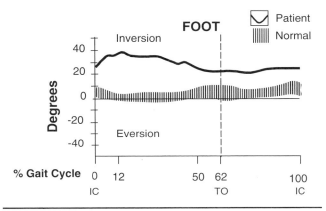

FIGURE 10-10. Forefoot Motion: Inversion of 28° at initial contact increasing to 40 degrees during mid-stance reducing to 20° throughout swing.

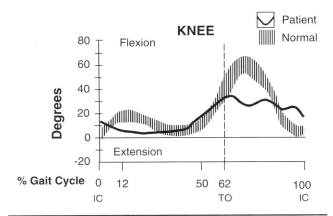

FIGURE 10-11. Stiff legged gait pattern with peak knee flexion reduced to 30 degrees in initial swing. Coupled with the equinovarus foot position, swing limb clearance is compromised.

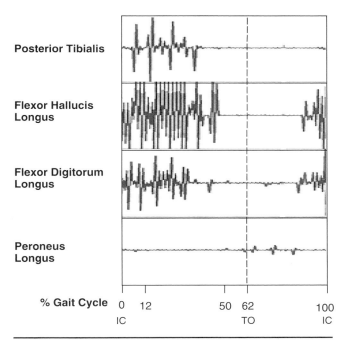

FIGURE 10-12. Premature EMG activity of the FHL and FDL without significant posterior tibialis activity suggests the toe flexors significantly contribute to forefoot varus.

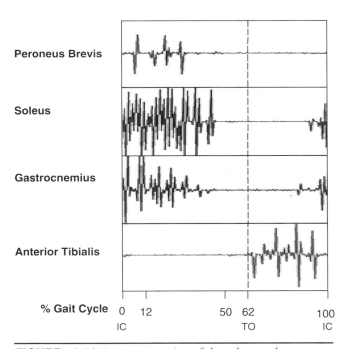

FIGURE 10-13. Premature action of the soleus and gastrocnemius prevent heel contact throughout stance. Lack of peroneals activity contributes to inversion throughout stance.

Interpretation:

Primitive synergistic patterns dominate with no selective motor control. Insufficient anterior tibialis activity, a PF contracture ($-30°$ DF PROM reducing to $-20°$ during weight bearing) and highly spastic gastroc & soleus (>5 sec of clonus) all contribute to equinovarus. Sparse EMG levels of posterior tibialis suggest it is not a primary varus contributor. Equinus is likely caused by the sustained and highly spastic soleus, gastrocnemius, and FHL. Low level continuous EMG indicates a combination of primitive motor control activation and contracture. The relatively high intensity toe flexor EMG suggests their activation and length is a major obstruction to forward progression. The marked subtalar and forefoot inversion may represent control error, but the EMG intensity of AT, PT and soleus was significantly less than the toe flexors. Reduced everter activity may also contribute to forefoot inversion. Inversion may also be the voluntary avoidance of weight bearing on the forefoot caused by toe clawing. Pain may also limit progression of the COP onto the forefoot.

Recommendations:
- Surgical:
  - Achilles tendon lengthening (with a medial emphasis) to neutral.
  - FHL transfer to the posterior-lateral calcaneus with the ankle in DF.
  - FDL release PL transfer to the lateral forefoot (cuboid) to supplement eversion. PT lengthened only if foot remains in fixed inversion after TAL & toe flexor release.

  Additional Recommendation: Kinesiologic EMG to determine cause of stiff legged gait with possible rectus femoris distal transfer to enhance knee flexion in swing for foot clearance.

- Physical Therapy
  - Post operative functional strengthening coupled with talocrural and subtalar mobilization
  - Balance and gait training with quad cane progressing to SPC to decrease risk for falls to improve community ambulation
  - Functional activities to promote independent household and community mobility
- Orthotics
  - Articulated AFO set in neutral for 6 months postoperatively to protect transfers.

CASE 4

Dx-Cerebral Palsy-Crouched Gait with Forefoot Contact Only (No Heel Contact)

This 4 year 9-month-old child diagnosed with spastic diplegia cerebral palsy is independently ambulatory with bilateral solid polypropylene AFOs and "tone inhibiting" footplate inserts. No previous surgeries were reported. During walking she exhibited an anterior pelvic tilt with excess pelvic rotation; flexion, adduction and medial rotation of the thigh; and knee flexion with persistent heel off during stance.

Chief Complaint: Decreased functional ambulation (distance and speed) at home & school.

Referring MD request: Evaluate for a possible heel cord lengthening, split anterior tibialis tendon transfer (SPLATT), posterior tibialis lengthening or transfer, and a hip adductor release.

Clinical Examination:

PROM:		
	DF (knee flexed)	20°
	DF (knee extended)	10°
	Eversion	30°
	Knee hyperextension	20°
	Hip extension	−20°
	SLR	70°

Strength Testing (In synergy)	Spasticity (EMG response)
Anterior Tibialis-Weak	None
Posterior Tibialis-Weak	+ (0.5 sec)
Soleus-Weak	+ (1.5 sec)
Gastrocnemius-Weak	+ (2.0 sec)
Adductor Longus-Weak	+ (>3.5 sec)

Gait Instrumentation: 3-D motion, stride, and kinesiologic EMG analyses during self selected paced walking.

Results

Foot Floor Contact: IC by forefoot (1st and 5th MT with toes), no heel contact throughout stance (Fig. 10-14)

Stride:		% Normal
Velocity:	44.5 m/min	69
Stride Length:	0.666 m	79
Cadence:	133	86

Motion:

Ankle: Neutral at initial contact progressing to 5 degrees of plantar flexion in mid-stance increasing to 15 degrees of PF degrees in terminal stance rapidly reaching 50 degrees in preswing (Fig. 10-15).

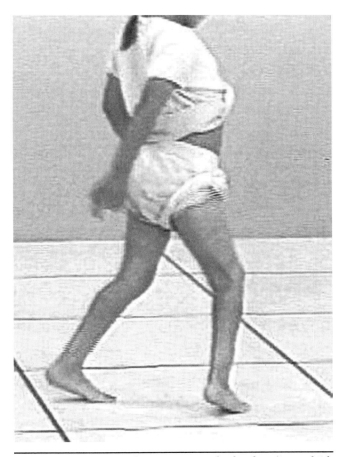

FIGURE 10-14. Foot Floor Contact: IC by forefoot (1st and 5th MT with toes), no heel contact in stance. Anterior rotation of the pelvis causes "apparent" medial hip rotation and medial foot progression angle. No heel contact throughout stance is caused by hip and knee flexion as the ankle is in a neutral position. Case 4: Cerebral Palsy: Crouched gait with "apparent" equinus.

Knee: Flexed 40 degrees at initial contact decreasing to 20 degrees in mid-stance, 40 degrees in terminal stance reaching a peak of 60 degrees in mid-swing.

Thigh Rotation: 40 degrees of medial rotation at initial contact decreasing to 25 degrees in loading, 35 degrees in mid-stance, decreasing to 10 degrees of external rotation in preswing. Thigh progressively medially rotates throughout swing to reach 40 degrees in terminal swing (Fig. 10-16).

Pelvic rotation: 20 degrees of medial rotation at initial contact increasing to 30 degrees during loading, reaching 8 degrees of lateral rotation in preswing (Fig. 10-17).

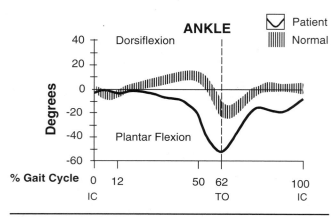

FIGURE 10-15. Ankle motion: Loading reduces the ankle to neutral that is maintained until late mid-stance with 50 degrees of plantar flexion in preswing decreasing to 10 degrees in terminal swing. Forefoot only contact is caused by excess knee and hip flexion rather than plantar flexion.

EMG:

Anterior Tibialis:	(67.8% MVC) premature onset & cessation
Soleus:	(66.5% MVC) premature onset & normal cessation
Gastrocnemius:	(28.3% MVC) premature onset & cessation
Posterior Tibialis:	(36.8% MVC) premature onset & cessation
Adductor Longus:	(6% MVC) normal onset & cessation

Interpretation: The persistent heel off posture implies equinus of the foot but the ankle is dorsiflexed to neutral at initial contact through loading response. Subsequent plantar flexion develops in late stance as advancement of the limb over the forefoot allows the knee to partially extend. The ankle position is caused by weight bearing on a markedly flexed knee that holds the tibia in a trailing

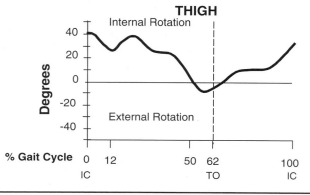

FIGURE 10-16. The "apparent" medial thigh rotation reflects pelvic rotation.

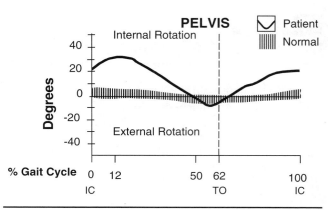

FIGURE 10-17. Medial rotation of the pelvis causes the "apparent" medial rotation of the thigh suggesting the lower extremity rotation is caused by excess anterior pelvic rotation.

position, while hamstring tightness is exaggerated by excessive hip flexion. The extreme ankle plantar flexion seen in preswing most likely represents a rebound response as unloading the foot releases energy in the stretched tissues. It signifies some gastrocsoleus contracture but correcting this by lengthening the entire Achilles tendon would result in excess dorsiflexion, as loading the flexed limb on the forefoot would continue to stretch the tendon. Knee flexion can be reduced by correcting the hip flexion contracture to make full hamstring length available. The "apparent" adduction and internal rotation of the limb and the medial foot progression angle are the result of the pelvic forward rotation rather than medial rotation of the hip caused by adductor activity. EMG testing of the medial hamstrings is recommended.

Recommendations:

- Surgical:
    - Iliopsoas: Aponeurotic lengthening
    - Possible medial hamstring lengthening (EMG recommended)
    - Soleus: Conservative lengthening of the aponeurosis to neutral. Preserve the gastrocnemius, and take caution to avoid overlengthening.
    - No posterior tibialis lengthening or transfer
    - No adductor surgery indicated
- Physical Therapy
    - Functional strengthening of the hip extensors, abductors, knee extensors, plantar flexor and dorsiflexors
    - Optimize motor control strategies to reduce pelvic rotation
    - Gait and balance training
    - Functional training for improved community ambulation and recreation
- Orthotic
    - Continue with bilateral solid polypropylene AFOs and "tone inhibiting" footplate inserts.

CASE 5

Dx-Post Polio Syndrome with Genu Recurvatum

This 48-year-old male with a diagnosis of post polio syndrome was a functional community ambulatory until he fractured his distal femur in a fall resulting in a femoral deformity requiring an osteotomy.

Chief Complaint: Pain in medial and posterolateral knee; weakness and fatigue in right limb with knee instability limiting community ambulation. He is currently wearing a KAFO with an articulated knee (0–145°) joint and ankle allowing free dorsiflexion with plantar flexion restricted to neutral.

Gait Instrumentation: Motion, stride, and kinesiologic EMG analyses during self-selected walking-Barefoot.

Strength	MMT	Torque	(% Normal)
Soleus/ Gastrocnemius	2–	Plantarflexion	0
Vastus Lateralis	3	Knee extension	8
Gluteus Medius	4	Abduction	45
Gluteus Maximus	3+	Hip Extension	30
Semimembranosus & BFLH	3+		

Foot floor contact: Initial contact with a flat foot avoiding the heel rocker thereby eliminating the flexor moment at the knee (Fig. 10-18). Prolonged heel contact throughout terminal stance into preswing.

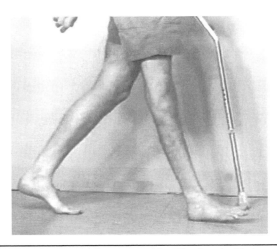

FIGURE 10-18. Initial contact with a flat foot in 10 degrees of plantar flexion that effectively eliminates the heel rocker reducing the knee flexion moment during loading. Patient has weak quadriceps (3/5) and uses available hyperextension as a passive extensor moment to stabilize the knee throughout stance. Case 5: Dx Post Polio Syndrome with genu recurvatum.

Stride:			% Normal
	Velocity:	54.5 m/min	67
	Stride Length:	1.331 m	88
	Cadence:	82 steps/min	76
	Single limb support:	Right	90.1

Motion:

Ankle: Excess plantar flexion in loading through midstance reversing to excess dorsiflexion in terminal stance causing knee instability.

Knee: Genu recurvatum throughout loading and midstance with rapid knee flexion in terminal stance (Fig. 10-19).

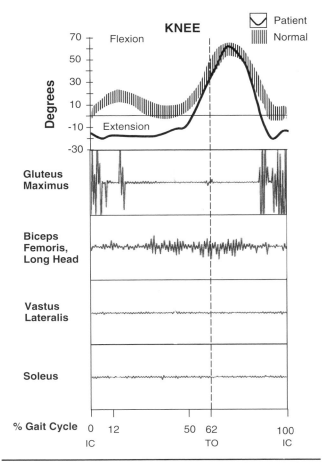

FIGURE 10-19. Knee hyperextension in stance for weight bearing stability with no EMG activity of the soleus or vastus lateralis. Gluteus maximus is active to control the knee in the presence of weak quadriceps.

EMG:

Upper and Lower Gluteus Maximus: Large motor units-onset normal with prolonged activity into mid-stance (Fig. 10-19)

> Vastus Lateralis: No EMG activity
> Soleus: No EMG activity

Interpretation: The primary deviation was knee hyperextension in early stance with knee collapse in late stance. The symptoms were aggravated by a knee extensor thrust into valgus and hyperextension. The mechanism for knee control was dynamic hip extension (intense gluteus maximus EMG) for stance stability caused by quadriceps weakness (3/5). Motor unit enlargement indicates more muscle fibers are activated simultaneously contributing to overuse and fatigue. With the patient dependent on the gluteus maximus for stability, orthotic restraint at the knee and ankle is essential to prevent joint deformity and pain.

Recommendations:
- No surgical recommendations.
- Physical Therapy
  Client education and guidance in modification of functional activities to avoid overuse. (J Perry recommendations for post polio syndrome [16,19]).

- Avoid activities causing fatigue that persists more than 10 minutes
- Interrupt active day by two rest periods
- Stop an activity before pain develops
- No resistive exercise causing muscle or joint pain
- Gait & balance training for independent functional community ambulation
- Orthotic:
  - KAFO: Lightweight

    Ankle: A dorsiflexion stop at 5 degrees to assist and protect a weak calf while reducing the flexor moment at the knee throughout stance. Free plantar flexion (to protect weak quads during IC and loading) to attenuate the effect of the heel rocker at initial contact. The goal is to prevent fatigue and overuse of quadriceps and hip extensors.

    Knee: freely mobile in flexion, restricted to 5 to 10 degrees of hyperextension with a posteriorly offset knee joint axis for added stability

CASE 6

Dx-Congenital Hip Dysplasia with Hip Pain During Jogging

This 17-year-old female was diagnosed with right congenital hip dysplasia

Chief complaint: Significant hip and low back pain when jogging which she performs for recreation and fitness.

Referring MD request: Evaluate for a possible total hip replacement

Past Medical History: Chiari osteotomy on the right hip 2.5 years ago to stabilize the hip joint

Clinical Examination:

True leg length discrepancy: 1 inch shorter on the right.
Strength Testing

Muscle Group	Grade MMT	Torque (% Normal)
TFL	3–	Abduction 58.5
Gluteus Medius	3–	
Adductor Longus	4	
Gluteus Maximus	5	Extension 79.8
Hamstrings	5	
DF, PF, Knee flexors & ext	5	

Gait Instrumentation: Motion, stride, and kinesiologic EMG analyses during self-selected and fast walking.

Results

Slight ipsilateral trunk lean and a contralateral pelvic drop throughout stance (Fig. 10-20)

Stride Characteristics with shoes & 1 inch lift

	Self selected	Fast
Velocity:	83% N	112% N
Stride length:	88% N	104% N
Cadence:	94% N	109% N
Single limb support:	101% N	116% N
Single limb stance:	Rt 100% N	L 115% N

Motion: Contralateral pelvic drop and a slight ipsilateral trunk lean in stance phase reducing the hip adduction moment (Fig. 10-21).

EMG:

Gluteus Medius: (31% MVC) premature onset and prolonged activity into terminal stance (Fig. 10-22)

Tensor Fascia Lata: (97.5% MVC) with premature onset and prolonged activity into initial swing (Fig. 10-22)

Upper & Lower Gluteus Maximus: no functionally significant activity despite high intensity EMG during torque testing.

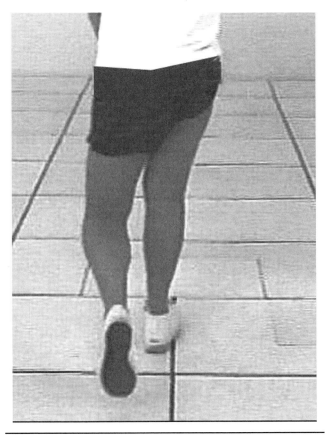

FIGURE 10-20. Stance phase on the right LE results in contralateral pelvic drop coupled with a slight ipsilateral trunk lean. One inch lift on the right equalizes SLS time. Case 6: Dx Congenital hip dysplasia.

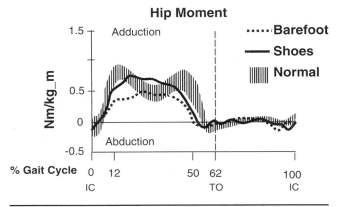

FIGURE 10-21. Right hip adductor moment reduced with an ipsilateral trunk lean decreasing the demand on the abductors. Joint reaction force is decreased which may reduce pain.

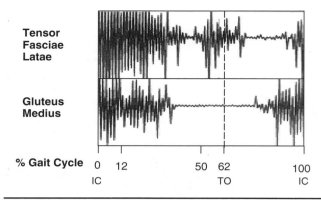

FIGURE 10-22. Gluteus medius and tensor fascia latae both displayed vigorous muscle activity and adequate strength to provide support if a total hip arthroplasty is elected at a later date if pain significantly limits function.

Interpretation: Both free and fast walking (with shoes and 1 inch lift) and muscle strength testing indicated a high level of function despite modest hip abduction instability and pain. Self selected velocity was 83% of normal with minimal asymmetry in single limb stance time (Rt-100% N versus L-115% N) signifying that hip pain did not sig-nificantly alter her ability to weight bear on the right limb. A valgus moment at the knee and a reduced adduction moment at the hip was consistent with a slight ipsilateral lateral trunk lean. There was also a contralateral pelvic drop in stance indicative of hip abductor weakness. Gluteus medius and tensor fascia lata both displayed vigorous muscle activity and adequate strength to provide support if a total hip arthroplasty is elected at a later date, if pain significantly limits function. Since the pain is experienced only during elective jogging and the Chiari procedure is functioning adequately, total hip replacement can be delayed.

Recommendations:

- Surgical
  - Joint replacement surgery is not indicated at this time
  - Right total hip arthroplasty if pain exacerbates and limits function
- Physical Therapy
  - Continue with 1 inch lift on right shoe
  - Strengthen right hip abductors (TFL & G medius– 58.5% normal) and hip extensors (80% normal)
  - Cardiovascular training for health promotion and fitness (UE ergometer and swimming)

ACKNOWLEDGMENTS

The authors wish to thank Judith Burnfield PT, PhD for the preparation of the figures and Alina Kaufman for her assistance with the references.

REFERENCES

1. Beasley WC. Quantitative muscle testing: principles and application to research and clinical services. *Arch Phys Med Rehabil*. 1961;42:398–425.
2. Brown L, Adams JM, Roller P, et al. Functional distances and velocities required of community ambulators in Ventura County. Masters Thesis. Northridge: California State University; June 2001.
3. Duncan PW, Badke MB. Determinants of abnormal motor control. In: Duncan PW, Badke MB, eds. *Stroke Rehabilitation, The Recovery of Motor Control*. Chicago: Year Book Medical Publishers; 1987:135–159.
4. Everett, D, Adams, J, Wolfe G, et al. The criterion-related validity of the Rancho Los Amigos observational gait analysis form in persons with cerebral vascular accident. Masters Thesis. Northridge: California State University; 2000.
5. Finley RF, Cody KA. Locomotive characteristics of urban pedestrians. *Arch Phys Med Rehabil*. 1970;51:423–426.
6. Gage JR. Gait analysis for decision-making in cerebral palsy. *Bull Hosp Joint Dis Orthop Inst*. 1983;43:147–163.
7. Greenberg M, Gronley J, Perry J, et al. Reliability and concurrent validity of Rancho Los Amigos Medical Center's observational gait analysis. California Chapter Conference Proceedings; Nov. 1996.
8. Kerrigan DC, Gronley J, Perry J. Stiff-legged gait in spastic paralysis: a study of quadriceps and hamstring activity. *Am J Phys Med Rehabil*. 1991;70(6):294–300.
9. Lyons K, Perry J, Gronley J, et al. Timing and relative intensity of hip extensor and abductor muscle action during level and stair ambulation: an EMG study. *Phys Ther*. 1983;63:1597–1605.
10. Mulroy S, Perry J, Gronley J. A comparison of clinical tests for ankle plantar flexion strength. *Trans Orthop Res Soc*. 1991;16:667.
11. Murray MP, Mollinger LA, Gardner GM, et al. Kinematic and EMG patterns during slow, free and fast walking. *J Orthop Res*. 1984;2(3):272–280.
12. Olney S, Winter D. Predictions of knee and ankle moments of force in walking from EMG and kinematic data. *J Biomech*. 1985;18:9–20.
13. Olney S. Hemiparetic gait following stroke. Part I: characteristics. *Gait Posture*. 1996;4:136–148.
14. Ounpuu S. Joint kinematics: methods, interpretation and treatment decision-making in children with cerebral palsy and myelomeningocele. *Gait Posture*. 1996;4:62–78.
15. Pathokinesiology Department, Physical Therapy Department, Rancho Los Amigos Medical Center. *Observational Gait Analysis Handbook*. Downey, CA: LAREI; 1989.
16. Perry J, Young S, Barnes G. Strengthening exercise for post-polio sequelae. *Arch Phys Med Rehab*. 1987;68:660.
17. Perry J. *Gait Analysis: Normal and Pathological Function*. Thorofare, NJ: Slack; 1992.
18. Perry J. Integrated function of the lower extremity including gait analysis. In: Cruess RL, Rennie WR, eds. *Adult Orthopedics*. New York: Churchill Livingston; 1984:1161–1207.
19. Perry J. Poliomyelitis. In: Nickel VL, Botte MJ, eds. *Orthopaedic Rehabilitation*. New York: Churchill Livingstone; 1992:493–520.
20. Richards CL. Hemiparetic gait following stroke. Part II: recovery and physical therapy. *Gait Posture*. 1996;4:149–162.
21. Sutherland D. An electromyographic study of the plantar flexors of the ankle in normal walking on the level. *J Bone Joint Surg*. 1966;48A(1):66–71.
22. Sutherland D. *Gait Disorders in Childhood and Adolescence*. Baltimore: Williams & Wilkins, 1984.
23. Sutherland D. The development of mature gait. *Gait Posture*. 1997;6:163–170.
24. Sutherland DH, Cooper L. The pathomechanics of progressive crutch gait in spastic diplegia. *Orthop Clin North Am*. 1978;9(1):143–154.
25. Waters RL, Garland DE, Perry J, et al. Stiff-legged gait in hemiplegia: surgical correction. *J Bone Joint Surg*. 1979;61A:927–934.
26. Waters RL, Lunsford BR, Perry J, et al. Energy-speed relationship of walking: standard tables. *J Orthop Res*. 1988;6(2):215–222.

Chapter 11

Lower Limb Prostheses: Implications and Applications

John W. Michael

In 1945, engineers and scientists at the University of California Biomechanics Laboratory were the first to objectively analyze the gait of amputees with lower limb prostheses. Their work provided the first comprehensive look at the biomechanical attributes of normal and amputee gait. Their concepts were illustrated with free body diagrams and theoretical descriptions of the forces thought to be involved in controlling a passive artificial limb using the remnant musculoskeletal system. Figure 11-1 is a reproduction of one such illustration (18). These constructs have proven invaluable in the decades that followed, shaping how prosthetists worldwide conceptualize their goals and practice their craft.

In more recent decades, as instrumented gait analysis laboratories became more widely available, a growing body of knowledge has increased our understanding of the fundamental characteristics of ambulation with an artificial limb. Available scientific evidence supports the majority of the concepts proposed by Inman and colleagues more than half a century ago, with only a few exceptions that will be noted later in this chapter.

FUNDAMENTAL ASSUMPTION

The fundamental assumption shared by rehabilitation experts is that grossly abnormal gait patterns are cosmetically and mechanically undesirable. An ample body of evidence supports this broad statement. For example, Waters et al. have shown that applying a plaster cast to block ankle movement in a normal subject decreases gait efficiency, while immobilizing the knee results in even more inefficient ambulation (37). Furthermore, eliminating motion at both the knee and ankle results in a gait that requires more energy than if only one joint or the other was restricted. Kaufman et al. have shown that an orthosis that locks the knee in extension throughout the entire gait cycle required a post-polio subject to consume more oxy-

gen per distance traveled per kilogram of body weight than one permitting unrestricted knee flexion during the swing phase (22). Thus, the primary goal of the clinician is to create prostheses and orthoses facilitating movements that approximate the kinematics and energetics of normal walking.

When interpreting amputee gait studies, it is important to note that no prosthetic components generate active propulsive motion at any of the lower limb joints. Due to the large torques developed during weight bearing, current electromechanical technology is unable to produce sufficient power in a lightweight, compact package to actively plantarflex the ankle or to actively extend the knee under load. This means that all prosthetic and orthotic components studied to date basically permit joint motion, or impede it, by limiting the range of motion or by applying resistance to decelerate movement.

From a biomechanical perspective, a free motion prosthetic component is analogous to the joint in an insensate biological limb with flaccid paralysis. The individual who walks with a hip disarticulation prosthesis having free motion hip, knee, and ankle components develops a gait pattern similar to that of the patient with a flail leg, making the study of amputee gait particularly relevant to the rehabilitation of individuals having limb paralysis. However, two primary differences between a paralyzed leg and a prosthetic limb must be kept in mind. First, the weight of a modern prosthesis is less than one-third that of a normal leg. Secondly, because each artificial joint is individually aligned and adjusted during walking trials, the prosthetist can optimize the biomechanical alignment of the artificial limb. Because the prosthetist can configure the artificial limb in an ideal manner, and because individuals with paralysis frequently have associated bony and soft tissue deformities, ambulation with an orthosis applied to a paralyzed leg may not be as effective in restoring normal walking as would a prosthesis. These factors may explain the observation that people with paralysis who wear an ankle-foot orthosis rarely compete in sports events that

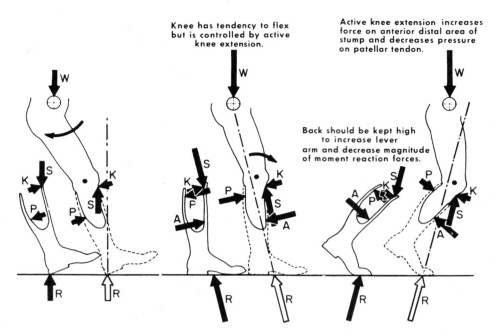

Knee has tendency to flex
but is controlled by active
knee extension.

Active knee extension increases
force on anterior distal area of
stump and decreases pressure
on patellar tendon.

Back should be kept high
to increase lever
arm and decrease magnitude
of moment reaction forces.

FIGURE 11-1. Anteroposterior forces in below-knee amputee wearing PTB prosthesis. *Left*, at heel contact. *Middle*, during midstance phase. *Right*, during push-off. W, body weight; S, support force; K, force on patellar ligament; P, posterior force; A, anterior force; R, floor reaction.

require running, while a number of amputees with modern transtibial prostheses do so and some learn to run faster than most nondisabled individuals.

More technologically advanced prosthetic components use various electromechanical methods to selectively add resistance to artificial joints to dampen undesired motion. Perhaps the best example is the use of a hydraulic cylinder linked to the knee joint that controls knee movement during swing phase. From a biomechanical perspective, prosthetic components that resist motion partially simulate muscles that are contracting eccentrically. However, there are two important distinctions from normal muscle. Current prosthetic components are not actively controlled by the amputee's neuromuscular system. The present state-of-the-art requires that the control be inherent in the mechanism itself, so even the most advanced microprocessor-controlled knee applies preestablished algorithms to simulate normal swing phase control. Equally important, prosthetic components that dampen movement should also absorb energy. The amputee must generate sufficient motion by using remaining hip flexor muscles to produce adequate swing phase function. The resistance within a prosthetic knee converts some of this kinetic energy into heat to limit excessive movement. This explains why ambulation with sophisticated prosthetic components may be more energy efficient than walking with more primitive devices, but no artificial limb is as efficient as an intact neuromuscular system.

One very important caveat is that some gait deviations are recognized clinically as necessary compensations for the musculoskeletal abnormalities inherent in limb amputation. Eliminating these aberrations may not result in a more effective gait pattern so long as the under-

lying deficiency still remains. For example, because the transfemoral residual limb no longer has functional knee extensors, people with this amputation who walk with a basic prosthetic knee mechanism quickly develop a characteristic "stiff knee" gait pattern throughout stance phase. The remaining hip extensor muscles are used to alter the ground reaction forces to create an external knee extension moment throughout stance, thus ensuring that the passive prosthetic knee will not buckle or collapse during weight bearing.

This gait deviation is a valuable compensation for the loss of active knee extension control, and without it the amputee could not walk using a basic artificial limb. Therefore, efforts to train the amputee to allow the knee to flex during early stance or to produce a more normal hip extensor muscle pattern while using such a simple prosthetic knee component would be inappropriate. This illustrates the concept that the optimal gait pattern for a particular amputee will not necessarily be fully normal and serves as a reminder that when evaluating amputee mobility, it is important not only to identify any gait abnormalities present but also to determine if they serve a useful clinical purpose.

AMPUTEE GAIT

Studies of amputee walking have consistently demonstrated characteristic disruptions in temporospatial, kinematic, kinetic, and metabolic gait parameters compared to normal walking. A key finding is that amputees typically spend less time bearing weight on the artificial limb and proportionately more time on the intact leg. This results in stride asymmetry with a shortened stance phase and more prolonged swing phase on the prosthesis (40). The typical amputee gait pattern is often characterized by more rapid unloading of the prosthetic limb in terminal stance combined with earlier loading of the contralateral limb (29). Amputees consistently demonstrate a slower than normal self-selected walking speed and transfemoral amputees often have a greater stride width, suggestive of a wider base of support to increase stability (21). Knee flexion during stance phase is markedly reduced on the prosthesis side (31) while hip extension, knee flexion, and ankle dorsiflexion of the opposite limb are increased from normal (3). Unilateral amputees demonstrate increased muscle activity on both the involved and contralateral side, with the pattern varying depending on whether the amputation is at the transtibial (19) or transfemoral level (20). This general pattern of compensating with the contralateral leg and with proximal muscles on the involved limb is believed to be one of the major causes for the increased effort required to walk with an artificial limb.

Level of Amputation

One of the principal findings reported in the literature is that more proximal amputations disrupt gait mechanics more extensively than distal amputations and increase the net energy cost to ambulate with a prosthesis over a given distance (9). These observations are the foundation for the surgical dictum to "preserve the functioning knee joint and spare all functional limb length."

It seems intuitive that as more biological joints are lost to amputation, the ability to actively control motion is further compromised, and available data consistently support this notion. Some reports in the literature also support the concept that *the shorter the bony remnant remaining, the more abnormal and inefficient the amputee's gait becomes.* For example, Gonzales et al. demonstrated that subjects with long transtibial amputations had a more energy efficient gait than individuals with short transtibial residual limbs (14). This suggests that a longer skeletal segment may provide the amputee with more leverage to control the prosthesis, which presumably leads to a more normal gait pattern.

Disarticulations are believed to offer characteristic biomechanical advantages over more proximal diaphyseal ablations, particularly when distal end weight bearing is possible. In addition to offering the longest possible bony lever arm for control of the artificial limb, disarticulation generally results in preservation of the full mass of all proximal muscle bellies, and the muscles are usually anchored distally under normal tension. Preserving all of the muscle's fibers and reattaching them at the normal resting length should allow the amputee to generate more force for prosthesis control than if the muscles had been transected and allowed to retract. To illustrate, Waters et al. have demonstrated that Syme ankle disarticulation amputees consume less energy than subjects with transtibial or higher amputations (39) and similar results have been shown for knee disarticulation compared to transfemoral amputation and for hip disarticulation amputation compared to transpelvic levels.

The biomechanical value of preserving remnants of the foot has recently been challenged and may prove to be an exception to the general rule that added bony length translates into more efficient gait. Several authors have suggested that the critical factor in partial foot amputation is the preservation of the metatarsal heads by disarticulation at the metatarsal-phalangeal junction. Recent gait studies have shown that once the metatarsal heads are disrupted, gait mechanics become grossly abnormal because the ability to actively push off is lost (30). Prostheses and orthoses studied to date have been unable to restore this ability for those with transmetatarsal and more proximal partial foot ablations (27).

Cause of Amputation

The cause of an amputation affects the quality of walking with a prosthesis. As a group, individuals with traumatic amputations have been shown to walk at a faster self-selected velocity, to have a lower net energy cost during ambulation, and to have a gait pattern that more closely approximates normal than do the group of individuals who have lost a limb as a result of vascular insufficiency (with or without associated diabetes mellitus). Amputation as a result of vascular disease tends to occur in older individuals, and many dysvascular amputees have associated comorbidities. These factors have been speculated to account, at least in part, for the difference in performance compared to traumatic amputees. Analyzing gait data according to the cause of the subject's limb loss helps to clarify differences between these two groups. Waters and Mulroy have published an excellent review of the energy costs of normal and pathologic gait discussing many of these factors (38). Figure 11-2 illustrates two general trends from the literature: individuals with more proximal amputations expend more energy to cover a given distance, as well as walk at progressively slower velocities than those with longer residual limbs.

PROSTHETIC COMPONENTS

A growing body of evidence has demonstrated that the functional components within the prosthesis can have a significant effect on the kinematics and kinetics of gait. The classic study by Doane and Holt was the first to conclude that the primary biomechanical distinction of the articulated, single axis foot was that it achieved foot flat

Amputee Walking: Relative Pace & Energy Consumption

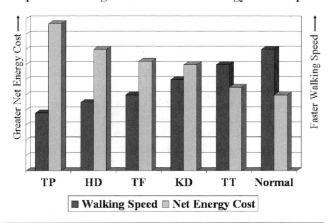

FIGURE 11-2. This overlay of two graphs, modified from Waters and Mulroy (1999), summarizes two important general trends from the literature on walking with a lower limb prosthesis. Individuals with higher amputation levels expend more net energy to walk a given distance than those having more distal amputations. In addition, their self-selected walking speed is progressively slower as the level of amputation becomes more proximal. TP = transpelvic amputation; HD = hip disarticulation amputation; TF = transfemoral amputation; KD = knee disarticulation amputation; TT = transtibial amputation; normal = nonamputee.

more rapidly than other tested alternatives (8), a conclusion borne out by subsequent researchers (7). To illustrate the importance of such findings, the primary indication today for the prescription of single axis ankle-foot mechanisms is to enhance prosthetic knee stability (25). This occurs because the net vertical ground reaction force vector quickly moves anteriorly at foot flat, from the back edge of the heel to the ankle mortise, thus creating an external moment on the prosthetic knee that stabilizes it in extension. The more rapidly this happens, the more stable the prosthetic limb.

A number of researchers have looked at prosthetic feet incorporating a plastic spring element within the forefoot, commonly referred to as "dynamic response" components. One consistent trend is that because they have a more flexible forefoot than earlier single axis or solid ankle cushion heel (SACH) feet, dynamic response feet allow a more normal range of passive ankle dorsiflexion in late stance (23), although the total range of motion is still less than normal. Particularly for those components whose design incorporates a spring that extends fully to the phalangeal region of the prosthetic foot, this seems to result in a longer stride length on the prosthetic side. Interestingly, dynamic response feet have also been shown to result in less vertical impact on the contralateral heel during loading response (1). This illustrates one of the primary advantages of instrumented gait analysis: it sometimes reveals effects that are unexpected and counterintuitive. Clini-

cians had not anticipated that prescription of a specific prosthetic component might reduce stresses on the surviving foot, which is known to be at risk for lesions in the case of the dysvascular amputee.

Research to date has not demonstrated any energy efficiency advantage for dynamic response feet when the amputee is walking on level surfaces at a relatively slow self-selected pace (32). However, during uphill walking or at more rapid cadences, dynamic response feet have been shown to reduce the net oxygen costs of ambulation compared to walking with less sophisticated mechanisms (24,36). However, it is important to recognize that ambulation with even the most advanced prosthetic ankle-foot devices still requires significantly more effort than normal walking. Gait studies have shown that amputee gait is characterized by a reduction in the magnitude of the second vertical ground reaction force peak (2), sometimes termed the A2 power burst, which occurs in the latter half of stance phase (4), as depicted in Figure 11-3. This illustrates that passive, spring keel prosthetic feet are unable to effectively restore this aspect of gait kinetics, which may contribute to the higher energy costs of amputee walking. Studies of normal subjects have established that individuals tend to choose a walking speed that is most energy efficient. It is possible that some of the increased effort required for amputees to ambulate a given distance is directly related to the slower cadence adopted by this population.

Childress' group at Northwestern University has done many of the more recent investigations of lower limb prosthetic components. One intriguing proposal from this laboratory has been that prosthetists dynamically align the ankle-foot mechanism to optimize its functional performance in view of each transtibial amputee's physical condition and individual gait pattern. It appears that the subjective changes the prosthetist makes to the angulation and linear position of the foot with respect to the prosthetic socket gives the prosthesis a "rollover characteristic" that approximates that of a normal ankle and foot (15).

Although prosthetic ankle-foot components have been studied extensively, less research has been conducted on the effect of prosthetic knee mechanisms on amputee gait. The growing clinical utilization of microprocessor-controlled devices should stimulate future research in this area. Basic prosthetic knee mechanisms with friction swing phase controls can only be optimized for a single cadence. Hicks et al. corroborated the clinical impression that such single axis constant friction prosthetic knees only swing at a fixed rate which is largely determined by the pendular effect of the shank (17). Their results showed that increasing or decreasing the amount of mechanical friction on the knee changed the magnitude of knee flexion in early swing but had very little effect on overall swing phase timing.

One important implication of this information is that studies of ambulation with a prosthesis should report on

FIGURE 11-3. This graph of the vertical ground reaction forces (GRF) generated during stance phase illustrates typical differences between amputee gait, shown as the solid line, and normal gait, shown as the dotted line. During the first half of stance phase, the prosthetic limb usually exhibits a somewhat lower maximum vertical GRF than normal, suggesting that the amputee is placing less load onto the artificial limb. During the latter half of stance phase, the second peak of the vertical GRF on the prosthetic limb is significantly lower than normal. This indicates that the prosthetic ankle-foot mechanism generates less propulsive force than the normal leg. Dynamic response prosthetic feet, which have forefoot springs, generate a higher second peak than less sophisticated components but do not exceed 100 percent of body weight; the intact limb generates about 120 percent of body weight during normal walking.

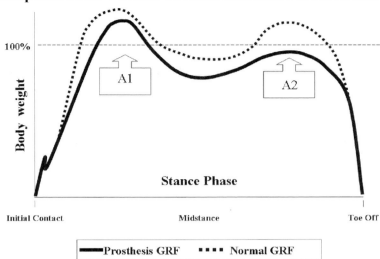

Amputee Gait: Vertical Ground Reaction Forces in Stance

the specific components being used. For example, if gait analysis shows that a group of transfemoral amputee subjects walked more slowly than a comparable transtibial group, it would be important to report that all of the TF subjects used a constant friction (one speed) knee. Similar results in a group that included TF subjects whose prostheses contained fluid-controlled knee mechanisms would be of particular interest, since hydraulic and pneumatic knees and particularly those that are microprocessor-controlled have been shown to permit amputees to walk safely throughout a range of cadences (17). Unfortunately, many of the gait studies of earlier decades did not report any information about the components within the prosthesis and therefore their results must be interpreted with caution.

SHOCK ABSORPTION

Inman and colleagues proposed that knee flexion during stance minimized the vertical displacement of the center of mass and therefore helped contribute to efficient ambulation. More recent studies have cast doubt on this assumption, suggesting that the primary benefit of knee flexion during loading response is to provide shock absorption (28). Current data also suggest that pelvic list, the second element in Inman's original six determinants of gait also contributes more to shock absorption than was originally believed (12). This increased appreciation for the role of shock absorption during normal walking has led to the development of prosthetic components that are intended to provide this function during amputee gait.

Within the past decade, several innovative prosthetic knee designs that allow controlled knee flexion during loading response have been developed. Gait analysis shows

that the range of knee flexion with these passive "stance flexion" components is less than normal and begins later in the stance phase, but these components clearly offer the potential for the amputee to walk without the stiff-legged gait that characterizes basic single axis devices (11). This emphasizes the point that gait data from subjects fitted with more technologically advanced knee components should be expected to differ significantly from earlier studies based on single axis, constant friction knee mechanisms. Some of the kinematic abnormalities identified in early gait studies, such as full knee extension throughout during early stance, were necessary compensations for the biomechanical limitations of the available components of that era.

Telescoping pylons, often termed "vertical shock systems" have become increasingly well accepted clinically, and preliminary research suggests that these components approximate the overall stiffness of the intact human leg. Gait analysis has shown that shock pylons can significantly reduce the loading on the residual limb during loading response (6) but may create a prosthesis that is functionally short under weight bearing (13). Further investigation is needed to better document the biomechanical implications of using these nonanatomic structures to provide shock absorption.

ADDITIONAL FACTORS

In the first edition of this text, Radcliffe and colleagues discussed a rationale for alignment of prosthetic knee devices based on the external moments created about the mechanical joint axis. Experimental evidence is now available to support this hypothesis, and at least one researcher has shown that a prosthesis that was subjectively considered "optimally aligned" by an experienced prosthetist and amputee subjects minimized the internal hip flexion and extension control moments generated on the affected side (26).

Moving the prosthetic knee one centimeter anterior or posterior to the subjectively determined "optimal" location in the sagittal plane increased the overall internal hip moments, suggesting that the amputee would exert more muscle force to control a knee that was malaligned. Moving the knee posteriorly resulted in an increase in the hip flexion moment, supporting Radcliffe's argument that more stable alignment would require increased force to "break" the knee to permit flexion during swing phase. Moving the knee anteriorly, which Radcliffe (33) proposed should make the knee less stable, required more hip extension force during loading response (5), presumably to prevent the prosthetic knee from collapsing.

Socket design is widely believed to be one of the most critical aspects of amputee rehabilitation, but very few gait studies have investigated the impact of this aspect of the artificial limb. Some authors have suggested that modern "ischial containment" transfemoral sockets result in a more energy-efficient gait than the earlier "quadrilateral" type (33), but the small number of subjects investigated limits the conclusions that can be drawn from such studies. Suspension mechanisms are also believed to be significant factors that influence use of the prosthesis, but very little data is available on the influence of suspension alternatives on prosthetic gait. These areas remain fertile ground for future investigations.

LIMITATIONS IN CURRENT STUDIES

Perhaps the greatest limitation to our current knowledge, present in almost all investigations of amputee gait published to date, is the small number of subjects studied. Major leg amputations are, fortunately, not a common problem and higher levels of loss occur less frequently than those below the knee joint. For example, hip disarticulation prostheses are only one or two percent of all artificial limbs fitted, so it is virtually impossible to recruit more than a handful of local subjects who walk with these devices for gait analysis. Transtibial amputation is the most common major lower limb loss and therefore this level has the largest number of subjects enrolled, as well as the greatest number of studies published. For most other levels, less than a dozen subjects have been studied at any one time.

Another factor making these studies challenging is that a certain level of physical fitness is required to walk for an extended period of time. Since most new amputations in the United States occur in individuals who are retirement age and older, and many have advanced vascular disease and associated cardiopulmonary restrictions, a substantial percentage of patients who use a prosthesis cannot complete the multiple trials necessary to participate in a scientific study. Many of those who do have the physical ability to walk for longer periods of time require balance aids such as canes, crutches, or a walker, which alter their gait mechanics.

As a practical matter, most published studies have a selection bias in that the subjects who participated were younger, more physically active individuals who required amputation due to trauma or tumor but who were otherwise healthy. Results from this population are not necessarily valid for the more typical elderly dysvascular amputee.

Finally, the technological sophistication of the components incorporated in the prosthesis has been shown to have a significant potential to influence the objective parameters measured during instrumented gait analysis. Most recently, microprocessor-controlled hydraulic and pneumatic prosthetic knee mechanisms have been shown to increase the efficiency of gait in tested subjects more than noncomputerized equivalents (10,35).

These limitations mean that current data on gait with a prosthesis, and the summary statements made in this chapter, are best viewed as suggestive evidence rather than verified fact. While it is likely that many of these findings will be corroborated by larger and better controlled future work, it is also quite possible that some of our beliefs will be shown to have significant limitations.

CONCLUSION

Free motion prosthetic joints have biomechanical characteristics that are quite similar to a limb with flail paralysis, except that the alignment and adjustments of the prosthetic components can be optimized for each individual patient. Altering the alignment or adjustment of the mechanisms and testing the results with observational or instrumented gait analysis can provide useful information. Adding resistance to prosthetic joints is similar to walking by using only eccentric muscle contractions. The passive nature of currently available prosthetic components provides a mechanically simple mechanism for walking that can seem surprisingly effective clinically but has significant limitations that instrumented gait analysis makes apparent. Insights from the growing body of evidence provided by modern gait analysis have spurred designers and clinicians to develop more sophisticated prosthetic components and advanced clinical methods intended to reduce the gap between normal and prosthetic walking.

REFERENCES

1. Barth DG, Schumacher L, Thomas SS. Gait analysis and energy cost of below-knee amputees wearing six different prosthetic feet. *J Prosthet Orthot* 1992;4:63–75.
2. Barth DG, Schumacher L, Thomas SS. Gait analysis and energy cost of below-knee amputees wearing six different prosthetic feet. *J Prosthet Orthot* 1992;4:63–75.
3. Bateni H, Olney SJ. Kinematic and kinetic variations of below-knee amputee gait. *Prosthet Orthot* 2002;14:2–10.
4. Bateni H, Olney SJ. Kinematic and kinetic variations of below-knee amputee gait. *J Prosthet Orthot* 2002;14:2–10.
5. Blumentritt S, Scherer HW, Michael JW. Transfemoral amputees walking on a rotary hydraulic prosthetic knee mechanism: a preliminary report. *J Prosthet Orthot* 1998;10:61–70.
6. Blumentritt S, Scherer HW, Wellershaus U. Design principles, biomechanical data and clinical experience with a polycentric knee offering controlled stance phase knee flexion: a preliminary report. *J Prosthet Orthot* 1997;9:18–24.
7. Culham EG, Peat M, Newell E. Below-knee amputation: a comparison of the effect of the SACH foot and single axis foot on electromyographic patterns during locomotion. *Prosthet Orthot Int* 1986;10:15–22.
8. Doane NE, Holt LE. A comparison of the SACH and single axis foot in the gait of unilateral below-knee amputees. *Prosthet Orthot Int* 1983;7:33–36.
9. Fisher GV, Gullickson G. Energy cost of ambulation in health and disability: a literature review. *Arch Phys Med Rehabil* 1978;59:124–133.
10. Gailey RS, Lawrence D, Burditt C. The CAT-CAM socket and quadrilateral socket: a comparison of energy cost during ambulation. *Prosthet Orthot Int* 1993;17:95–100.
11. Gard SA, Childress DS. The effect of pelvic list on the vertical displacement of the trunk during normal walking. *Gait Posture* 1997;5:233–238.
12. Gard SA, Childress DS. What determines the vertical displacement of the body during normal walking? *J Prosthet Orthot* 2001;13:64–67.
13. Gard SA, Konz RJ. The effect of a shock absorbing pylon on the gait of persons with unilateral transtibial amputation. *J Rehabil Res Dev* 2003;40:109–124.
14. Gonzales EG, Corcoran PJ, Reyes RL. Energy expenditure in below-knee amputees: correlation with stump length. *Arch Phys Med Rehabil* 1974;55:111–118.
15. Hafner BJ, Sanders JE, Czerniecki JM, Fergason J. Transtibial energy-storage-and-return prosthetic devices: a review of energy concepts and a proposed nomenclature. *J Rehabil Res Dev* 2002;39:1–11.
16. Hansen AH, Childress DS, Knox EH. Prosthetic foot roll-over shapes with implications for alignment of trans-tibial prostheses. *Prosthet Orthot Int* 2000;24:205–215.
17. Hicks R, Tashman S, Cary JM. Swing phase control with knee friction in juvenile amputees. *J Orthop Res* 1985;3:198–201.
18. Inman VT, Ralston HJ, Todd F. *Human Walking*. Baltimore/London: Williams & Wilkins 1982;140.
19. Isakov E, Bruger H, Krajnik J. Knee muscle activity during ambulation of trans-tibial amputees. *J Rehabil Med* 2001;33:196–199.
20. Jaegers SMHJ, Arendzen JH, De Jongh HJ. An electromyographic study of the hip muscles of transfemoral amputees in walking. *Clin Orthop* 1996;328:119–128.
21. James U, Oberg K. Prosthetic gait pattern in unilateral above-knee amputees. *Scand J Rehabil Med* 1973;5:35–50.
22. Kaufman KR, Irby SE, Mathewson JW. Energy-efficient-knee-ankle-foot orthosis: a case study. *J Prosthet Orthot* 1996;8:79–85.
23. MacFarlane PA, Nielsen DH, Shurr DG. Mechanical gait analysis of transfemoral amputees: SACH foot versus the Flex-Foot. *J Prosthet Orthot* 1997;9:144–151.
24. MacFarlane PA, Nielsen DH, Shurr DG. Transfemoral amputee physiological requirements: comparison between SACH foot walking and Flex-Foot walking. *J Prosthet Orthot* 1997;9:138–143.
25. Michael J. Modern prosthetic knee mechanisms. *Clin Orthop* 1999;361:39–47.
26. Michaud SB, Gard SA, Childress DS. A preliminary investigation of pelvic obliquity patterns during gait in transtibial and transfemoral amputees. *J Rehabil Res Dev* 2000;37:1–10.
27. Murphy AT, Burgess-Limerick. Influence of partial foot amputation on sagittal gait mechanics and locomotor function. *Abstract from 7th Annual Gait and Clinical Movement Analysis Society Conference*, April 16-29, 2002 [available online at www.motionanalysis.com/pdf/gcmas2002/murphy.pdf]
28. Murray MP, Mollinger LA, Sepic SB, Gardner GM, Linder MT. Gait patterns in above-knee amputee patients: hydraulic swing control versus constant-friction knee components. *Arch Phys Med Rehabil* 1983;64:339–345.
29. Nissan M. The initiation of gait in lower limb amputees: some related data. *J Rehabil Res Dev* 1991;28:1–12.
30. Pinzur MS, Wolf B, Havel RM. Walking pattern of midfoot and ankle disarticulation amputees. *Foot Ankle Int* 1997;18: 635–638.
31. Powers CM, Rao S, Perry J. Knee kinetics in trans-tibial amputee gait. *Gait & Posture* 1998;8:1–7.
32. Powers CM, Torburn L, Perry J. Influence of prosthetic foot design on sound limb loading in adults with unilateral below-knee amputations. *Arch Phys Med Rehabil* 1994;75:825–829.
33. Radcliffe CW. Functional considerations in the fitting of above-knee prostheses. *Artificial Limbs* 1955;2:35–60.
34. Schmalz T, Blumentritt S, Jarasch R. Energy expenditure and biomechanical characteristics of lower limb amputee gait: the influence of prosthetic alignment and different prosthetic components. *Gait Posture* 2002:16:255–263.
35. Taylor MB, Clarke E, Offord EA. A comparison of energy expenditure by a high level trans-femoral amputee using the Intelligent Prosthesis and conventionally damped prosthetic limbs. *Prosthet Orthot Int* 1996;2:116–121.
36. Torburn L, Perry J, Ayyappa E. Below-knee amputee gait with dynamic elastic response prosthetic feet: a pilot study. *J Rehabil Res Dev* 1990;27:369–384.
37. Waters RL, Campbell J, Thomas L, Hugos L, Davis P. Energy costs of walking in lower extremity prosthetic casts. *J Bone Joint Surg Am* 1982;64: 896–899.
38. Waters RL, Mulroy S. The energy expenditure of normal and pathological gait. *Gait and Posture* 1999;9:207–231.
39. Waters RL, Perry J, Antonelli D. Energy cost of walking of amputees: influence of level of amputation. *J Bone Joint Surg* 1976;58A:42–46.
40. Zuniga EN, Leavitt LA, Calvert JC. Gait patterns in above-knee amputees. *Arch Phys Med Rehabil* 1972;53:373–382.

Chapter 12

Simulation of Walking

Frank C. Anderson, Allison S. Arnold, Marcus G. Pandy,
Saryn R. Goldberg, and Scott L. Delp

Many elements of the neuromusculoskeletal system interact to enable walking. Scientists fascinated by human movement have performed an extensive range of studies to describe these elements, e.g., to identify the processes involved in neuromuscular activation, characterize the mechanics of muscle contraction, describe the geometric relationships between muscles and bones, and quantify the motions of joints. Clinicians who treat walking abnormalities in individuals with cerebral palsy, stroke, and other neuromusculoskeletal disorders have examined the electromyographic (EMG) patterns, gait kinematics, and ground reaction forces of literally thousands of patients, both before and after treatment interventions. However, synthesizing detailed descriptions of the neuromusculoskeletal system with gait measurements to create an integrated understanding of normal gait, to identify the sources of pathologic gait, and to establish a scientific basis for treatment planning remains a major challenge.

Using experiments alone to meet this challenge has two fundamental limitations. First, important variables, including the forces generated by muscles, are not readily accessible in experiments. Second, even when variables can be measured accurately, it is often difficult to establish cause-effect relationships. As a result, elucidating the functions of muscles from experiments is not straightforward. For example, ground reaction forces (see Chapter 4) can be measured and used to estimate the accelerations of the body's center of mass. However, force plate measurements alone offer little insight into how muscles contribute to these accelerations, and therefore to the critical tasks of supporting and propelling the body forward. EMG recordings (see Chapter 6) can indicate *when* a muscle is active, but examination of EMG recordings does not allow one to determine which motions of the body arise from a muscle's activity. Indeed, determining how individual muscles contribute to observed motions is not necessarily intuitive, as explained below, because a muscle can accelerate joints that it does not span and body segments that it does not touch (105).

A theoretical framework is needed, in combination with experiments, to advance our understanding of neuromusculoskeletal function during walking, e.g., to uncover the principles that govern the coordination of muscles during normal gait, to determine how neuromuscular impairments contribute to abnormal gait, and to predict the functional consequences of treatments. It is imperative that this framework reveals the cause-effect relationships between neuromuscular excitation patterns, muscle forces, ground reaction forces, and motions of the body. A dynamic simulation of walking that integrates facts about the anatomy and physiology of the neuromusculoskeletal system and the mechanics of multi-joint movement provides such a framework.

What is a dynamic simulation of movement, and how can it complement experimental studies of walking? A dynamic simulation is, in essence, a solution to a set of equations that describe how the forces acting on a system cause motions of the system over time, as governed by the laws of physics. A "muscle-driven" dynamic simulation of walking, therefore, describes how the forces produced by muscles (and other sources of force, such as gravity) contribute to motions of the body segments during the gait cycle.

The process for developing, testing, and analyzing a muscle-driven simulation of movement involves four stages (Figure 12-1). Stage 1 is to create a computer model that characterizes the dynamic behavior of the neuromusculoskeletal system with sufficient accuracy to answer specific research questions. The models that we, and others have developed typically include detailed descriptions of musculoskeletal geometry and equations that describe the activation and force production of muscles and the multi-joint dynamics of the body. Stage 2 is to find a set of muscle excitations which, when applied to the model, generate a simulation that reproduces the movement of interest. Stage 3 is to verify that the simulation is indeed representative of the movement of interest by comparing the results of the simulation to experimental data. Stage 4 is to analyze the simulation to answer the research or clinical questions posed.

193

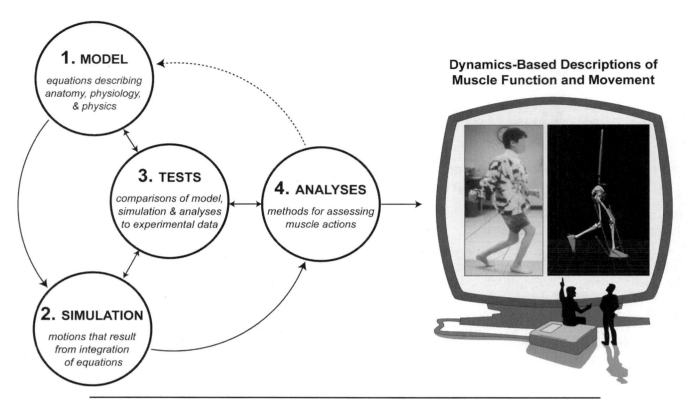

FIGURE 12-1. Stages involved in creating and analyzing a simulation of walking. A rigorous assessment of muscle function during walking requires (1) a model of neuromusculoskeletal dynamics, typically formulated as a set of equations that relate accelerations of the limb segments to the forces generated by muscles and other external forces, such as the force of gravity, (2) a simulation of the gait cycle, obtained by applying a set of muscle excitations to the model and integrating the equations of motion forward in time, (3) tests to verify that the simulation is sufficiently accurate to answer specific research questions, generally performed by comparing aspects of the model and simulation to experimental data, and (4) analyses of the simulation to determine how individual muscles generate forces and contribute to motions of the body.

A muscle-driven dynamic simulation provides unique capabilities that complement experimental approaches. Simulations provide estimates of important variables, such as muscle and joint forces, which are difficult to measure experimentally. Simulations also enable cause-effect relationships to be explained. For instance, the contribution that a muscle makes to the ground reaction force can be calculated. A simulation also allows "what if?" studies to be performed in which, for example, the excitation pattern of a muscle can be changed and the resulting motion can be observed. These capabilities provide new ways to characterize the functions of muscles during walking and other tasks.

Why are simulations needed to characterize the functions of muscles during walking? Simulations are needed because experimental approaches to infer a muscle's actions, based on the muscle's attachments, EMG activity, and measured motions of the body, do not explain how the forces produced by the muscle accelerate the body segments and contribute to motions of the joints. When a muscle applies a force to a segment, that segment is ac-

celerated (Figure 12-2). The acceleration of the segment is resisted by the inertia of adjoining segments, giving rise to intersegmental forces at the joints. These intersegmental forces are transmitted from one segment to another due to the "coupled" multi-articular nature of the body. The transmission of these intersegmental forces, often referred to as *dynamic coupling*, means that a force applied to one body segment accelerates all body segments, not just the segment to which the force is applied. The relative magnitudes of the intersegmental forces at the joints depend, in part, on the mass and inertial properties of the segments being accelerated. For example, intersegmental forces at the hip that arise from accelerations of the thigh are generally greater than intersegmental forces at the metatarsophalangeal joints that arise from accelerations of the toes because the thigh is more massive than the toes. The magnitudes and directions of the intersegmental forces also depend on the applied muscle force and the configuration of the body.

How significant are the intersegmental forces induced by muscles during walking? In particular, are these forces

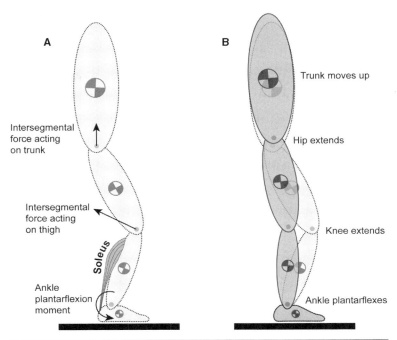

FIGURE 12-2. Dynamic actions of soleus during single-limb stance (knee flexion angle is exaggerated for the purpose of illustration). (**A**) The force applied by soleus, a uniarticular muscle spanning the ankle, not only generates an ankle plantarflexion moment (circular black arrow), but also induces intersegmental forces throughout the body. The magnitudes and directions of these intersegmental forces depend on the force applied by the muscle, the moment arms of the muscle, the inertial properties of the segments, and the configuration of the body. In this example, the force applied by soleus produces a counter-clockwise angular acceleration of the shank. This acceleration requires the location of the knee joint to accelerate to the left and upward. The inertia of the thigh resists this acceleration, resulting in an intersegmental force at the knee (straight black arrow). The intersegmental force at the knee accelerates the thigh, which in turn induces an intersegmental force at the hip (straight black arrow), and so on. (**B**) As a consequence of the intersegmental forces induced by soleus, soleus accelerates not only the ankle, but all the joints of the body. At the body position shown, soleus accelerates the ankle toward plantarflexion, the knee toward extension, the hip toward extension, and the trunk upward. Over time, these accelerations give rise to changes in position. Thus, due to dynamic coupling, soleus does not function solely as an "ankle plantarflexor"—in many situations, it likely does much more. In similar fashion, other muscles induce intersegmental forces and accelerate joints that they do not span.

large enough to influence our interpretation of the muscles' actions? The answer to this question, in many cases, is yes. Due to dynamic coupling, a muscular moment generated at one joint induces accelerations of that joint and other joints— including joints that the muscle does not span. These "muscle-induced" accelerations are generally small at joints far removed from the muscle; however, the induced accelerations of nearby joints can be substantial. For example, soleus exerts only an ankle plantarflexion moment, yet Zajac and Gordon (105) have demonstrated that soleus can accelerate the knee into extension more than it accelerates the ankle into plantarflexion. During the stance phase of normal gait (Figure 12-2), soleus accelerates both the knee and the ankle toward extension (9,45,56), an action commonly termed the *plantarflexion – knee extension couple* (33). The plantarflexion moment exerted by soleus during stance also accelerates

the hip toward extension (9,45,58) and provides vertical support for the trunk (6,56,106). Based on this work and other examples, we believe that the effects of dynamic coupling must be considered when attempting to determine the functional roles of muscles during gait. Using a muscle-driven dynamic simulation, the intersegmental forces that result from a muscle's force can be calculated, and the resulting motions of the body segments can be quantified.

The remainder of this chapter summarizes our experiences with the development and analysis of muscle-driven simulations of human walking. There are many plausible approaches, and this chapter is not intended to be a comprehensive review. Rather, the chapter describes the development (Stages 1 and 2) and testing (Stage 3) of a particular simulation—a three-dimensional dynamic simulation of normal gait (5). Three studies are reviewed in which this simulation was analyzed (Stage 4) to gain new insights into the functions of individual muscles during walking. The chapter concludes by summarizing some of the limitations of current modeling, simulation, and analysis techniques. Consideration of these limitations suggests future research.

STAGE 1: CREATING A DYNAMIC MODEL OF THE MUSCULOSKELETAL SYSTEM

In a muscle-driven dynamic simulation, elements of the neuromusculoskeletal system are modeled by sets of differential equations that describe muscle activation dynamics, musculotendon contraction dynamics, musculoskeletal geometry, and skeletal dynamics (Figure 12-3). These equations characterize the time-dependent behavior of the musculoskeletal system in response to neuromuscular excitation. Formulating these equations is the necessary first stage in generating a simulation (see also Pandy (67) for a review).

Muscles do not generate forces instantaneously in response to neuromuscular excitation (see also Chapter 6). Muscle activation dynamics, the time course of Ca^{++}-mediated activation of the contractile apparatus as modu-

lated by motor unit action potentials, can be modeled by relating the time rate of change of muscle activation ($\dot{a}$) to muscle activation (a) and excitation (u):

$$\dot{a} = (u^2 - ua)/ \cdot \tau_{act} + (u - a)/\tau_{deact}, \tag{1}$$

where τ_{act} and τ_{deact} are the time constants for activation and deactivation, respectively (62). Excitation and activation levels in Eq. 1 are allowed to vary continuously between zero (no excitation and activation) and one (full excitation and activation). Activation levels serve as inputs to the equations for musculotendon contraction dynamics that estimate muscle forces.

Musculotendon contraction dynamics, the time course of muscle force generation as determined by the energetics of cross bridge formation, the sliding of actin filaments, and the dynamics of tendon, can be modeled by relating the time rate of change of muscle force ($\dot{f}_M$) to musculotendon length (l_{MT}), musculotendon shortening velocity ($\dot{l}_{MT}$), and muscle activation (a):

$$\dot{f}_M = f(l_{MT}, \dot{l}_{MT}, a), \tag{2}$$

where the function $f(l_{MT}, \dot{l}_{MT}, a)$ characterizes the force-length-velocity properties of muscle and the force-length properties of tendon (66,107). The contraction dynamics of a particular muscle can be estimated by scaling the function by five parameters: maximum isometric muscle

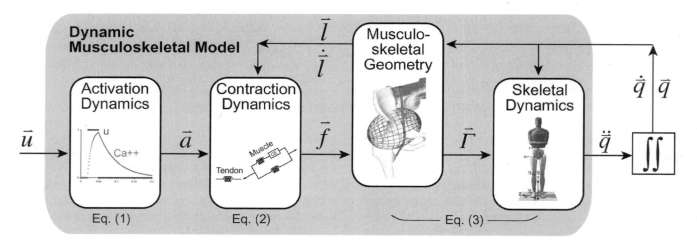

FIGURE 12-3. Elements of a muscle-driven simulation of walking. When a dynamic musculoskeletal model (shaded region) is driven by muscle excitations ($\vec{u}$), the resulting motions of the body, ($\ddot{\vec{q}}, \dot{\vec{q}}, \vec{q}$) can be calculated. The equation for muscle activation dynamics relates the muscle excitations to muscle activations ($\vec{a}$). The equations for musculotendon contraction dynamics relate the muscle activations to muscle forces (f); the muscle forces depend on musculotendon lengths and shortening velocities ($\vec{l}, \dot{\vec{l}}$). The muscle forces are transmitted to the skeleton resulting in joint torques ($\vec{\Gamma}$), which accelerate the limb segments according to the equations of motion that govern the multi-joint dynamics of the body. These accelerations ($\ddot{\vec{q}}$) depend on the mass and inertial characteristics of the limb segments, Coriolis and centrifugal forces, gravity, muscle forces, and any external forces produced when the body interacts with the environment. Equations 1–3 are numerically integrated forward in time to produce a simulation.

force and the corresponding muscle fiber length, maximum shortening velocity, pennation angle, and tendon slack length (i.e., the length at which tendon begins to transmit force when stretched). When applied to the skeleton, musculotendon forces act to accelerate the body segments.

The accelerations of the body segments in response to muscle forces and other loads can be computed from a description of the musculoskeletal geometry and the equations of motion that govern the multi-joint dynamics of the body:

$$\ddot{\vec{q}} = \vec{I}^{-1}(\vec{q}) \cdot \{\vec{G}(\vec{q}) + \vec{C}(\vec{q},\dot{\vec{q}}) + \vec{R}(\vec{q}) \cdot \vec{f}_M + \vec{F}_E(\vec{q},\dot{\vec{q}})\}. \tag{3}$$

In this set of equations, $\vec{q}$, $\dot{\vec{q}}$, and $\ddot{\vec{q}}$ are the generalized coordinates (e.g., joint angles), velocities, and accelerations of the model, respectively. $\vec{I}^{-1}$ is the inverse of the system mass matrix, which specifies the mass and inertial properties of the body segments. $\vec{G}$ is a vector of forces arising from gravity. $\vec{C}$ is a vector of forces arising from Coriolis and centrifugal forces, which are generated from the rotations of the body segments (e.g., like the forces encountered when swinging an object around in circles at the end of a rope). $\vec{R}$ is a matrix of muscle moment arms, and $\vec{f}_M$ is a vector of muscle forces. The muscle moment arms, or lever arms, determine the joint moments that result from application of the muscle forces. $\vec{F}_E$ is a vector of external forces that characterize the interactions with the environment.

We have used this general approach to create a model to simulate walking (4,5). The skeleton was represented as a 10 segment, 23 degree-of-freedom linkage (Figure 12-4). The pelvis was modeled as a rigid segment that was free to translate and rotate with respect to the ground. The remaining nine segments branched in an open chain from the pelvis. Segment masses, centers of masses, and moments of inertia were derived based on the regression equations reported by McConville et al (52) and anthropometric measures obtained from five healthy adult males. The equations of motion (Eq. 3) for the model were generated using a software package called SD/Fast (PTC, Needham, Massachusetts). Interactions between the feet and the ground were characterized using a series of spring-damper units distributed under the sole of each foot (i.e.,$\vec{F}_E$ in Eq. 3). Torques representing the actions of ligaments were applied to the joints to prevent the joints from hyperextending during a simulation.

The model was driven by 54 musculotendon actuators. The path (i.e., line of action) of each actuator was specified based on anatomical landmarks (25). When an actuator wrapped around a bone or other muscles, via points and/or via cylinders were introduced to represent the path more accurately (26,35). Muscle activation dynamics were described using Eq. 1 with activation and deactivation

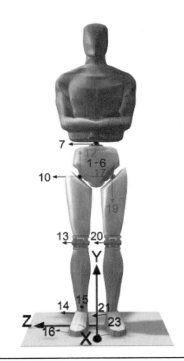

FIGURE 12-4. Skeletal degrees of freedom of the model. The head, arms, and torso were represented as a single rigid segment that articulated with the pelvis via a ball-and-socket joint located at approximately the third lumbar vertebra. Each hip was modeled as a ball-and-socket joint, each knee as a hinge joint, each ankle-subtalar joint as a universal joint, and each metatarsal joint as a hinge joint. Figure adapted from Anderson and Pandy (7).

time constants of 22 and 200 msec, respectively (66,107). Musculotendon contraction dynamics were described using Eq. 2 with musculotendon parameters based on data reported in the literature (18,25,31,97,107). Values of maximum isometric force and tendon slack length were adjusted for each actuator so that the isometric torque-angle curves for each joint in the model approximated the average torque-angle curves measured for five subjects (4). The model was completed when Eqs. 1–3 were formulated for the 54 musculotendon actuators and the 10 segment, 23 degree-of-freedom linkage.

STAGE 2: GENERATING A MUSCLE-DRIVEN SIMULATION OF WALKING

To generate a simulation of movement, the differential equations of a dynamic model are integrated forward in time (Figure 12-3). If the simulation is driven by muscles, a set of muscle excitations (i.e., u in Eq. 1) must be applied. A set of initial state variables (i.e., joint angles, joint angular velocities, muscle forces, and muscle activations at the initial time step) must also be specified. Integration of the equations yields the time histories of all state variables in the model, including the muscle activations, musculotendon forces, and joint angles.

Finding a set of muscle excitations that produces a coordinated movement can be challenging. This is especially true for a movement as complex as walking. Not only must many degrees of freedom be controlled (e.g., 23 in the case of the musculoskeletal model described above), but also the time-dependent, nonlinear force-generating properties of muscle must be taken into account. To meet this challenge, dynamic optimization can be used (e.g., 4,5,23,44,55,56,65,103).

Dynamic optimization is a mathematical approach for finding a set of control values (e.g., the time histories of muscle excitations) for a dynamic system (e.g., a dynamic musculoskeletal model) that minimizes or maximizes a time-dependent performance criterion, possibly subject to constraints. To simulate walking or other multi-joint movements, a variety of performance criteria can be formulated. One approach is to solve an optimal tracking problem (e.g., 23,56). In this approach, the performance criterion is specified based on the difference between simulated and experimentally determined quantities, such as joint angles, joint powers, and ground reaction forces. By minimizing the performance criterion over the period of the simulation, the model is driven explicitly to reproduce experimental data. In other formulations, a set of muscle excitations might be found that minimizes or maximizes the model's performance of some hypothesized motor goal.

We have used this goal-based approach, in combination with the musculoskeletal model described above, to generate a muscle-driven simulation of walking (5). We hypothesized that the locomotor patterns of healthy individuals result from minimizing metabolic energy expenditure per unit distance traveled. This hypothesis is supported by measurements of metabolic energy consumption and observations of preferred walking speeds (76). The performance criterion (J) was therefore formulated as follows:

$$J = \frac{\int_0^{t_f} \dot{E}^M_{total}}{X_{cm}(t_f) - X_{cm}(t_i)} + penalty\ terms, \qquad (4)$$

where $\dot{E}^M_{total}$ is the rate at which total metabolic energy is consumed in the model and $X_{cm}(t_i)$ and $X_{cm}(t_f)$ denote the position of the model's center of mass at the initial and final times of the simulated gait cycle, respectively. The penalty terms were appended to increase the value of the performance criterion if any of the joints hyperextended during a simulation. $\dot{E}^M_{total}$ was computed by adding the basal metabolic heat rate of the whole body to the activation heat rate, maintenance heat rate, shortening heat rate, and the mechanical work rate of each muscle in the model. These rate terms were computed from the muscle activations, forces, shortening velocities, and other states

of the model (16). To enforce repeatability of the gait cycle, we specified a number of terminal constraints. Specifically, the values of the joint angular displacements, joint angular velocities, muscle forces, and muscle activations at the end of the simulation were required to be the same as the values at the beginning. The values of the state variables at the beginning of the simulation were based on averaged experimental data.

Thus, the dynamic optimization problem that we solved was to find time histories of the muscle excitations that minimized J (Eq. 4) and met the constraints imposed to enforce repeatability. To solve this problem, we implemented a parameter optimization algorithm on parallel supercomputers (8,62). We applied the resulting muscle excitations to the dynamic model, integrated the equations of motion forward in time, and generated a simulation of walking. The locomotor pattern predicted by the optimal solution (Figure 12-5) successfully reproduced the salient features of normal gait.

STAGE 3: TESTING THE ACCURACY OF DYNAMIC SIMULATIONS

Before a simulation of movement can be analyzed, the simulation and the underlying model should be tested. In particular, it is important to verify that the dynamic behavior of the neuromusculoskeletal system is represented with sufficient fidelity to answer the research questions posed. For example, if the actions of individual muscles are of interest, the model should accurately characterize the muscle moment arms for the ranges of body positions assumed by the model during the simulation. Confidence in the muscle moment arms can be gained by comparing the moment arms predicted by the model to the moment arms determined experimentally from image data (e.g., 43) or from cadaveric specimens (e.g., 13,24). Confidence in the moment-generating capacities of muscles can be gained by comparing the maximum isometric joint moments generated by the model to the moments generated by human subjects (e.g., 4).

A simulation of movement can be tested by comparing quantities predicted by the simulation to quantities determined experimentally in the laboratory. For instance, the muscle excitation patterns, joint angles, joint moments, and ground reaction forces from a simulation of walking can be compared to EMG, kinematic, and kinetic data obtained from gait analysis. The similarity between predicted and measured values of metabolic energy consumption can also be assessed.

We have made detailed comparisons of the walking simulation, described above, to experimental data from five subjects (5). In most cases, the joint angles predicted by the simulation were within one standard deviation of the joint angles measured for the subjects. The simulated and

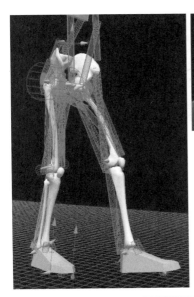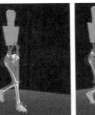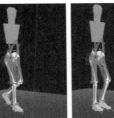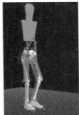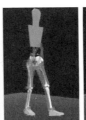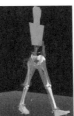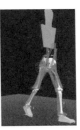

FIGURE 12-5. Snapshots of the muscle-driven simulation of walking obtained by solving a dynamic optimization problem.

measured ground reaction forces and muscle excitations also compared favorably (e.g., Figure 12-6). These tests provide some confidence that our simulation of walking reproduces the dynamics of normal gait (5).

STAGE 4: ANALYZING A SIMULATION OF WALKING

Once a muscle-driven simulation of movement is generated and tested, the simulation can be analyzed in several ways. Qualitatively, the motions produced from a particular set of muscle excitations can be visualized. Quantitatively, the contributions of individual muscles to the joint moments, joint angular accelerations, ground reaction forces, segmental energies, and other variables of interest can be determined. It is through the rigorous analysis and interpretation of such data that the value of a simulation can be realized.

The following examples demonstrate how a dynamic simulation can be analyzed to extract information about the actions of individual muscles during movement. Example 1 describes a method for decomposing the ground reaction force. We used this method to determine which muscles contribute to the vertical ground reaction force, and therefore to the vertical support of the body, during walking. Example 2 describes a technique for calculating the instantaneous angular accelerations of the joints induced by individual muscles during movement. We used this technique to determine which muscles are responsible for generating knee extension during the single-limb stance phase. Example 3 describes a method for quantifying how individual muscles (or other elements of a model)

influence the motions of the body segments over time. We used this method to determine which muscles have the greatest potential to diminish knee flexion velocity prior to toe-off, a possible cause of stiff-knee gait. All three examples were generated using the dynamic optimization solution for walking described above.

Example 1: Decomposition of the Ground Reaction Force to Quantify Contributions to Support

The vertical ground reaction force is measured routinely, and its characteristic shape is well known for normal walking (Figure 12-6A). Because achieving adequate vertical support is one of the basic requirements of walking (42), quantifying how muscles contribute to the vertical ground reaction force, and therefore to the vertical acceleration of the center of mass, is an important part of our basic understanding of gait mechanics.

Several studies have examined how the shape of the ground reaction force is influenced by muscle activity (48,53,56,63,64,68,72,88,100). There has been broad consensus that the second maximum observed in the vertical ground reaction force is due largely to the forces exerted by the plantarflexors during late stance. However, an explanation for the shape of the ground reaction force during early stance and midstance has been less definitive. Muscles that potentially contribute have been inferred from experiments based on similarities between net joint moments and the shape of the ground reaction force (100), changes in the ground reaction force after the administration of nerve blocks (88), and the timing of muscle activity (72). However, without a theoretical framework for attributing portions of the ground reaction force to the forces produced by individual muscles, determining the relative

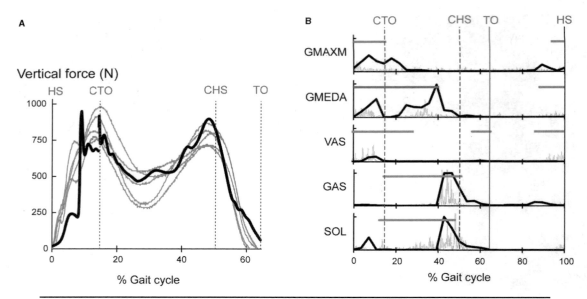

FIGURE 12-6. Tests of the muscle-driven simulation of walking. (**A**) The vertical ground reaction force generated during the simulation (*black line*) is representative of the ground reaction forces measured from five subjects during normal gait (*gray lines*). (**B**) The muscle excitation histories predicted by the dynamic optimization solution (black lines) compare favorably with EMG data recorded from one subject (gray lines) and with EMG data reported in the literature (horizontal gray bars) (75). The marked kinematic events are contralateral toe-off (CTO), contralateral heel-strike (CHS), toe-off (TO), and heel-strike (HS). (Figure adapted from Anderson and Pandy [5].)

contributions of muscles to the shape of the ground reaction force is difficult.

A number of studies (48,53,56) have used models of gait dynamics to estimate how muscles and other sources of force, such as gravity, contribute to the ground reaction force. This example summarizes the analyses we have performed to identify which sources of force make the largest contributions to the vertical ground reaction force, and therefore to support of the body during walking (6).

When interpreting experimental data obtained from gait analysis, it is often appealing to think of the ground reaction force as existing of its own accord, as a force to be balanced by net joint moments. Physically, however, the reverse is the case. "Reaction" forces, including the ground reaction force, arise as a consequence of "action" forces that act on and within the body. When muscles or other sources of force act on the body, they accelerate each foot with respect to the ground. Over time, these accelerations result in motion. When this motion brings a foot into contact with the ground, the foot and the ground deform (e.g., the compression of the sole of a shoe, or the depression of a wooden floor). Reaction forces are generated as a result of these deformations.

A muscle-driven dynamic simulation enables the cause-effect relationships between action forces, such as the forces produced by muscles, and reaction forces, such as the ground reaction force, to be established. Specifically, the ground reaction force generated during a simulation, $\vec{f}_E$, can be attributed to the Coriolis and centrifugal, grav-

ity, ligament, and muscle forces that are applied:

$$\vec{f}_E = \vec{f}_E^C + \vec{f}_E^G + \vec{f}_E^L + \vec{f}_E^M, \tag{5}$$

where $\vec{f}_E^C$, $\vec{f}_E^G$, $\vec{f}_E^L$, and $\vec{f}_E^M$ are the contributions made to the ground reaction force by the Coriolis and centrifugal, gravity, ligament, and muscle forces, respectively. During walking, deformations of the foot and ground are small (i.e., typically much less than 1 cm), and $\vec{f}_E^C$, $\vec{f}_E^G$, $\vec{f}_E^L$, and $\vec{f}_E^M$ can be computed by assuming rigid contact between each foot and the ground. That is, when a foot contacts the ground, the component of the ground reaction force caused by a particular action force can be estimated by applying that action force to the model in isolation and calculating the reaction force needed to prevent the portion of the foot in contact with the ground from accelerating. The reaction force induced by a muscle, $\vec{f}_E^{M_i}$, for example, can be computed as the force necessary to prevent the foot from accelerating when muscle M_i alone acts on the body. We have used this method, in conjunction with our walking simulation, to generate a decomposition of the vertical ground reaction force throughout the stance phase (6).

Muscles made the largest contribution to vertical support in our simulation, accounting for 50% to 95% of the vertical ground reaction force generated in stance (Figure 12-7A, Muscle+Ligaments). The hip and knee extensors (gluteus maximus, posterior portion of gluteus medius, and vasti) were the main contributors to support in early stance, although prior to foot-flat the ankle dorsiflexors made important contributions as well (Figure 12-7B). The hip abductors (anterior and posterior portions of gluteus medius and minimus) were the main contributors to support in midstance (Figure 12-7C). The ankle plantarflexors (primarily soleus and gastrocnemius) were the main contributors to support in late stance (Figure 12-7D). The passive transmission of force through the joints and bones in resistance to gravity accounted for 20% to 50% of the ground reaction force when the foot was flat on the ground, but made much smaller contributions before foot-flat and after heel-off (Figure 12-7A, Gravity). Coriolis and centrifugal forces acted to reduce the ground reaction force, but these contributions were far less than the contributions made by muscles or gravity (Figure 12-7A, Coriolis and Centrifugal).

Thus, by analyzing the cause-effect relationships between muscle forces and ground reaction forces during walking, a quantitative picture of how muscles contribute to the shape of the vertical ground reaction force has emerged. The first maximum in the ground reaction force results from the actions of the hip and knee extensors; the second maximum from the ankle plantarflexors. These muscles, along with the hip abductors, are the predominant contributors to vertical support during normal gait. The skeleton offers some support in resistance to gravity, but this support is less than 50% of body weight.

The methodology described in this example has numerous applications. By analyzing a simulation of a patient's abnormal gait, for instance, it may be possible to link deviations in the ground reaction force to the actions of particular muscles, perhaps identifying the cause of the patient's gait abnormality. In addition, as described in the next example, performing a decomposition of the ground reaction force is necessary for calculating the accelerations of the joints induced by individual muscles.

Example 2: Induced Acceleration Analysis to Quantify Muscle Actions in Single-Limb Stance

Children with cerebral palsy frequently walk with excessive knee flexion during the stance phase. This movement abnormality, called crouch gait, is problematic because it increases patellofemoral force (69), impedes toe clearance, and dramatically increases the energy requirements of walking (19,81,87). The persistent knee flexion typically worsens if left uncorrected (32,89) and can lead to altered patellofemoral joint mechanics and chronic knee pain (17,50,82,90).

Unfortunately, the biomechanical causes of crouch gait are often unclear, making it challenging to determine the most appropriate treatment. In some cases, abnormally "short" or "spastic" hamstrings are presumed to limit knee extension, and surgical lengthening of the hamstrings is performed (1,17,29,70). In other cases, diminished plantarflexion strength is thought to be a factor, and ankle-foot orthoses are prescribed (34,79). Other hypothesized causes

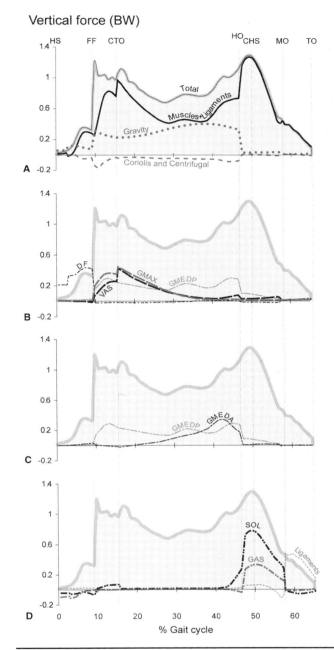

FIGURE 12-7. Decomposition of the ground reaction force during normal gait. (**A**) Contributions made to the ground reaction force by muscle and ligament forces (Muscles + Ligaments), Coriolis and centrifugal forces (Coriolis and Centrifugal), and resistance to gravity provided by the bones and joints of the skeleton (Gravity). Contributions made to the ground reaction force (**B**) during early stance by the dorsiflexors (DF), vasti (VAS), gluteus maximus (GMAX), the posterior portion of gluteus medius and minimus (GMEDP), (**C**) during mid-stance by the posterior and anterior portions of gluteus medius and minimus (GMEDA and GMEDP, respectively), and (**D**) during late stance by soleus (SOL), gastrocnemius (GAS), and the ligaments (Ligaments). The marked kinematic events are heel-strike (HS), foot-flat (FF), contralateral toe-off (CTO), heel-off (HO), contralateral heel-strike (CHS), metatarsal-off (MO), and toe-off (TO). (Figure adapted from Anderson and Pandy [(6)].

of crouch gait include malrotation of the femur, tibia, and foot (34,85), tight hip flexors (17,60,77,80), weak hip extensors (98), weak knee extensors (15,22,34), and poor balance (32).

Successful treatment of crouch gait is difficult, in part, because the factors that contribute to knee extension during normal gait are not well understood, and because the potential of individual muscles to produce knee flexion or extension during the stance phase is unknown. Knee motions are influenced not only by muscles that cross the knee, but also by muscular moments that are generated at other joints. To understand how knee extension is achieved during normal gait, and to elucidate the factors that potentially contribute to crouch gait, the effects of dynamic coupling must be considered. That is, the intersegmental forces that arise from a muscle's force must be computed, and the resulting multi-joint accelerations of the body must be evaluated.

We have used the simulation of walking, described above, to quantify the angular accelerations of the knee induced by the gluteus maximus, hamstrings, vasti, soleus, and other muscles during single-limb stance (9). This example illustrates how a simulation can be analyzed to reveal the dynamic actions of individual muscles during movement.

We determined the muscle-induced accelerations of the knee using the equations of motion for the model (Eq. 3) and the decomposition of the ground reaction force described in Example 1. At each time step in the simulation, a muscle's contributions to the instantaneous accelerations of the generalized coordinates ($\ddot{\vec{q}}_{M_i}$) were computed by applying that muscle's force ($\vec{f}_{M_i}$), as generated during the simulation, and the corresponding portion of the ground reaction force induced by that muscle ($\vec{f}_E^{M_i}$):

$$\ddot{\vec{q}}_{M_i} = \ddot{I}(\vec{q})^{-1} \cdot \left\{ \ddot{R}(\vec{q}) \cdot \vec{f}_{M_i} + \ddot{E}(\vec{q}) \cdot \vec{f}_E^{M_i} \right\} \qquad (6)$$

All other forces in the model were set to zero. $\ddot{E}$ is a matrix that converts the foot-ground spring forces into generalized forces (46).

Two descriptions of the muscle actions during single-limb stance were examined. First, the angular accelerations of the knee induced by individual muscles were quantified to determine which of the muscles enabled knee extension in the simulation of normal gait. Second, the muscle-induced accelerations of the knee per unit force were calculated to assess the "dynamic potential" of each muscle to accelerate the knee toward flexion or extension. This measure of a muscle's actions (obtained by setting $\vec{f}_{M_i} = 1N$, computing the corresponding $\vec{f}_E^{M_i}$, and substituting these quantities into Eq. 6) does not depend on the muscle excitations or forces applied during the simulation; rather, it reflects the influence of a muscle's moment arms and the inertial properties of the body. Hence, this analysis

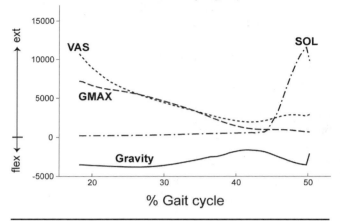

FIGURE 12-8. Contributions of vasti (VAS), gluteus maximus (GMAX), soleus (SOL), and gravity to the angular accelerations of the knee during the single-limb stance phase of normal gait. Gravity, together with its contribution to the ground reaction force, accelerated the knee toward flexion. The effects of gravity were resisted by muscles crossing the hip, knee, and ankle.

evaluated the relative potential of a muscle to generate (or limit) knee extension if, for example, the muscle was activated inappropriately or was producing excessive passive force.

Examination of the muscle-induced accelerations showed that the gluteus maximus, vasti, soleus, and posterior portion of the gluteus medius made substantial contributions to knee extension during normal gait (Figure 12-8). Per unit force, the gluteus maximus had greater potential than the vasti to accelerate the knee toward extension (Figure 12-9). These data suggest that diminished force in the hip extensors, knee extensors, or ankle plantarflexors

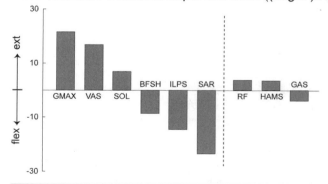

FIGURE 12-9. Angular accelerations of the knee per unit force, averaged over the single-limb stance phase (17%–50% of the gait cycle), induced by gluteus maximus (GMAX), vasti (VAS), soleus (SOL), biceps femoris short head (BFSH), iliopsoas (ILPS), sartorius (SAR), rectus femoris (RF), hamstrings (HAMS), and gastrocnemius (GAS).

may contribute to crouch gait, and strengthening these muscles, particularly the gluteus maximus, may help to improve both hip and knee extension. Abnormal forces generated by spasticity or contracture of the iliopsoas may also cause crouch gait in some cases, since these muscles have a large potential to accelerate the knee toward flexion (Figure 12-9).

The potential of the biarticular hamstrings, rectus femoris, and gastrocnemius muscles to induce angular accelerations of the knee during single-limb stance was small relative to other muscles (Figure 12-9). This was caused by dynamic coupling. Each of these muscles generated a moment about the knee and a moment about an adjacent joint, and these moments induced opposing accelerations of the knee. For example, the knee flexion moment generated by hamstrings acted to accelerate the knee toward flexion, but the hip extension moment generated by hamstrings acted to accelerate the knee toward extension. During the stance phase, in fact, the hamstrings had the potential to weakly accelerate the knee toward *extension* in our model. This occurred because the hamstrings' hip extension moment accelerated the knee toward extension more than the hamstrings' knee flexion moment accelerated the knee toward flexion. This unexpected result suggests that abnormally short or spastic hamstrings, a reputed cause of crouch gait, may not be the direct source of excessive knee flexion in some patients.

Our analysis of the muscle-induced accelerations of the knee, as described in this example, has clarified some of the actions of muscles during walking and has identified factors that are likely to contribute to excessive knee flexion in persons with cerebral palsy. This work emphasizes the need to consider how muscular forces contribute to multijoint movement when attempting to identify the causes of a patient's abnormal gait. Another method for characterizing the actions of muscles during movement is described in the next example.

Example 3: Perturbation Analysis to Quantify Muscle Actions in Double Support

Knee flexion velocity at toe-off is an important factor in generating swing-phase knee flexion during normal gait (53,73). Low knee flexion velocity at toe-off is a potential contributor to stiff-knee gait, a movement abnormality associated with stroke and cerebral palsy in which swing-phase knee flexion is diminished. Stiff-knee gait is commonly attributed to excessive activity of the rectus femoris, which is thought to limit knee flexion by producing an excessive knee extension moment during swing (71,91). However, we have shown that many individuals with stiff-knee gait do not exhibit excessive knee extension moments during swing phase, but instead walk with a low knee flexion velocity at toe-off (38). During normal gait, just prior to toe-off, knee flexion velocity increases dramatically during double support. If the muscles that produce angular accel-

erations of the knee during double support were known, then perhaps treatments to correct stiff-knee gait could be designed more effectively.

Comparisons of EMG recordings and measured gait kinematics have suggested that gastrocnemius, popliteus, and occasionally gracilis contribute to knee flexion during the late stance phase (72). Rectus femoris (72) and, in some cases, vasti (101) are also active during this period and are thought to limit knee flexion. However, the potential of these and other muscles to produce knee flexion or extension during walking cannot be deduced from kinesiologic observations alone. We have used the muscle-driven simulation of walking, described above, to identify the muscles that influence knee flexion velocity during double support and to determine which muscles have the greatest potential to alter this velocity (37).

In a muscle-driven simulation, joints are accelerated because of muscle forces. If a muscle's force is altered, or "perturbed," by a small amount during a simulation, the resulting changes in the motions of the joints can be quantified (i.e., by reintegrating the equations of motion forward in time). This technique, called perturbation analysis, is useful for investigating how individual muscles or other elements of a model influence the angular displacements and velocities of the joints. We used this technique in this example.

We quantified the actions of individual muscles in our simulation by systematically perturbing each muscle's force in double support and calculating the resulting changes in peak knee flexion velocity (Figure 12-10). We altered the muscle forces in two ways. First, we increased the force in each muscle by a percentage of the muscle's unperturbed force. The resulting change in knee flexion velocity depended on the muscle's unperturbed force and characterized how much that muscle's force influenced peak knee flexion velocity during the simulation. Second, we increased the force in each muscle by a fixed amount in Newtons. Using this approach, the resulting change in knee flexion velocity per unit force was independent of the muscle's unperturbed force, and characterized the potential of the muscle to influence knee flexion velocity based on the muscle's moment arms and the inertial properties of the body.

Analysis of the simulation revealed that iliopsoas and gastrocnemius were the largest contributors to peak knee flexion velocity during double support (Figure 12-11A). Each of these muscles exerted relatively large forces in the simulation, and each had a large potential to increase knee flexion velocity (Figure 12-11B). The forces generated by vasti, soleus, and rectus femoris, by contrast, decreased knee flexion velocity (Figure 12-11A). Vasti decelerated knee flexion the most. This is because vasti had the largest potential to decrease knee flexion velocity (Figure 12-11B), and because these muscles developed passive forces during double support. Soleus also exerted large forces

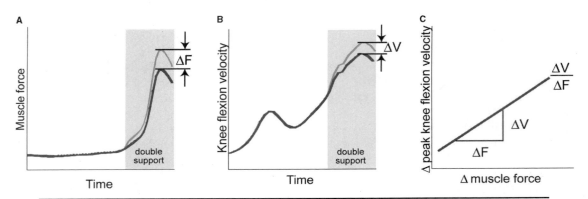

FIGURE 12-10. Steps to assess muscle function in a perturbation analysis. (**A**) A perturbation in an individual muscle force was introduced during the period of double support. (**B**) A dynamic simulation was performed with this altered muscle force and the resulting change in peak knee flexion velocity during double support was observed. (**C**) After repeating steps A) and B) for a range of perturbation sizes, the change in peak knee flexion velocity was plotted vs. the size of the force perturbation. The resulting slope was computed for different muscles to assess the relative influence of these muscles on knee flexion velocity.

during double support, but had a small potential relative to vasti to decrease knee flexion velocity (Figure 12-11B).

The muscles with the greatest potential to increase knee flexion velocity during double support, per unit force, were sartorius and gracilis (Figure 12-11B). When activated, these muscles generate hip flexion moments and knee flexion moments, both of which promote knee flexion. Biceps femoris short head, a uniarticular knee flexor, also had a relatively large potential to increase knee flexion velocity.

These analyses have advanced our understanding of muscle function during normal gait, and have helped to identify several possible causes of stiff-knee gait. In particular, our results suggest that insufficient force in iliopsoas or gastrocnemius, or excessive force in vasti or rec-

tus femoris could limit knee flexion velocity during double support, and cause swing-phase knee flexion to be diminished. The stance-phase actions of these and other muscles, such as gracilis, should be considered before performing muscle-tendon surgery to treat stiff-knee gait.

CHALLENGES AND FUTURE DIRECTIONS

The first muscle-driven simulation of walking was developed more than three decades ago by Chow and Jacobson (21). Their dynamic model consisted of a single leg confined to the sagittal plane that was driven by four

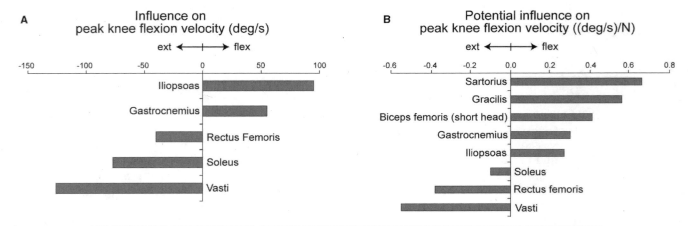

FIGURE 12-11. The muscles with the most influence and the most potential to influence peak knee flexion velocity. (**A**) The influence of selected muscles on the peak knee flexion velocity during double support. The influence was calculated as the slope of the change in peak knee flexion velocity (ΔV) vs. perturbation size as a percentage of unperturbed muscle force (ΔF) throughout the period of double support. (**B**) The potential influence of selected muscles on the peak knee flexion velocity during double support. These values characterize the change in peak knee flexion velocity (ΔV) due to a 1 N change in muscle force (ΔF) throughout the period of double support. (Figure adapted from Goldberg, et al.) (37).

idealized muscles. Nearly two decades passed before Davy and Audu (23) and then Yamaguchi and Zajac (104) published significantly advanced muscle-driven simulations of walking. Over the last few years, there has been a dramatic increase in the number and complexity of walking simulations, enabled, in large part, by new modeling software and increases in computer speed. To date, simulations of normal gait have been developed and analyzed to estimate the forces produced by muscles (e.g., 7), to determine how individual muscles support the body (56,58), accelerate the joints (44,45), and distribute energy among the limb segments (58,59), and to evaluate theories of neuromotor control (36,40,61,92,106). Muscle-driven simulations have also been created and used to evaluate exercise protocols for persons with spinal cord injury (84) and patients with patellofemoral pain (57), to examine the influence of foot positioning and joint compliance on the occurrence of ankle sprains (102), to assess computational prototypes of knee implants (74), and to investigate causes of stiff-knee gait (3,37,73,78). These studies, and the examples presented in this chapter, demonstrate the utility of muscle-driven simulations for elucidating the functions of muscles during movement and, potentially, improving the outcomes of treatments for persons with neuromusculoskeletal impairments.

Although models of the musculoskeletal system have become more sophisticated and novel approaches for analyzing simulations have been developed, rigorous dynamics-based techniques for determining which impairments contribute to the abnormal gait patterns of persons with neuromusculoskeletal disorders do not exist. We believe that the limitations of current models and analyses must be addressed before simulations can be widely used to guide treatment decisions for patients. Some of the important issues to be resolved in future studies are outlined below.

Modeling Challenges

Models that more accurately and efficiently characterize the musculoskeletal geometry and the joint kinematics of individual subjects need to be developed. This is imperative because the results of simulations are often sensitive to the accuracy with which the lengths and moment arms of muscles can be estimated. Studies of muscle function during walking have typically relied on "generic" models of adult subjects with normal musculoskeletal geometry. We have modified generic models to represent bone deformities (10-12), osteotomies (30,83), and tendon transfer surgeries (27). However, more work is needed to understand how variations in musculoskeletal geometry due to size, age, deformity, or surgery might influence the predictions of a model, and to determine when, and under what conditions, simulations based on generic models are applicable to individual patients. One approach might be to develop subject-specific models from magnetic resonance images or ultrasonography scans (e.g., 43,51,86,99). However, this approach may not always be practical. An alternative approach that combines medical images with generic musculoskeletal models, we believe, offers a promising, tractable way to construct models that are representative of patients. For instance, it may be possible to transform a generic model to represent a range of individuals with cerebral palsy using multi-dimensional scaling techniques, algorithms for deforming bones, and a few subject-specific parameters derived from image data or experimental measurements (11,20). We have begun to develop and evaluate such models (10,11), and we believe that additional efforts are warranted.

The equations for musculotendon dynamics that we have used in simulations must be further tested. While existing models capture many features of muscle force generation in unimpaired subjects, they do not account for adaptations that can occur in persons with neuromuscular disorders or alterations that might occur after surgery. We have developed models that attempt to account for decreases in the muscle fiber lengths that may occur with contracture (28). However, muscle-tendon models that account for structural changes in the extracellular matrix that may occur with chronic spasticity (49), or alterations in force transmission due to scar tissue (14) are not yet generally available. Muscle-tendon models that characterize the effects of pathology, surgery, and other treatment modalities on the time course of muscle force generation are needed to assess the impact of these effects on movement and neuromotor control.

Simulation Challenges

Using dynamic optimization to determine the muscle excitation patterns needed to simulate complex three-dimensional movements, such as walking, incurs great computational expense. The dynamic optimization solution for normal walking presented in this chapter required over 5000 computer processor hours to compute, and relied heavily on the use of parallel supercomputers (5). Although approaches for solving dynamic optimization problems are improving (41,47,54,96), this process is still very slow— at best, a solution for pathological gait might be obtained in a few days or a week. If dynamic simulations are to guide treatment decisions, then efficient computational algorithms for generating subject-specific simulations must be developed.

Fortunately, alternatives to dynamic optimization are emerging. Adaptations of traditional robotics control techniques appear to be particularly promising (e.g., 93,95). A technique called computed muscle control, for example, has been used to generate a simulation of bicycle pedaling approximately 100 times faster than conventional dynamic optimization approaches (93). We believe that this technique will soon enable subject-specific simulations of walking to be generated in a few minutes.

Perhaps the most profound limitation of the simulation of walking described in this chapter is its exclusion of the nervous system. The simulation was performed open loop; that is, the muscle excitations were not modulated by reflexes. This is true of most dynamic simulations of movement generated to date, particularly those involving the lower extremity. However, simulations that are driven by neural networks and/or central pattern generators, that include simplified models of the nervous system, are being developed (e.g., 39,61,92). The incorporation of accurate representations of sensory-motor control (e.g., 94) into dynamic simulations of abnormal movements is one of the most critical challenges to be overcome if models are to be developed that can predict the outcomes of treatments.

Analysis Challenges

Characterizing the functions of muscles and extracting the principles that govern muscle coordination from dynamic simulations is nontrivial. Three approaches for quantifying the actions of muscles were illustrated in this chapter, but each of these analyses has limitations. Our method for decomposing the ground reaction force, as performed in Example 1, assumes rigid contact between the foot and the ground. To the extent that contact is not rigid, a portion (usually a small portion) of the reaction force cannot be explained (2). Calculations of muscle-induced accelerations, as performed in Example 2, rely on an accurate decomposition of the ground reaction force, and depend on the degrees of freedom that are included (or not included) in the model. Perturbation analysis, as performed in Example 3, provides an intuitive method for assessing how a muscle influences movement (i.e., not just accelerations, but also velocities and positions) by altering muscle force and quantifying the changes in movement over time. However, the results of perturbation analyses can be misleading if the perturbations in muscle force are too large or if the time windows over which perturbations are applied are too long. We believe that improved methods for analyzing simulations will evolve by applying these and other techniques to a range of research problems and critically evaluating the results.

Experimental observations and a theoretical framework are needed to establish a scientific basis for the treatment of gait abnormalities. Before a simulation of walking can be used to make treatment decisions, the simulation and the underlying model must be tested. If possible, simulation results should be compared with experimental data to verify that a particular simulation is of sufficient fidelity to answer the clinical question being posed. Sensitivity studies must be performed to determine whether the conclusions drawn from analysis of a simulation are sensitive to variations in model parameters, especially if a direct comparison with experimental data is not feasible. Ultimately, controlled clinical studies are required to determine if the insights gained from simulations can indeed improve treatment outcomes.

Experiments and Theory

We believe that a comprehensive explanation for how muscles are coordinated to produce gait is emerging. This belief is supported by the convergence of findings between some experimental and theoretical studies. For instance, it was no surprise in Example 1 that the plantarflexors are largely responsible for the second maximum in the vertical ground reaction force (Figure 12-7D); this was inferred previously from several experimental studies, and a number of simulations have confirmed a cause-effect relationship. Other results from our simulation-based analyses of walking are more surprising. For example, our finding that hamstrings weakly accelerate the knee toward extension during stance (Example 2, Figure 12-9) was unexpected. It is the unexpected findings from simulations, and the reconciliation of these findings with what we believe we already know from experiments, that have the potential to deepen our understanding of walking.

With the development, analysis, and testing of muscle-driven dynamic simulations, we are now in a position to establish quantitative, cause-effect relationships between the neuromuscular excitation patterns, muscle forces, ground reaction forces, and motions of the body that are observed in the laboratory. Coupled with high quality experimental measurements, dynamic simulations will be used to elucidate how the elements of the neuromusculoskeletal system interact to produce movement and, we hope, improve the outcomes of treatments for persons with movement disorders.

REFERENCES

1. Abel MF, Damiano DL, Pannunzio M, Bush J. Muscle-tendon surgery in diplegic cerebral palsy: Functional and mechanical changes. *J Pediatr Orthop* 1999;19:366–375.
2. Anderson FC, Arnold AS, Delp SL. Reaction forces induced by muscles in the presence of compliant contact. *Proceedings from the 4th World Congress of Biomechanics*, 2002.
3. Anderson FC, Goldberg SR, Pandy MG, Delp SL. Contributions of muscle forces and toe-off kinematics to peak knee flexion during the swing phase of normal gait: An induced position analysis. *J Biomech* 2004;37:731–737.
4. Anderson FC, Pandy MG. A dynamic optimization solution for vertical jumping in three dimensions. *Comput Methods Biomech Biomed Engin* 1999;2:201–231.
5. Anderson FC, Pandy MG. Dynamic optimization of human walking. *J Biomech Eng* 2001;123:381–390.
6. Anderson FC, Pandy MG. Individual muscle contributions to support in normal walking. *Gait Posture* 2003;17:159–169.
7. Anderson FC, Pandy MG. Static and dynamic optimization solutions for gait are practically equivalent. *J Biomech* 2001;34:153–161.
8. Anderson FC, Ziegler JM, Pandy MG, Whalen RT. Application of high-performance computing to numerical simulation of human movement. *J Biomech Eng* 1995;117:155–157.

9. Arnold AS, Anderson FC, Pandy MG, Delp SL. Muscular contributions to hip and knee extension during the stance phase of normal gait: A framework for investigating the causes of crouch gait. In press.

10. Arnold AS, Blemker SS, Delp SL. Evaluation of a deformable musculoskeletal model for estimating muscle-tendon lengths during crouch gait. *Ann Biomed Eng* 2001;29:263–274.

11. Arnold AS, Delp SL. Rotational moment arms of the medial hamstrings and adductors vary with femoral geometry and limb position: Implications for the treatment of internally-rotated gait. *J Biomech* 2001;34:437–447.

12. Arnold AS, Komattu AV, Delp SL. Internal rotation gait: A compensatory mechanism to restore abduction capacity decreased by bone deformity? *Dev Med Child Neurol* 1997;39:40–44.

13. Arnold AS, Salinas S, Asakawa DJ, Delp SL. Accuracy of muscle moment arms estimated from MRI-based musculoskeletal models of the lower extremity. *Comput Aided Surg* 2000;5:108–119.

14. Asakawa DJ, Blemker SS, Rab G, Bagley A, Delp SL. Three dimensional muscle tendon geometry after rectus femoris transfer. *J Bone Joint Surg Am* 2004;86–A:348–354.

15. Beals RK. Treatment of knee contracture in cerebral palsy by hamstring lengthening, posterior capsulotomy, and quadriceps mechanism shortening. *Dev Med Child Neurol* 2001;43:802–805.

16. Bhargava LJ, Pandy MG, Anderson FC. A phenomenological model for estimating metabolic energy consumption in muscle contraction. *J Biomech* 2004;37:81–88.

17. Bleck EE. *Orthopaedic Management in Cerebral Palsy*. London: Mac Keith Press, 1987.

18. Brand RA, Pedersen DR, Friederich JA. The sensitivity of muscle force predictions to changes in physiologic cross-sectional area. *J Biomech* 1986;19:589–596.

19. Campbell J, Ball J. Energetics: Application to the study and management of locomotor disabilities. Energetics of walking in cerebral palsy. *Orthop Clin North Am* 1978;9:374–377.

20. Chao EYS, Lynch JD, Vanderploeg MJ. Simulation and animation of musculoskeletal joint system. *J Biomech Eng* 1993;115:562–568.

21. Chow C, Jacobson D. Studies of human locomotion via optimal programming. *Math Biosci* 1971;10:239–306.

22. Damiano DL, Vaughan CL, Abel MF. Muscle response to heavy resistance exercise in children with spastic cerebral palsy. *Dev Med Child Neurol* 1995;37:731–739.

23. Davy DT, Audu ML. A dynamic optimization technique for predicting muscle forces in the swing phase of gait. *J Biomech* 1987;20:187–201.

24. Delp SL, Hess WE, Hungerford DS, Jones LC. Variation of rotation moment arms with hip flexion. *J Biomech* 1999;32:493–501.

25. Delp SL, Loan JP, Zajac FE, Topp EL, Rosen JM. An interactive graphics-based model of the lower extremity to study orthopaedic surgical procedures. *IEEE Trans Biomed Eng* 1990;37:757–767.

26. Delp SL, Loan JP. A computational framework for simulation and analysis of human and animal movement. *IEEE Comput Sci Eng* 2000;2:46–55.

27. Delp SL, Ringwelski DA, Carroll NC. Transfer of the rectus femoris: Effects of transfer site on moment arms about the knee and hip. *J Biomech* 1994;27:1201–1211.

28. Delp SL, Statler K, Carroll NC. Preserving plantar flexion strength after surgical treatment for contracture of the triceps surae: A computer simulation study. *J Orthop Res* 1995;13:96–104.

29. DeLuca PA, Ounpuu S, Davis RB, Walsh JH. Effect of hamstring and psoas lengthening on pelvic tilt in patients with spastic diplegic cerebral palsy. *J Pediatr Orthop* 1998;18:712–718.

30. Free SA, Delp SL. Trochanteric transfer in total hip replacement: Effects on the moment arms and force-generating capacities of the hip abductors. *J Orthop Res* 1996;14:245–250.

31. Friederich JA, Brand RA. Muscle fiber architecture in the human lower limb. *J Biomech* 1990;23:91–95.

32. Gage JR, Schwartz M. Pathological gait and lever-arm dysfunction. In: Gage JR, ed. *The Treatment of Gait Problems in Cerebral Palsy*. London: Mac Keith Press, 2004;180–204.

33. Gage JR. *Gait Analysis in Cerebral Palsy*. London: Mac Keith Press, 1991.

34. Gage JR. Treatment principles for crouch gait. In: Gage JR, ed. *The Treatment of Gait Problems in Cerebral Palsy*. London: Mac Keith Press, 2004;382–397.

35. Garner BA, Pandy MG. The obstacle-set method for representing muscle paths in musculoskeletal models. *Comput Methods Biomech Biomed Engin* 2000;3:1–30.

36. Gerritsen KG, van den Bogert AJ, Hulliger M, Zernicke RF. Intrinsic muscle properties facilitate locomotor control: A computer simulation study. *Motor Control* 1998;2:206–220.

37. Goldberg SR, Anderson FC, Pandy MG, Delp SL. Muscles that influence knee flexion velocity in double support: Implications for stiff-knee gait. *J Biomech* 2004;37:1189–1196.

38. Goldberg SR, Ounpuu S, Delp SL. The importance of swing phase initial conditions in stiff-knee gait. *J Biomech* 2003;36:1111–1116.

39. Hase K, Miyashita K, Ok S, Arakawa Y. Human gait simulation with a neuromusculoskeletal model and evolutionary computation. *J Vis Comput Animat* 2003;14:73–92.

40. Hase K, Yamazaki N. Computer simulation study of human locomotion with a three-dimensional entire-body neuro-musculoskeletal model (I. Acquisition of normal walking). *JSME Int J Ser C* 2002;45:1040–1072.

41. Higginson JS, Neptune RR, Anderson FC. Simulated parallel annealing within a neighborhood for optimization of biomechanical systems. *J Biomech* 2005;38:1938–1942.

42. Inman VT, Ralston HJ, Todd F. *Human Walking*. Baltimore: Williams & Wilkins; 1981.

43. Ito M, Akima H, Fukunaga T. In vivo moment arm determination using b-mode ultrasonography. *J Biomech* 2000;33:215–218.

44. Jonkers I, Stewart C, Spaepen A. The complementary role of the plantarflexors, hamstrings and gluteus maximus in the control of stance limb stability during gait. *Gait Posture* 2003;17:264–272.

45. Jonkers I, Stewart C, Spaepen A. The study of muscle action during single support and swing phase of gait: Clinical relevance of forward simulation techniques. *Gait Posture* 2003;17:97–105.

46. Kane T, Levinson D. *Dynamics: Theory and application*. New York: McGraw-Hill; 1985.

47. Kaplan ML, Heegaard JH. Predictive algorithms for neuromuscular control of human locomotion. *J Biomech* 2001;34:1077–1083.

48. Kepple TM, Siegel KL, Stanhope SJ. Relative contributions of the lower extremity joint moments to forward progression and support during gait. *Gait Posture* 1997;6:1–8.

49. Lieber RL, Steinman S, Barash IA, Chambers H. Structural and functional changes in spastic skeletal muscle. *Muscle Nerve* 2004;29:615–627.

50. Lloyd-Roberts GC, Jackson AM, Albert JS. Avulsion of the distal pole of the patella in cerebral palsy. *J Bone Joint Surg Br* 1985;67B:252–254.

51. Maganaris CN. In vivo measurement-based estimations of the moment arm in the human tibialis anterior muscle-tendon unit. *J Biomech* 2000;33:375–379.

52. McConville JT, Clauser CE, Churchill TD, Cuzzi J, Kaleps I. *Anthropometric Relationships of Body and Body Segment Moments of Inertia*. Report AFAMRL-TR-80-119. Air Force Aerospace Medical Research Laboratory, Wright-Patterson AFB, Ohio, 1980.

53. Mochon S, McMahon TA. Ballistic walking: An improved model. *Math Biosci* 1980;52:241–260.

54. Neptune R. Optimization algorithm performance in determining optimal controls in human movement analyses. *J Biomech Eng* 1999;121:249–252.

55. Neptune RR, Hull ML. Evaluation of performance criteria for simulation of submaximal steady-state cycling using a forward dynamic model. *J Biomech Eng* 1998;120:334–341.

56. Neptune RR, Kautz SA, Zajac FE. Contributions of the individual ankle plantar flexors to support, forward progression and swing initiation during walking. *J Biomech* 2001;34:1387–1398.

57. Neptune RR, Kautz SA. Knee joint loading in forward versus backward pedaling: Implications for rehabilitation strategies. *Clin Biomech* 2000;15:528–535.

58. Neptune RR, Zajac FE, Kautz SA. Muscle force redistributes segmental power for body progression during walking. *Gait Posture* 2004;19:194–205.

59. Neptune RR, Zajac FE, Kautz SA. Muscle mechanical work requirements during normal walking: The energetic cost of raising the body's center-of-mass is significant. *J Biomech* 2004;37:817–825.

60. Novacheck T, Trost J, Schwartz M. Intramuscular psoas lengthening improves dynamic hip function in children with cerebral palsy. *J Pediatr Orthop* 2002;22:158–164.

61. Ogihara N, Yamazaki N. Generation of human bipedal locomotion by a bio-mimetic neuro-musculo-skeletal model. *Biol Cybern* 2001;84:1–11.

62. Pandy MG, Anderson FC, Hull DG. A parameter optimization approach for the optimal control of large-scale musculoskeletal systems. *J Biomech Eng* 1992;114:450–460.

63. Pandy MG, Berme N. Quantitative assessment of gait determinants during single stance via a three-dimensional model: Part 1. Normal gait. *J Biomech* 1989;22:717–724.

64. Pandy MG, Berme N. Quantitative assessment of gait determinants during single stance via a three-dimensional model: Part 2. Pathological gait. *J Biomech* 1989;22:725–733.

65. Pandy MG, Garner BA, Anderson FC. Optimal control of non-ballistic muscular movements: A constraint-based performance criterion for rising from a chair. *J Biomech Eng* 1995;117:15–26.

66. Pandy MG, Zajac FE, Sim E, Levine WS. An optimal control model for maximum-height human jumping. *J Biomech* 1990;23:1185–1198.

67. Pandy MG. Computer modeling and simulation of human movement. *Ann Rev Biomed Eng* 2001;3:245–273.

68. Pandy MG. Simple and complex models for studying muscle function in walking. *Philos Trans R Soc Lond B Biol Sci* 2003;358:1501–1509.

69. Perry J, Antonelli D, Ford W. Analysis of knee-joint forces during flexed-knee stance. *J Bone Joint Surg Am* 1975;57A:961–967.

70. Perry J, Newsam C. Function of the hamstrings in cerebral palsy. In: Sussman MD, ed. *The Diplegic Child: Evaluation and Management.* Rosemont, IL: American Academy of Orthopaedic Surgeons, 1992;299–307.

71. Perry J. Distal rectus femoris transfer. *Dev Med Child Neurol* 1987;29:153–158.

72. Perry J. *Gait analysis: Normal and pathological function.* Thorofare, NJ: Slack Incorporated, 1992.

73. Piazza SJ, Delp SL. The influence of muscles on knee flexion during the swing phase of gait. *J Biomech* 1996;29:723–733.

74. Piazza SJ, Delp SL. Three-dimensional dynamic simulation of total knee replacement motion during a step-up task. *J Biomech Eng* 2001;123:599–606.

75. Rab GT, Muscle. In: Rose J, Gamble JG, eds. *Human Walking.* 2nd ed. Baltimore: Williams and Wilkins, 1994;101–121.

76. Ralston HJ. Energetics of human walking. In: Herman RM, Grillner S, Stein PSG, Stuart DG, eds. *Neural Control of Locomotion.* New York: Plenum Press, 1976;77–98.

77. Reimers J. Static and dynamic problems in spastic cerebral palsy. *J Bone Joint Surg Br* 1973;55-B:822–827.

78. Riley PO, Kerrigan DC. Torque action of two-joint muscles in the swing period of stiff-legged gait: A forward dynamic model analysis. *J Biomech* 1998;31:835–840.

79. Rodda J, Graham HK. Classification of gait patterns in spastic hemiplegia and spastic diplegia: A basis for a management algorithm. *Eur J Neurol* 2001;8(suppl 5):98–108.

80. Roosth HP. Flexion deformity of the hip and knee in spastic cerebral palsy: Treatment by early release of spastic hip-flexor muscles. *J Bone Joint Surg Am* 1971;53-A:1489–1510.

81. Rose J, Gamble J, Medeiros J, Burgos A, Haskell W. Energy expenditure index of walking for normal children and for children with cerebral palsy. *Dev Med Child Neurol* 1990;32:333–340.

82. Rosenthal RK, Levine DB. Fragmentation of the distal pole of the patella in spastic cerebral palsy. *J Bone Joint Surg Am* 1977;59A:934–939.

83. Schmidt DJ, Arnold AS, Carroll NC, Delp SL. Length changes of the hamstrings and adductors resulting from derotational osteotomies of the femur. *J Orthop Res* 1999;17:279–285.

84. Schutte LM, Rodgers MM, Zajac FE. Improving the efficacy of electrical stimulation-induced leg cycle ergometry: An analysis based on a dynamic musculoskeletal model. *IEEE Trans Rehab Eng* 1993;1:109–125.

85. Schwartz M, Lakin G. The effect of tibial torsion on the dynamic function of the soleus during gait. *Gait Posture* 2003;17:113–118.

86. Sheehan FT, Zajac FE, Drace JE. Using cine phase contrast magnetic resonance imaging to non-invasively study in vivo knee dynamics. *J Biomech* 1998;31:21–26.

87. Stout JL, Koop S. Energy expenditure in cerebral palsy. In: Gage JR, ed. *The Treatment of Gait Problems in Cerebral Palsy.* London: Mac Keith Press, 2004;146–164.

88. Sutherland DH, Cooper L, Daniel D. The Role of the Ankle Plantar Flexors in Normal Walking. *J Bone Joint Surg Am* 1980;62-A:354–363.

89. Sutherland DH, Cooper L. The pathomechanics of progressive crouch gait in spastic diplegia. *Orthop Clin North Am* 1978;9:143–154.

90. Sutherland DH, Davids JR. Common gait abnormalities of the knee in cerebral palsy. *Clin Orthop* 1993;288:139–147.

91. Sutherland DH, Santi M, Abel MF. Treatment of stiff-knee gait in cerebral palsy: A comparison by gait analysis of distal rectus femoris transfer versus proximal rectus release. *J Pediatr Orthop* 1990; 10: 433–441.

92. Taga G. A model of the neuro-musculo-skeletal system for anticipatory adjustment of human locomotion during obstacle avoidance. *Biol Cybern* 1998;78:9–17.

93. Thelen DG, Anderson FC, Delp SL. Generating forward dynamic simulations of movement using computed muscle control. *J Biomech* 2003;36:321–328.

94. van der Helm FCT, Rozendaall LA. Musculoskeletal systems with intrinsic and proprioceptive feedback. In: Winters JM, Crago PE, eds. *Biomechanics and Neural Control of Posture and Movement.* New York: Springer-Verlag, Inc., 2000;164–174.

95. van der Helm FCT, van Soest AJ. Planning of human motions: How simple must it be? In: Winters JM, Crago PE, eds. *Biomechanics and Neural Control of Posture and Movement.* New York: Springer-Verlag, Inc., 2000;373–381.

96. van Soest AJK, Casius LJR. The merits of a parallel genetic algorithm in solving hard optimization problems. *J Biomech Eng* 2003; 125:141–146.

97. Wickiewicz TL, Roy RR, Powell PL, Edgerton VR. Muscle architecture of the human lower limb. *Clin Orthop* 1983;275–283.

98. Wiley ME, Damiano DL. Lower-extremity strength profiles in spastic cerebral palsy. *Dev Med Child Neurol* 1998;40:100–107.

99. Wilson DL, Zhu Q, Duerk JL, Mansour JM, Kilgore K, Crago PE. Estimation of tendon moment arms from three-dimensional magnetic resonance images. *Ann Biomed Eng* 1999;27:247–256.

100. Winter DA. Overall principle of lower limb support during stance phase of gait. *J Biomech* 1980;13:923–927.

101. Winter DA. *The Biomechanics and Motor Control of Human Gait: Normal, Elderly, and Pathological.* Waterloo, Ontario, Canada: Waterloo Biomechanics, 1991.

102. Wright IC, Neptune RR, van den Bogert AJ, Nigg BM. The influence of foot positioning on ankle sprains. *J Biomech* 2000;33:513–519.

103. Yamaguchi GT, Zajac FE. A planar model of the knee joint to characterize the knee extensor mechanism. *J Biomech* 1989;22:1–10.

104. Yamaguchi GT, Zajac FE. Restoring unassisted natural gait to paraplegics via functional neuromuscular stimulation: A computer simulation study. *IEEE Trans Biomed Eng* 1990;37:886–902.

105. Zajac FE, Gordon ME. Determining muscle's force and action in multi-articular movement. *Exerc Sport Sci Rev* 1989;17:187–230.

106. Zajac FE, Neptune RR, Kautz SA. Biomechanics and muscle coordination of human walking part II: Lessons from dynamical simulations and clinical implications. *Gait Posture* 2003;17:1–17.

107. Zajac FE. Muscle and tendon: Properties, models, scaling, and application to biomechanics and motor control. *Crit Rev Biomed Eng* 1989;17:359–411.

Chapter 13

The Next Step: Restoring Walking After Paralysis

Ronald J. Triolo and Rudi Kobetic

Loss of the ability to walk as a result of paralysis following spinal cord injury (SCI) can compromise the ability to work, engage in social or leisure activities, pursue an education or participate in other activities associated with an independent and productive lifestyle. Long periods of immobility after SCI can cause degenerative changes of almost every major organ system including the bones, joints, heart, lungs, and skin. However, if the damage to the nervous system is confined to the upper motor neurons, then the peripheral nerves (alpha motor neurons) can often be excited with small electric currents to cause the muscles they innervate to contract. Functional electrical stimulation (FES) refers to a developing assistive technology that can generate purposeful, useful movements of the extremities through such electrical activation of paralyzed or spastic muscles. In selected individuals with SCI, standing and walking can be achieved by coordinating the actions of weak, paralyzed, or uncontrollable muscles with each other and with remaining voluntary movement.

This chapter describes the status of motor system neural prostheses (technologies that facilitate or restore movement by replacing or augmenting the damaged or dysfunctional nervous system) for standing and walking for individuals paralyzed by low cervical (tetraplegia) or thoracic (paraplegia) SCI. In these systems, FES can support the body against gravity to prevent collapse and provide forward progression through the actions of the electrically activated musculature. Balance is provided through voluntary interactions with walkers, crutches, or other walking aids. Such neural prostheses have the potential to postpone or prevent medical complications secondary to paralysis and to improve the independence of people with SCI by providing a means to exercise, stand, step, and negotiate physical barriers.

For an individual with complete absence of motor and sensory function below the level of injury, smooth, energy efficient, and cosmetically appealing walking with FES presents many technical challenges. These challenges include the lack of higher level descending command inputs, absence of feedback from natural or body-mounted sensors, inability to isolate and fully activate target muscles, reverse order of motor unit recruitment with electrical stimulation, muscle deconditioning and rapid fatigue, as well as critical issues related to stimulus timing and modification during the gait cycle. Although all major muscles of the trunk, hips, knees, and ankles can be activated with electrical stimulation, walking with FES is not normal and requires various compensatory mechanisms such as bracing and walking aids.

The state of the art in standing and walking with FES via transcutaneous, intramuscular end implanted electrode technologies are reviewed in this chapter. Current research directions addressing the many challenges to achieving natural and energy efficient lower extremity function after paralysis, through more efficient methods for interfacing with the nervous system and controlling stimulation are identified.

MUSCULAR RESPONSES TO ELECTRICAL STIMULATION

Contractile Properties

The contractile properties of the electrically activated muscles are a large determinant of the quality of standing and walking possible with FES. In general, muscles that are paralyzed after spinal cord injury are atrophied and composed mostly of fast-twitch fibers (29). When electrically activated, such muscles produce less than normal force and fatigue quickly.

The force of a muscle contraction is related to the net charge delivered to the nerve. The net force output and speed of the contraction increases with increasing stimulus current amplitude, pulse duration, and frequency. Muscle fibers in the intact neuromuscular system are recruited in an asynchronous fashion, generally beginning with slow-twitch, fatigue resistant fibers and progressing toward the fast-twitch fibers when additional forces are required. This recruitment order is reversed with FES, which elicits contractions in the larger fast-twitch motor units first, because of their lower threshold to depolarization by an external electric field. Electrical stimulation also produces a synchronous contraction of all supra-threshold motor units. Furthermore, muscle composition after SCI tends to shift from slow to predominantly fast fiber types. These phenomena combine to produce nonlinearities (delays, thresholds, strength, and fatigability) in the recruitment properties of stimulated muscle that complicate control and coordination.

Muscle contraction and relaxation properties are critical in the synthesis of walking with electrical stimulation because event times and relative phasing between bursts of muscle activities during the gait cycle are on the order of tenths of a second. Muscle contraction rise time is dependent on the frequency of stimulation (15) and on the muscle fiber type composition. Typical rise times, from the first stimulus to 90% of maximal moment developed at a joint, are on the order of 100 to 300 msec. Therefore, stimulation must be initiated before a desired joint moment is required to make the stimulation effective. Computer simulations of gait in paraplegics using electrical stimulation show great sensitivity to on/off timing of muscle activity (81). This has been confirmed by our observations where a delay in muscle activation as small as 20 msec produced a visually noticeable effect on walking.

Half relaxation time, the time from last stimulus to a 50% decrease in the joint moment, was found to correlate with the percentage of fast-twitch type II fibers in the muscle. Estimated values of half relaxation times are 240 msec for slow-twitch fibers and 57 msec for fast-twitch fibers (56). An electrically stimulated paralyzed muscle can have a half relaxation time in this range of values depending on conditioning; the time is longer when the muscle is fatigued. Relaxation time has been found to increase both with increases in the stimulation frequency (15) and with the onset of muscle fatigue (21).

Strength and Endurance

Reconditioning of the paralyzed muscle is required before initiating walking with electrical stimulation to reverse the effects of disuse and improve stimulated strength and fatigue resistance to the levels required to generate safe and effective standing and stepping motions. Although no optimal program to maximize both strength and endurance of paralyzed muscle has been established, some general trends have emerged. An electrical exercise program of isotonic muscle contraction of 30 minutes per day, with a 1:1 duty cycle (4 sec on and off times) at a stimulation frequency of 20 Hz produced a strength increase in most individuals with SCI. However, only a few individuals experienced an increase in endurance with this protocol (7). Other studies demonstrated that exercise at a stimulation frequency of 10 Hz was effective in increasing endurance (60). With an exercise protocol of 30 minutes of stimulation per day at a frequency varying from 16 to 30 Hz, we observed a significant increase in the strength and fatigue resistance of paralyzed muscle within 3 months of training. Electrical exercise was a mix of isometric, eccentric, isokinetic, and isotonic contractions that more closely approximates muscle activity in an individual with an intact nervous system.

The well-conditioned electrically stimulated muscle will retain a stable fiber type composition with predictable fatigue properties (60). At a constant stimulus frequency, fatigue causes a shift in recruitment properties manifesting in an elevated threshold of pulse duration required to elicit a contraction as well as a decreased maximum output. This shift in the recruitment curve is an ongoing process during stimulation until it reaches some steady state position. During the rest period, this process is reversed. Similarly, at constant stimulus pulse duration the muscle undergoes frequency dependent fatigue and recovery (23). A negligible increase in the knee moment has been observed during isometric contraction of the quadriceps muscles at stimulation frequencies above 50 Hz both in normal and paralyzed human muscle (15,22).

Relevant measures of fatigue and/or endurance include the number of repetitions above a target joint moment and the amount of moment remaining during continuous stimulation. During cyclic stimulation at various on/off stimulation times the peak isokinetic moment at the knee settles to a steady state value within the first 10 minutes and remains constant for more than 1 hour. The normalized steady state moment is strongly related to the amount of rest time between the cycles. Thus, the shorter the off-time the lower the amount of usable moment available to produce a desired function at the joint. During continuous stimulation, there is a marked reduction in isometric moment within the first 2 minutes of stimulation. The remaining steady state moment is dependent on stimulation frequency. The available moment at the knee during continuous quadriceps stimulation is a good indicator of the subject's ability to stand.

The moment produced by electrical stimulation of a paralyzed muscle about a particular joint varies greatly among different subjects. The strength of an electrically activated contraction is a function of many factors such as electrode position and its ability to recruit all muscle fibers at a safe maximal level of stimulation. Other factors include the frequency of stimulation, which has negligible effect above 50 Hz in a well-conditioned electrically activated muscle (15), and antagonistic or synergistic muscle activity. Caution must be used when measuring maximal isometric or eccentric contraction in paraplegic individuals, especially in those with considerable osteoporosis (10). Ultimately, the strength of contraction depends primarily on the state of muscle atrophy and the position of the

TABLE 13-1 Isometric Joint Moments*

Action	Moment (N-m)	Angle (Degree)
Trunk extension	70	0
Hip flexion	60	0
Hip extension	70	45
Hip abduction	40	0
Hip adduction	30	0
Knee extension	80	45
Knee flexion	15	90
Ankle plantar flexion	55	15 (dorsi)
Ankle dorsiflexion	15	15 (plantar)

*Average values of joint moments at specified angles obtained from six conditioned volunteers with paraplegia with electrical stimulation at maximum pulse width of 150 μsec and maximum frequency of 50 Hz.

electrode. Well-conditioned muscles produce from 30% to 60% of normal joint moment. Table 13-1 presents average values of stimulated joint moments. Except for ankle plantar flexion and hip abduction, measured moments were sufficient to sustain independent normal speed walking as predicted by computer simulation (81).

ELECTRICAL STIMULATION TECHNOLOGIES

Walking with FES after complete paraplegia requires the application of depolarizing electric fields to the nerves that innervate the muscles required for the desired movement. These fields are applied either transcutaneously through electrodes placed on the skin surface, or via implanted electrodes in closer proximity to the targeted neural structures.

Transcutaneous Stimulation

Transcutaneous (surface) stimulation achieves strong contractions of large muscle groups served by superficial nerves, but lacks selectivity and is unable to access deeper muscles. Furthermore, surface electrodes need to be reapplied each time such a system is to be used, compromising day-to-day repeatability of the stimulated responses, and the management of external cables rapidly becomes difficult as the number of stimulus channels increases. As few as two surface stimulation channels per leg can produce standing and reciprocal stepping motions through a combination of direct activation of the quadriceps muscles via a pair of surface electrodes on the anterior thigh and the triggering of a flexion withdrawal reflex via a second pair of electrodes over the dermatomes of the peroneal, sural or saphenous sensory nerves (6,25,28). Standing is achieved by simultaneously activating the quadriceps bilaterally in response to a command input, such as the simultaneous depression of switches on the handles of a rolling walker or crutches. A stride is pro-

duced by maintaining activation to the quadriceps of the stance limb while initiating a flexion withdrawal in the contralateral limb. Depression of the crutch- or walker-mounted switch on the swing limb side stimulates the afferent sensory fibers and triggers a spinal reflex arc that causes hip, knee, and ankle flexion in response to the electrical stimulus. To complete the advancement phase of the stride, activation of the knee extensors on the swing limb is initiated while the reflex is still active and flexing the hip. The stimulus producing the flexion reflex is then removed, leaving the user in double-limb support once again with bilateral quadriceps stimulation. It has been reported that some paralyzed subjects walk at speeds approaching one quarter of normal, and can ascend a curb or step with surface stimulation.

Complicating issues with this system include active flexion at the hip generated by the rectus femoris muscle that compromises erect standing posture and results in an anterior pelvic tilt with compensatory lordosis, or excessive weight on the arms to remain upright. In addition, not all patients will exhibit a flexion withdrawal reflex that is strong or repeatable enough for stepping. The reflex can habituate with repeated activation, limiting the number of steps that can be taken.

Intramuscular Stimulation

Intramuscular electrodes with percutaneous leads that exit the skin are thin, helically coiled, and insulated multistranded stainless steel wires similar to kinesiologic EMG recording electrodes. These devices can be introduced with a hypodermic needle. The uninsulated stimulating tip is placed near the target nerve, thus bypassing cutaneous sensory fibers and providing improved selectivity and access to deep muscles (51). The configuration of a stainless steel helix around a polypropylene core provides strain relief to reduce fatigue fracture of the wire and allows movement with surrounding tissue (66). Leads from multiple electrodes distributed about the lower extremities, pelvis, and trunk can be routed subcutaneously to a common exit site for convenient connection to an external stimulator. Monopolar cathodic stimulation is commonly employed with the anode placed on the skin surface over a bony prominence. Once implanted, such electrodes can remain in the body as long as they produce strong, isolated contractions. The integrity of an electrode is monitored by the strength, selectivity, and recruitment properties of the muscle contraction it elicits as well as its electrical impedance. The most frequent reason for electrode failure in the first few weeks after implantation is spontaneous movement away from the motor point, which alters the contractile response. Another cause is breakage beneath the skin with loss of the uninsulated section. This results in high electrical impedance since the surface area for delivery of charge is reduced (55). An average survival rate of the intramuscular electrode is 70% at 1 year, and many have remained functional for more than 5 years.

Chronically indwelling helically coiled fine wire intramuscular electrodes with percutaneous leads have allowed researchers to synthesize complex lower extremity motions (45) by activating numerous muscle groups with up to 48 separate channels of stimulation under the control of a programmable microprocessor-based external stimulator (12). Users select one of a series of movement patterns by scrolling through a menu of options presented on a liquid-crystal display via switches on a command ring worn on the index finger. Preprogrammed patterns of stimulation to the appropriate muscles are synchronized with the gait cycle by successive switch depressions for each step, or by insole mounted pressure sensors that detect contact and loading. The quality of the motions produced with this system depends on the availability, strength, and endurance of the paralyzed muscles; the ability of the therapist or engineer to specify patterns of stimulation for ambulation; and the subject's experience with the device. Some well-trained subjects are able to walk 300 meters repeatedly at 30 m per minute with this system (44). Although such systems are best suited for temporary therapeutic applications, or to simulate the actions of a completely implanted system, with the proper care and maintenance FES systems for walking based on intramuscular electrodes with percutaneous leads can remain operational and safe for functional use for many years (2).

Implanted Systems

Implanted systems utilizing electrodes placed on or around the target nerve (epineural), sutured or inserted to the muscle near the nerve entry point (epimysial and intramuscular), and connected to surgically implanted pulse generators provide many major advantages over surface and percutaneous stimulation. Advantages of this pacemaker-like approach include improved convenience, cosmetics, reliability, maintenance, and repeatability (42). Multichannel implanted systems for walking after paraplegia provide standing and swing-through gait (13,34). Exercise and standing functions have been reported with a cochlear implant modified to deliver 22 channels of stimulation to the lower extremities (18), and a 12-channel system for intradural stimulation of the L2-S2 motor roots (64).

Because of their ability to activate muscles inaccessible to surface stimulation, intramuscular electrodes with percutaneous leads have been valuable tools to simulate the action of completely implanted FES systems. Researchers at the Cleveland FES Center utilized these devices to complete three studies essential to proceeding with clinical trials of implanted FES technology. First, multichannel percutaneous systems were employed to devise a standardized procedure and set of rules for specifying and adjusting patterns of stimulation for reciprocal walking (45). This codified the process of generating stimulus profiles in such a way as to be repeatable by other clinicians or researchers. Next, experiments with subjects with multichannel percutaneous systems defined the minimal muscle set required to achieve stable standing and repeatable stepping (47). This provided a set of primary target muscles for implantation. Finally, the locations and stimulated responses of intramuscular electrodes with percutaneous leads were used to guide the establishment of the surgical approaches required to access the motor points of the target muscles (69). Cadaver and intraoperative tests confirmed the insight provided by the experience with percutaneous electrodes. To date, these approaches have been used to install surgically implanted lower extremity systems for standing, transfers, and short distance mobility in the vicinity of the wheelchair to 19 volunteers with complete thoracic or incomplete low-cervical injuries (46,77).

The implanted components of these systems include an eight-channel receiver-stimulator, illustrated in Figure 13-1, and epimysial (3) and surgically-implanted intramuscular (53) electrodes. The implant is a passive pacemaker-like device that receives power and command signals from a wearable external control unit (70). To achieve standing, epimysial electrodes are installed bilaterally in the vastus lateralis (to achieve knee extension without hip flexion), the semimembranosus (and alternately the posterior portion of the adductor magnus), and the gluteus maximus, while intramuscular electrodes are inserted at the lumbar spinal roots to activate the erector spinae muscles. The entire system can be implanted in a single surgical procedure and allows recipients to rise from a seated position, perform one-handed reaching tasks to retrieve objects from wheelchair inaccessible shelves and achieve swing-through gait with a walker (16,17).

Standing and stepping with completely implanted systems can be achieved without braces for persons with complete paraplegia with 16 channels of stimulation (the four listed above for standing, plus the tibialis anterior, tensor fascia lata, sartorius and hamstrings, bilaterally). These systems rely on two eight-channel devices as depicted in Figure 13-2. Users of the standing systems with complete thoracic level injuries below the level of T4 can have the second implant installed to activate the additional muscles required for walking in a second surgical procedure. Figure 13-3 shows reciprocal gait with a rolling walker using the 16-channel dual-implant system. System recipients trigger each step via successive depressions of a ring-mounted thumb switch. Walking speeds of up to 10 m per minute at cadences of 26 steps per minute were achieved with this approach (46).

Hybrid Systems

Hybrid systems combine bracing with FES in an attempt to overcome the disadvantages of stimulation or orthoses alone for providing ambulation after SCI. The

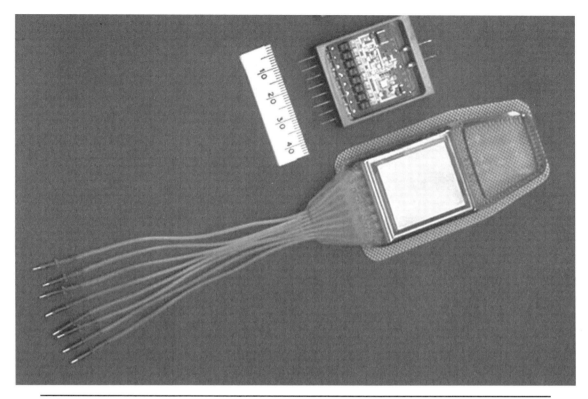

FIGURE 13-1. The eight-channel implanted receiver-stimulator (IRS-8) developed at Case Western Reserve University and Cleveland Department of Veterans Affairs Medical Center. The electronics shown at the top are hermetically sealed in a titanium package that serves as a common system anode. Eight leads provide in-line connections to stimulating electrodes implanted in or on the target muscle or around the target nerve.

advantages of orthoses lie primarily in their ability to constrain the motions of the joints, reduce the degrees of freedom of movement and provide mechanical stability. For static activities such as quiet standing, individuals with paraplegia can assume a stable posture with little or no muscular exertion by locking the knees of a brace and hyperextending the hips, thus avoiding the fatigue associated with continuous stimulation. FES is quite effective at introducing large impulsive forces to move the body forward through activation of large lower extremity muscles, which would reduce the upper extremity exertion required for walking in conventional braces. Combining FES and bracing in a hybrid orthosis offers an opportunity to take advantage of the positive aspects of each technology and minimize the potential shortcomings. To date, hybrid systems remain primarily exercise devices with limited functionality (4,5,38,61,62,67).

One such system is an FES-powered reciprocating gait orthosis (RGO) (32,48). Adding FES to a standard RGO improved walking distance from 100 to 800 m, reduced energy expenditure by 15%–30%, improved balance on inclines, and provided unassisted rising (72). There was a significant reduction in heart rate (8) and in physiologic cost index (PCI) when walking by adding FES, but no change in cadence, step length or velocity was noted (37). After

14 weeks of training with 3 hours of walking per week, significant reduction in spasticity, total cholesterol and low density lipids, hydroxyproline to creatinine ratio, and increased knee extensor torque were evident (73). The addition of FES to the gluteals during stance when using the long leg braces resulted in a 36% reduction in the crutch force (52), a 30% reduction in PCI (74), and provided forward propulsion by driving the stance leg into extension.

By incorporating joint locks or brakes, standing and stance-limb stability against collapse can be accomplished with minimal muscle stimulation. Numerous examples of such systems have been prototyped and tested, yet few have proven clinically viable (30,39,41,59). A hybrid orthosis that utilized surface FES and incorporated closed-loop, computer-controlled magnetic particle brakes at the hip and knee is reported to have been successful in regulating desired position and velocity of the joints during gait (19,26). The muscle fatigue was significantly reduced when compared with FES-only gait (27). Major drawbacks of this system were size, weight, ease of donning and doffing, and cosmetics of the brace. With fully locked joints, the power requirements were prohibitive for practical use out of the laboratory.

A controlled knee joint that provides stability during stance phase and allows freedom during swing has been

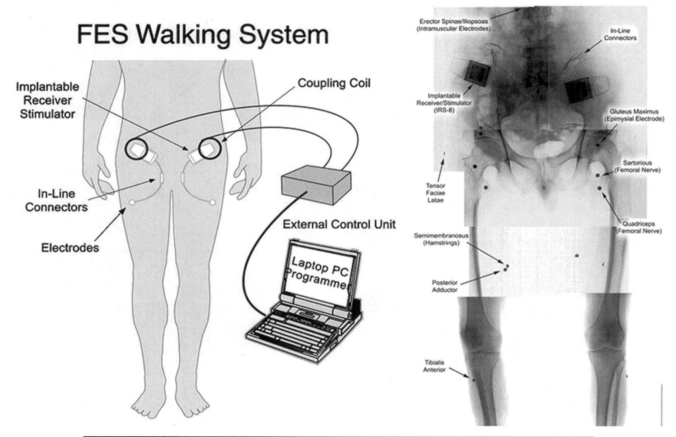

FIGURE 13-2. A schematic presentation of the FES walking system is shown on the left. Stimulus patterns are created on a personal computer and downloaded to a wearable external control unit that transmits power and stimulus information to the implanted components. On the right is a radiograph of 16-channel implanted walking system consisting of two receiver-stimulators, 14 epimysial and two intramuscular electrodes.

designed based on a wrap-spring clutch (36). This system provided significant reduction in oxygen consumption during walking when compared to a locked knee brace (35). The hybrid combination of a brace with an isocentric reciprocator and lockable knee joints resulted in gait that was slower, but with less forward trunk lean than walking with FES alone (43).

SYNTHESIS OF GAIT WITH ELECTRICAL STIMULATION

Muscle Functions and Interactions

The 48-channel percutaneous stimulation system employed at our center has provided an excellent opportunity to study human functional musculoskeletal anatomy and develop control strategies that mimic the human central nervous system. Muscles are generally targeted for implantation for their primary actions, although they often have secondary and tertiary motor functions that need to be counterbalanced with additional channels of stimulation. The process of balancing the actions of the stimulated mus-

cles at the joint level can often be simplified by recruiting multiple muscles with a single electrode. For example, one precisely located electrode can produce balanced dorsiflexion by stimulating the deep peroneal nerve to activate the tibialis anterior and peroneus tertius while minimizing the extensor digitorum longus and extensor hallucis longus. Similarly, one judiciously placed electrode can recruit the soleus and both heads of the gastrocnemius to maximize the plantarflexion moment. Tibialis posterior recruitment is usually avoided because it causes foot inversion. The gluteus minimus is usually activated with the tensor fascia lata, although it is possible to implant the tensor without the gluteus minimus. Muscles with multiple innervations are difficult to recruit with a single peripherally placed electrode, although they can be accessed with electrodes located at the spinal roots above the lumbarsacral plexus. For example, second and third lumbar motor root stimulation recruits the iliopsoas but may also include undesirable stimulation of the adductors and quadriceps, which are to be avoided.

Muscles not only accelerate the joint or joints that they span, but can also induce accelerations at other joints (82).

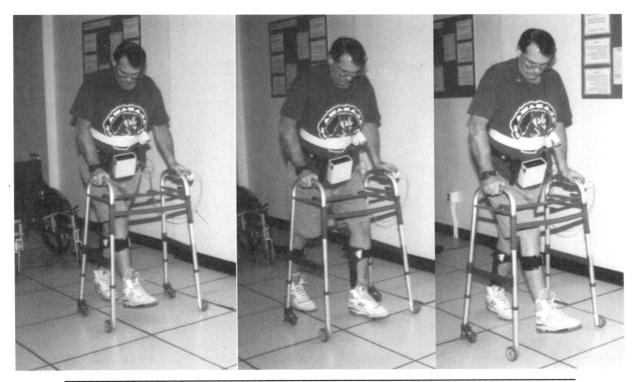

FIGURE 13-3. A subject stepping with a 16-channel implanted FES walking system using a hand switch to initiate each step and a walker for balance. The external control unit is attached to his belt and ankle foot orthoses protect against ankle injury.

Therefore, the action of a stimulated muscle depends on the posture and motion of the entire musculoskeletal system at the time it is activated, rather than solely by its direct anatomical connections. For example, gluteus maximus acts as an extensor of the hip and an external rotator of the femur. During stance, gluteus maximus rotates the femur posteriorly, thereby extending the knee. Thus, during walking the concept of a total extension moment at the hip, knee, and ankle may be more useful than considering the moment produced by individual muscles at their respective joints (80,82). Biarticulate muscles may produce flexion at one joint and extension at another. For example, semimembranosus produces flexion at the knee and extension at the hip; rectus femoris produces flexion at the hip and extension at the knee. These dual functions at two joints are difficult to separate when using electrical stimulation. Other muscles have dual (antagonistic) functions at the same joint depending on position. For example, gracilis and adductor longus act as hip flexors to about 30 degrees of hip flexion, but at greater angles they become hip extensors (75).

Stimulation Patterns

General templates for patterns of stimulation for stepping after complete paralysis have been developed through a process of trial and error based on the well-studied EMG activity during normal gait. These patterns can be customized for the unique responses from individual electrodes. Multichannel computer-controlled stimulators have been developed that can control pulse duration, frequency and current amplitude on a pulse by pulse basis with a resolution of 1 msec. Conditional jumps to specialized patterns of stimulation, or other control actions such as delays and wait states, have been implemented based on volitional switch closures, insole pressure sensors or information from other body-mounted sensors.

Figure 13-4 illustrates a typical temporal pattern of stimulation for generating stepping motions in individuals with complete SCI. The shaded areas in the figure show when the stimulation is delivered to the muscles. The amplitude of the shaded bars corresponds to the durations of individual pulses with a maximum set at 150 μsec. Ramping up and down of the bars indicates increasing and decreasing the width of each successive pulse. The pattern is divided into "tics" representing a generalized time base over which stimulus pulse widths and interpulse intervals are varied for each electrode throughout the gait cycle. In this example, the gait cycle is divided into 100 tics. Control actions occur at "breakpoints" (BPs) that divide the stimulation pattern into segments and allow the definition of how command inputs are to be interpreted. For example, progression through the pattern can continue uninterrupted, and can be delayed at a BP in order to await trigger input signals from switches or insole-mounted foot-floor contact sensors before initiating the next step.

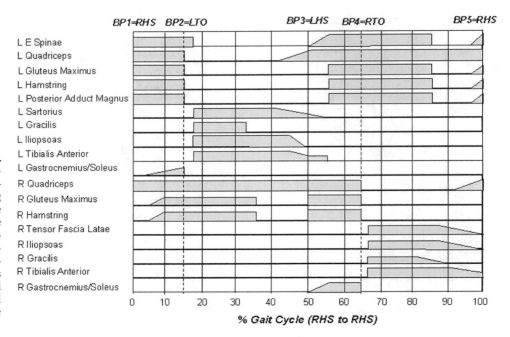

FIGURE 13-4. A graphical presentation of an 18-channel stimulation pattern for the walking illustrated in Figure 13-5. Pulse duration versus time through one gait cycle is indicated by the magnitude of the shaded areas. Stimulus pulse duration can be modulated from 0 to 150 microseconds and frequency can be modulated between 16 and 30 pulses/second continuosly for a given pulse amplitude.

Walking speed can also be varied by scaling the amount of time between BPs.

Breakpoint 1 (**BP1**) in the stimulation pattern represents right heel strike (RHS). At this point, stimulation is provided to the right and left quadriceps to keep the knees extended and to the left hip and trunk extensors to maintain posture. The processor can remain at **BP1** until the subject presses the finger switch indicating readiness for the next step or can continue uninterrupted in well trained users, as was the case in this example. The period between **BP1** and **BP2** corresponds to weight shifting to the right leg and renewal of momentum for progression accomplished by activation of the right hip and trunk extensors and left plantar flexors. Following **BP2**, stimulation to the left knee and hip extensors was turned off, and the left hip flexors and ankle dorsiflexors were activated. Left toe off (LTO) occurred shortly thereafter. Just before **BP3**, the left hip flexors were turned off, and at the same time knee extensors were activated in preparation for the left heel strike (LHS). Left ankle dorsiflexors remained active to prevent slapping of the foot at heel strike. A second burst of stimulation was provided to the right hip and trunk extensors to maintain posture, but then turned off shortly during the latter part of stance phase to delay the onset of muscle fatigue. Left hamstrings may be activated earlier at **BP3** to reduce extension moment on the knee and prevent hyperextension. At **BP3**, the right step was initiated without a delay. Pulse width and frequency of stimulation to the left hamstrings, posterior portion of adductor magnus and gluteus maximus, and the right plantar flexors were increased to produce a strong and rapid contraction to help transfer weight to the left leg and to move the body forward. At **BP4**, the right hip and trunk extensors

and plantar flexors were turned off and right swing was initiated. The stimulation was provided to tensor fascia lata, iliopsoas, and gracilis to produce hip flexion, and tibialis anterior to dorsiflex the ankle for the foot-floor clearance during swing. At the end of right swing, the flexors were turned off and knee extensors were activated in preparation for heel strike. The pattern then looped from **BP5** back to **BP1** to repeat the entire gait cycle.

The timing of the stimulation depends on the speed of walking and on the type of control used. When each step was initiated by a hand switch, the left hip extensors were activated before **BP3** to maintain hip stability and posture while the user prepared for the next step. Similarly, the right hip extensors were activated before the **BP5**.

MECHANICS OF WALKING WITH FES

The kinematics of electrically stimulated walking vary depending on the availability, strength, and conditioning of paralyzed muscles, the therapist's ability to synthesize gait, and the subject's experience. Although maximal forces are not required during normal gait (24), reduced muscle strength in the major muscle groups of the trunk and lower extremities will reduce speed (11), symmetry (58), and stability of gait and increase the energy cost (65). Muscles acting at the hip and ankle joints are particularly sensitive to strength reductions, and the forces at these joints have a significant correlation to walking speed (11). In stimulated gait, elimination of hip or trunk extensors or plantar flexors reduces walking speed. Hamstring elimination reduces speed by up to half. Removal of the posterior adductor causes a wide stance with side sway, and removal of the

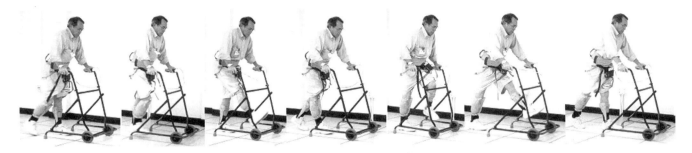

FIGURE 13-5. A paraplegic subject (T–9, ASIA A) walking with a percutaneous FES system connected to a belt-worn stimulator cycling through the activation pattern shown in Figure 13-4. Different phases of the gait cycle are illustrated.

erector spinae reduces speed and requires increased arm support. The salient mechanical features of stepping with FES illustrated in Figure 13-5 are summarized below to illustrate the similarities and differences with normal gait:

Initial Contact: The stance phase begins with initial foot contact. In FES walking, the heel strikes the floor after an exaggerated swing phase with the foot in slight plantar flexion. The knee is fully extended, and the hip is flexed up to 50 degrees. Neutral ankle position is difficult to achieve in some individuals because of heel cord tightness, even with maximal activity of the pretibial muscles. The knee is extended by the activity of the quadriceps in late swing. Extensors of the knee move the leg into excessive hip flexion before heel contact, but the hip angle at initial contact is somewhat controlled by hamstring, gluteus maximus, and posterior adductor activity.

Weight Acceptance: In this period of double limb support, the leading leg progresses from initial heel strike to total foot contact with the floor. The ankle moves into further plantar flexion even though restrained by maximum pretibial muscle stimulation. In some individuals with SCI, maximum pretibial stimulation is undesirable since it may cause a withdrawal reflex resulting in knee and hip flexion. During the loading phase, the knee tends to slightly hyperextend instead of flex. In the early part of this phase, the ground reaction vector (GRV) passes behind the ankle joint and in front of the knee and hip, generating moments that plantar flex the foot and extend the knee. Knee extension is partly caused by the hip extensors that produce posterior rotation of the thigh. Weight acceptance on the leading leg is not completed until halfway into midstance. With the body weight still behind the stance foot and excessive forward lean on the trunk, the hip flexes, resulting in loss of forward momentum and hampering weight transfer of the leading leg. At contralateral toe-off, the GRV passes in front of the ankle and remains in front of the knee and hip. This produces a dorsiflexion moment at the ankle and a flexion moment at the hip. The knee remains in forced extension. Weight transfer to the stance leg is delayed, and brief forces of up to 22% of body weight are exerted on each arm through the walking aid.

Midstance: Single limb support is initiated in midstance with the foot in total contact with the floor. A substantial amount of weight is accepted on the supporting leg in this phase. The GRV remains in front of the ankle, knee, and hip throughout, indicating that the ankle is passively forced into dorsiflexion throughout midstance without pretibial stimulation. As the heel rises the ankle dorsiflexes up to $\sim$ 10 degrees. Midstance knee extension causes excessive vertical fluctuation of the center of mass requiring extra hip and trunk extensor force to bring the body forward over the stance leg. As a result, much metabolic energy is wasted. The knee remains locked in extension as the GRV passes in front of the knee. Quadriceps are active during midstance, and the hip extensors are relaxed before their second burst of activity during terminal stance. When hip extensor stimulation is stopped, a slight knee flexion occurs because of the flexion moment at the knee. The GRV remains behind the knee for the rest of stance.

In subjects with weak hip and trunk extensors, the hip flexes in midstance rather than extending, interfering with the body's forward momentum. Increased hip flexion effectively lengthens the swing leg and interferes with toe clearance, shortening step length and making weight transfer difficult. Much of the body weight must be absorbed through the arms to prevent falling. The GRV passes lateral to the subtalar joint and medial to the knee and hip joint in the frontal plane. This indicates that an eversion moment is occurring at the ankle and an adduction moment at the hip. In this phase, stimulation of the posterior portion of the adductor magnus produces hip extension, and erector spinae and gluteus medius produce hip abduction.

Terminal Stance: This phase begins with heel rise and terminates with double limb support. Activity of the plantar flexors is initiated to generate the push-off force and to prevent excessive dorsiflexion because of the passive moment created by the GRV positioned in front of the ankle. This is a critical point during FES-induced gait. If the plantar flexors act too soon, they tend to raise the body instead of propelling it. This effectively shortens the swing leg and prevents proper swing foot contact. In addition, activity of the swing leg hip extensors will rotate the leg backward, reducing its effective step length and interfering with weight transfer. A push-off delayed into double stance is less effective in weight transfer. With the body weight far posterior and with loss of momentum, the hip of the weight-accepting leg will tend to flex, and much of the body weight must be supported by the arms. A second burst of stimulation is delivered to the hip and trunk extensors. It helps to stabilize the hip and trunk, especially at the opposite heel strike. The GRV is now behind the hip, helping the active hip extensors. The knee remains in slight flexion with the GRV behind it. Knee collapse is prevented by active knee and hip extensors.

Preswing: Regulation of the knee and ankle is critical for weight transfer to the other leg and for initiation of swing. A stiff knee of the stance leg can effectively shorten the swing leg, making transfer more difficult. Similarly, if the body weight has not progressed far enough forward, the stance knee will collapse and interrupt weight transfer. Proper control of knee flexion is difficult with pre-programmed stimulation and depends on the relaxation properties of the extensor muscles and the contraction properties of the knee flexors. Knee flexion is achieved by stimulation of the sartorius and gracilis. Knee flexion magnitude is slightly less than normal and varies between 30 and 40 degrees. Even though the GRV is far behind the knee, the residual knee extension moment during quadriceps relaxation resists flexion. However, an observable improvement in forward progression is achieved with even 5 to 10 degrees of knee flexion compared with a stiff knee. The ankle continues to plantar flex and reaches 10 degrees before toe-off. Plantar flexor stimulation is discontinued halfway into this phase, but the relaxation moment continues to create further plantar flexion for the next 100 msec. Early deactivation of hip extensors results in internal leg rotation and foot inversion. Hip flexion is initiated by the sartorius, gracilis, tensor fascia lata, and iliopsoas. Neutral is reached before toe-off.

Initial Swing: This phase is initiated at toe-off. Knee flexion is produced by contraction of the sartorius and gracilis and is often initially inadequate, resulting in toe drag and poor swing phase mechanics. The stance leg must be cleared as the leg swings through. Excessive in-toeing of the swing leg can catch easily. Because the gracilis also strongly adducts, balance from the tensor fascia lata and the gluteus minimus or medius is needed to clear the stance leg. The tensor fascia lata medial thigh rotation also balances the sartorius external rotation. Stimulation of the contralateral abductors will give additional toe and leg clearance.

Midswing: Maximum knee flexion in FES-generated gait is nearly normal. At peak knee flexion, hip flexion is normal and continues to overshoot to 60 degrees. This exaggerated flexion is caused by acceleration of the leg resulting from stimulation of the quadriceps while hip flexors are deactivated. Energy is wasted because muscle action is used to overcome gravity for an unnecessary motion,

but a benefit is that a vigorous leg swing provides needed progressional momentum during terminal stance of the opposite leg.

Terminal Swing: An overly flexed hip is extended by gravitational forces of the leg and activity of the hamstrings to control step length in preparation for foot contact.

Energy Expenditure

The metabolic energy currently required for ambulation with FES is still too high to make it a practical alternative to the wheelchair. The goal is to bring the energy requirement to below 50% of the individual's maximum aerobic capacity. At that level of energy consumption, walking can be sustained for hours (79).

Average maximum aerobic capacity of untrained female and male individuals with paraplegia was determined to be 16 and 25 mL O_2/kg per minute, respectively (14). Trained males with paraplegia averaged 28 mL O_2/kg per minute (14), whereas individuals with thoracic SCI using lower extremity stimulation plus an arm ergometer while seated reached a maximal aerobic capacity of 36 mL O_2/kg per minute (20). At this fitness level, prolonged walking with FES should require no more than 18 mL O_2/kg per minute. However, walking with FES at 30 m per minute currently averages 28 mL O_2/kg per minute. This far exceeds the goal of 50% maximum aerobic capacity, as well as the nominal value of 8 mL O_2/kg per minute for normal able-bodied gait (54).

A subject lying supine on a mat using a pattern of stimulation designed to produce walking motions without weight bearing or ground contact consumes 20 mL O_2/kg per min (54). Therefore, 8 mL of O_2/kg per minute are typically used by the voluntarily controlled arm and trunk muscles for support, balance, and propulsion via a walker or crutches. Progressive addition of the muscle groups to the walking stimulation pattern in the supine position results in a lower energy requirement for the full set of muscles than if all muscle groups were initiated at once. This suggests that a warm up prior to walking might reduce the energy demand. Finer control of stimulation to reduce reliance on the upper extremities and more efficient generation of stepping motions are needed to reduce energy consumption to reasonable levels.

RESEARCH DIRECTIONS AND FUTURE DEVELOPMENTS

The quest for efficient and effective methods of reanimating the paralyzed musculature to restore standing and walking function to individuals with spinal cord injuries continues in research laboratories and clinics around the world (57). Research and development efforts are focused on expanding the capabilities of implanted systems through additional channels of stimulation, new electrode configurations, more natural command and control sources, and advanced techniques for automatic control and regulation of movement (1,78).

A new family of implanted stimulation devices is being developed and readied for clinical testing at our center as the common platform for the next-generation of neural prostheses (71). The most important improvements offered by this new technology is the capability to provide up to 16 independent channels of nerve or muscle-based stimulation, and the capability to telemeter information from implanted sensors to an external controller that can utilize it to modulate stimulation in a closed-loop fashion (76). Such devices have been successfully implemented clinically to process information from implanted joint angle transducers consisting of a Hall-effect sensor array and magnet packaged in threaded titanium capsules that are inserted into the bones on either side of the joint (9,40), and to modulate stimulation based on feedback from multiple channels of EMG data acquired from muscles under volitional control as sensed by implanted recording electrodes. This ability to derive "afferent" information about body position or voluntary muscle activity and exploit it to alter the "efferent" stimulation delivered to a large number of paralyzed muscles offers the potential for unprecedented improvements in the quality of standing and walking motions and more interactive, intimate, and intuitive control of neural prostheses (71).

Preliminary success has also been reported in the use of "natural sensors" to control stimulation, such as can be accomplished by recording the electroneurogram (ENG) from an afferent nerve serving the mechanoreceptors in the plantar surface of the foot or the joint afferents of the knee (76). A recording cuff electrode placed around the appropriate sensory nerve can sense the biopotentials related to the mechanical events of foot-floor contact, weight acceptance, or loading response. Appropriately processed ENG signals can then be used to trigger, terminate, or modulate stimulation to the muscles required for the corresponding phase of the gait cycle. Such techniques have been applied clinically to produce active dorsiflexion during swing and control plantarflexion during initial stance to correct footdrop, improve swing limb clearance, and prevent foot slap with initial contact in individuals with hemiparesis (9). Similar methods can be applied to individuals with partial paralysis resulting from incomplete SCI to seamlessly coordinate the actions of stimulated muscles with intact volitional movements.

Other improvements to our ability to synthesize smooth, cosmetically acceptable, and energy efficient gait after paralysis will result from the development and application of new nerve-based electrode technologies and stimulation techniques that can completely and selectively activate all of the motor units in a targeted muscle or block unwanted and counterproductive activity because of spasticity in antagonist muscles. The muscle-based electrodes currently employed in neural prostheses for walking achieve selectivity at the expense of full activation of all available motor units by virtue of their location in the periphery (typically at a single nerve entry point to the targeted muscle). On the other hand, nerve-based electrodes can achieve maximal recruitment because of their intimate contact with the nerve above the point where it branches into multiple motor points, usually at the expense of selectivity. Since all distal muscles are represented by distinct fascicles in the proximal nerve trunk, an effective nerve electrode must also be able to selectively recruit only the desired fascicles within a multifascicular nerve. Selective activation of subpopulations of axons in a synergistic nerve trunk can delay the effects of fatigue by switching between different muscles or portions of a muscle while maintaining a constant net moment about the joint. This intermittent "sequential" or "cyclical" stimulation reduces the effective duty cycle of each muscle fiber, allows some recovery from fatigue, and has been shown to improve endurance for locking the knee in extension (63).

Further advantages of selective stimulation are realized by implanting a cuff electrode proximally where the nerve contains axons to multiple muscles that produce different functions. A single multicontact electrode that can selectively activate individual fascicles within a nerve trunk is highly desirable as it could simplify implant surgery while simultaneously providing access to an increased number of muscles. This approach has the potential to profoundly improve neural prosthesis implementation by streamlining the implant procedure, obviating the need to distribute and manage multiple lead wires to various points in the periphery, eliminating the time-consuming process of exposing and deploying an individual electrode on each of many target muscles, and activating muscles that are too small or inaccessible for muscle-based electrodes. While such a system can enhance the performance of standing neural prostheses, it will be even more important for achieving the advanced functions of stepping and stair climbing in the future.

CONCLUSION

Walking with FES for individuals with motor and sensory complete SCI requires the cooperative effort of people from diverse disciplines including surgery, engineering, and therapy. Although the feasibility of ambulation with FES has been established experimentally and through computer simulation, much work remains to be done to more efficiently interface with the nervous system. New and deeper understanding of the response of paralyzed muscle to electrical stimulation are required to advance the performance of lower extremity neural prostheses. More effective means of controlling the motion of individual joints and multisegmental body structures are needed to make FES-generated gait energy efficient and clinically practical. Improved activation and deactivation of muscles should reduce unnecessary stimulation, improve balance, and reduce energy requirements.

Functional electrical stimulation provides an opportunity to activate and utilize muscles no longer under direct volitional control (40). In complete spinal cord injury, FES allows short distance walking, stair climbing, maneuverability in small spaces, and other functional activities. This technology has the potential to provide patients with partial spinal cord injuries with enhanced function and less need for conventional bracing.

In addition to their applications after complete thoracic SCI, implanted stimulation systems will soon be clinically available to restore or improve walking or transfers in people with partial paralysis or spasticity (68) from spinal cord injury, stroke, head injury, cerebral palsy, multiple sclerosis, and Parkinson's disease. More complex multichannel systems incorporating sensory feedback for closed loop control will require much more development and testing before they can be readied for widespread clinicalk use.

ACKNOWLEDGMENTS

The authors acknowledge the contribution of the Cleveland FES Center, a consortium consisting of the Louis Stokes Cleveland Department of Veteran Affairs Medical Center, Case Western Reserve University and MetroHealth Medical Center. Some of the work described was supported by the Rehabilitation R&D service of the US Department of Veterans Affairs, the Office of Orphan Product Development of the United States Food and Drug Administration and the National Institutes of Health (NINDS and NIBIB). Further recognition is due to Dr. E. Byron Marsolais, the General Clinical Research Center (GCRC) at Metro Health Medical Center, and all the research participants, engineers, therapists, physicians, and technicians who have worked on this project over the past 30 years for their invaluable contributions.

REFERENCES

1. Abbas JJ, Riener R. Using mathematical models and advanced control systems techniques to enhance neuroprosthesis function. *Neuromodulation* 2001;4:187–195.
2. Agarwal S, Kobetic R, Nandurkar S, Marsolais EB. Functional electrical stimulation for walking in paraplegia: 17 year follow-up of 2 cases. *J Spinal Cord Med* 2003;26:86–91.
3. Akers JM, Peckham PH, Keith MW, Merritt K. Tissue response to chronically stimulated implanted epimysial and intramuscular electrodes. *IEEE Trans Rehabil Eng* 1996;5:207–220.
4. Andrews BJ, Baxendale RH, Barnett R, Phillips GF, Paul JP, Freeman PA. A hybrid orthosis for paraplegics incorporating feedback control. *Proc 9th Symp ECHE*, 1997;297–311.
5. Andrews BJ, Baxendale RH, Barnett R, et al. Hybrid FES orthosis incorporating closed loop control and sensory feedback. *Biomed Eng* 1988;10:189–195.
6. Bajd T, Kralj A, Turk R. Standing up of a healthy subject and a paraplegic patient. *J Biomech* 1982;15:1–10.
7. Bajd T, Kraij A, Turk R, Benko H, Sega J. The use of a four-channel electrical stimulator as an ambulatory aid for paraplegic patients. *Phys Ther* 1983;63:1116–1120.

8. Beillot J, Carre F, Le Claire G, et al. Energy consumption of paraplegic locomotion using reciprocal gait orthosis. *Eur J Appl Physiol* 1996;73:376–381.
9. Bhadra N, Peckham PH, Keith MW, et al. Implementation of an implantable joint-angle transducer. *J Rehabil Res Dev* 2002;39(3):411–422.
10. Biering-Sorensen F, Bohr H. Bone mineral content of the lumbar spine and lower extremities years after spinal cord lesion. *Paraplegia* 1988;26:293–301.
11. Bohannon RW. Relevance of muscle strength to gait performance in patients with neurologic disability. *J Neuro Rehabil* 1989;3:97–100.
12. Borges G, Ferguson K, Kobetic R. Development and operation of portable and laboratory electrical stimulation systems for walking in paraplegic subjects. *IEEE Trans Biomed Eng* 1989;36:798–800.
13. Brindley GS, Polkey CE, Rushton DN. Electrical splinting of the knee in paraplegia. *Paraplegia* 1979;16:248.
14. Burkett LN, Chisum J, Stone W, Fernhall B. Exercise capacity of untrained spinal cord injured individuals and the relationship of peak oxygen uptake to level of injury. *Paraplegia* 1990;28:512–521.
15. Carroll SG, Triolo RJ, Chizeck HJ, Kobetic R, Marsolais EB. Tetanic response of electrically stimulated paralyzed muscle at varying interpulse intervals. *IEEE Trans Biomed Eng* 1989;36:644–653.
16. Davis JA, Triolo RJ, Uhlir JP, et al. Surgical technique for installing an 8-channel neuroprosthesis for standing. *Clin Orthop Rel Res* 2001;2001:237–252.
17. Davis JA, Triolo RJ, Uhlir JP, Bieri C, Rohde L, Lissy D. Preliminary performance of a surgically implanted neuroprosthesis for standing and transfer. *J Rehabil Res Dev* 2001;38:609–617.
18. Davis R, Eckhouse R, Patrick JF, Delehanty A. Computer-controlled 22-channel stimulator for limb movement. *Acta Neurochirurgica Suppl* 1987;39:117–120.
19. Durfee W, Goldfarb M. Controlled-brake orthosis, U.S. Patent 5 476 441,1995.
20. Edwards BG, Marsolais EB. Metabolic responses to arm ergometry and functional neuromuscular stimulation. *J Rehabil Res Dev* 1990;27:107–114.
21. Edwards RHT, Hill DK, Jones DA. Heat production and chemical changes during isometric contractions of the human quadriceps muscle. *J Physiol (Lond)* 1975;251:303–315.
22. Edwards RHT, Young A, Hosking GP, Jones DA. Human skeletal muscle function: Description of tests and normal values. *Clin Sci Mol Med* 1977;52:283–290.
23. Edwards RHT. Human muscle function and fatigue. In: Human muscle fatigue: Physiological mechanisms. *Ciba Found Symp* 1981;82:1–18.
24. Ericson MO, Nisell R, Ekholm J. Quantified electromyography of lower-limb muscles during level walking. *Scand J Rehabil Med* 1986;18:159–163.
25. Gallien P, Brissot R, Eyssette M, Tell L, Barat M, Wiart L, Petit H. Restoration of gait by functional electrical stimulation for spinal cord injured patients. *Paraplegia* 1995;33:660–664.
26. Goldfarb M, Durfee WK. Design of a controlled-brake orthosis for FES-aided gait. *IEEE Trans Rehabil Eng* 1996;1:13–24.
27. Goldfarb M, Korkowski K, Harrold B, Durfee WK. Preliminary evaluation of a controlled-brake orthosis for FES-aided gait. *IEEE Trans Rehabil Eng* 2003;11:241–248.
28. Graupe D, Kohn K. *Functional Electrical Stimulation for Ambulation by Paraplegics*. Malabar FL: Krieger Publishing Co; 1994;1–26.
29. Grimbv G, Broberg C, Krotkiewska 1, Krotkiewski M. Muscle fiber composition in patients with traumatic cord lesion. *Scand J Rehabil Med* 1976;8:37–42.
30. Harrison R, Lemaire E, Jeffreys Y, Goudreau L. Design and pilot testing of an orthotic stance-phase control knee joint. *Orthopadie Technik;* 2001;2–4.
31. Haugland MK, Sinkjær T. Cutaneous whole nerve recordings used for correction of footdrop in hemiplegic man. *IEEE Trans Rehabil Eng* 1995;3:307–317.
32. Hirokawa S, Grimm M, Thanh LE, et al. Energy consumption in paraplegia ambulation using the reciprocating gait orthosis and electrical

stimulation of the thigh muscles. *Arch Phys Med Rehabil* 1990;71:687–694.

33. Hoffer JA, Stein RB, Haugland MK, et al. Neural signals for command control and feedback in functional neuromuscular stimulation [review]. *J Rehabil Res Dev* 1996;33:145–157.

34. Holle J, Frey M, Gruber H, Kern H, Stohr H, Thoma H. Functional electrostimulation of paraplegics. experimental investigations and first clinical experience with an implantable stimulation device. *Orthopaedics* 1984;7:1145–1160.

35. Irby SE, Kaufman KR, Mathewson JW, Sutherland DH. Automatic control design for a dynamic knee-brace system. *IEEE Trans Rehabil Eng* 1999a;7:135–139.

36. Irby SE, Kaufman KR, Wirta RW, Sutherland DH. Optimization and application of a wrap-spring clutch to a dynamic knee-ankle-foot orthosis. *IEEE Trans Rehabil Eng* 1999;7:130–134.

37. Isakov E, Douglas R, Berns P. Ambulation using the reciprocating gait orthosis and functional electrical stimulation. *Paraplegia* 1992;30:239–245.

38. Jaeger RT, Yarkony GM, Roth EG. Standing by a combined orthotic/electrical stimulation system in thoracic paraplegic. *Proc IC-CAART*, Montreal, 1988:336–337.

39. Jaspors P, Van Petegem W, Van der Perre G, Peeraer L. Optimisation of a combined ARGO-FES system: adaptation of the knee mechanism to allow flexion of the knee during the swing phase. *IEEE/EMBS Conference*, Montreal, 1995.

40. Johnson MW, Peckham PH, Bhadra N,et al. An implantable transducer for two-degree-of-freedom joint angle sensing. *IEEE Trans Biomed Eng* 1999;7:349–359.

41. Kagaya H, Shimada Y, Sato K, Satom, Iizuka K, Obinata G. An electrical knee lock system for functional electrical stimulation. *Arch Phys Med Rehabil* 1996;77:870–873.

42. Kilgore KL, Peckham PH, Keith MW, et al. An implanted upper extremity neuroprosthesis: A five patient follow-up, *J Bone Joint Surg Am* 1997;79A:533–541.

43. Kobetic R, Marsolais EB, Davy D, Gaudio R, Triolo R. Development of a hybrid gait orthosis: a case report. *J Spinal Cord Med* 2003;26:254–258.

44. Kobetic R, Marsolais EB, Samame P, Borges G. The next step: artificial walking. In: Rose J, Gamble JG, eds. *Human Walking.* 2nd ed. Baltimore: Williams & Wilkins; 1994:225–252.

45. Kobetic R, Marsolais EB. Synthesis of paraplegic gait with multichannel functional neuromuscular stimulation. *IEEE Trans Rehabil Eng* 1994;2:66–79.

46. Kobetic R, Triolo RJ, Uhlir J, et al. Implanted functional electrical stimulation system for mobility in paraplegia: A follow-up case report. *IEEE Trans Rehabil Eng* 1999;7:390–398.

47. Kobetic R, Triolo RJ. Muscle selection and walking performance of multichannel FES systems for ambulation in paraplegia. *IEEE Trans Rehabil Eng* 1997;5:23–29.

48. Larson PF, Douglas RD, Petrofsky JS, Phillips CA. Walking assistance system, U.S. Patent 4 697 808,1987.

49. Marsolais EB, Kobetic R, Barnicle K, Jacobs J. FNS application for restoring function in stroke and head-injury patients. *J Clin Eng* 1990;15:489–496.

50. Marsolais EB, Kobetic R. Functional electrical stimulation for walking in paraplegia. *J Bone Joint Surg* 1987;69-A:728–733.

51. Marsolais EB, Kobetic R. Implantation techniques and experience with percutaneous intramuscular electrodes in the lower extremities. *J Rehabil R & D* 1986;23:1–8.

52. McClelland M, Andrews BJ, Patrick JH, Freeman PA, El Masri WS. Augmentation of the Oswestry parawalker orthosis by means of surface electrical stimulation: gait analysis of three patients. *Paraplegia* 1987;25:32–38.

53. Memberg WD, Peckham PH, Keith MW. A surgically-implanted intramuscular electrode for an implantable neuromuscular stimulation system. *IEEE Trans Biomed Eng* 1994;2:80–91.

54. Miller PC, Kobetic R, Lew RD. Energy cost of walking and standing using functional electrical stimulation. *Rehabilitation Engineering Society of North America, 13th Annual Conference on Rehabilitation Technology*, Washington DC, 1990:155–156.

55. Mortimer JT, Kaufman D, Roessmann U. Intramuscular electrical stimulation: Tissue damage. *Ann Biomed Eng* 1980;8:235–244.

56. Moulds RFW, Young A, Jones DA, Edwards RHT. A study of the contractility, biochemistry and morphology of an isolated preparation of human skeletal muscle. *Clin Sci Mol Med* 1977;52:291–297.

57. Munih M, Ichie M. Current status and future prospects for upper and lower extremity motor system neuroprostheses. *Neuromodulation* 2001;4:176–186.

58. Murray MP, Cuten GN, Sepic SB, Gardner GM, Baldwin JM. Function of triceps surae during gait. *J Bone Joint Surg* 1978;60- A:473–475.

59. Myers WN, Shadoan MD, Frobes JC, Baker KJ, Darron CR. Selectively lockable knee brace, U.S. Patent 5 490 831,1996.

60. Peckham PH, Mortimer JT, Marsolais EB. Alteration in the force and fatigability of skeletal muscle in quadriplegic humans following exercise induced by chronic electrical stimulation. *Clin Orthop Relat Res* 1976;114:326–334.

61. Petrofsky JS, Phillips CA, Douglas R, Larson P. A computer-controlled walking system: The combination of an orthosis with functional electrical stimulation. *J Clin Eng* 1986;11:121–133.

62. Popovic D, Schwirtlich L. Hybrid powered orthoses. In: Popovic D, ed. *Advances in External Control of Human Extremities IX.* Yugoslav Committee for ETAN, Yugoslavia; 1987:95–104.

63. Pournezam M, Andrews BJ, Baxendale RH, et al. Reduction of muscle fatigue in man by cyclical stimulation. *J Biomed Eng* 1988;10:196–200.

64. Rushton DN, Perkins TA, Donaldson N, et al. LARSI: How to obtain favorable muscle contractions. Proceedings of the Second Annual IFESS Conference (IFESS '97) and Neural Prosthesis: Motor Systems 5 (NP '97), Burnaby, British Columbia, Canada, 16–21 Aug., 1997:163–164.

65. Saunders JB, Inman VT, Eberhart HD. The major determinants in normal and pathologic gait. *J Bone Joint Surg* 1953;35-A:543–558.

66. Scheiner A, Polando G, Marsolais EB. Design and clinical application of a double helix electrode for functional electrical stimulation. *IEEE Trans Biomed Eng* 1994;41:425–431.

67. Schwirtlich L, Popovic D. Hybrid orthosis for deficient locomotion. In: Advances in External Control of Human Extremities VIII edited by Dejan Popovic, Yugoslav Committee for Electronics and Automation, Belgrade. 1984:23–32.

68. Scott TR, Haugland M. Command and control interfaces for advanced neuroprosthetic applications. *Neuromodulation* 2001;4:165–175.

69. Sharma M, Marsolais EB, Polando G, et al. Implantation of a 16-channel functional electrical stimulation walking system. *Clin Ortho* 1998;347:236–242.

70. Smith B, Peckham PH, Keith MW, Roscoe DD. An externally powered, multichannel implantable stimulator for versatile control of paralyzed muscle. *IEEE Trans Biomed Eng* 1987;34:499–508.

71. Smith B, Tang Z, Johnson M, et al. An externally powered, multichannel, implantable stimulator-telemeter for control of paralyzed muscle. *IEEE Trans Rehabil Eng* 1998;45:463–475.

72. Solomonow M, Baratta R, Hirokawa S, et al. The RGO Generation II: Muscle stimulation powered orthosis as a practical walking system for thoracic paraplegics. *Orthopedics* 1989;12:1309–1315.

73. Solomonow M, Reisin E, Aguilar E, Baratta RV, Best R, D'Ambrosia RD. Reciprocal gait orthosis powered with electrical muscle stimulation (RGO II). Part II: medical evaluation of 70 paraplegic patients. *Orthopedics* 1997a;20:411–418.

74. Stallard J, Major RE. The influence of orthosis stiffness on paraplegic ambulation and its implication for functional electrical stimulation (FES) walking systems. *Prosthet Orthot Int* 1995;19:108–114.

75. Steindier A. *Kinesiology of the Human Body.* 5th ed. Springfield: Charles C Thomas; 1977:316.

76. Tang Z, Smith B, Schild JH, Peckham PH. Data transmission from an implantable biotelemeter by load-shift keying using circuit configuration modulator. *IEEE Trans Biomed Eng* 1995;42:525–528.

77. Triolo RJ, Bieri C, Uhlir J, Kobetic R, Scheiner A, Marsolais EB. Implanted FNS systems for assisted standing and transfers for individuals with cervical spinal cord injuries: Clinical case reports. *Arch Phys Med & Rehabil* 1996;77:1119–1128.

78. Troyk PR, Donaldson N. Implantable FES stimulation systems: what is needed? *Neuromodulation* 2001;4:196–204.

79. Waters RL, Lunsford BR. Energy expenditure of normal and pathologic gait: Application to orthotic prescription. In: *Atlas of Orthotics*. 2nd ed. St. Louis: Mosby; 1985:151–159.

80. Winter DA. *Biomechanics and Motor Control of Human Movement*. 2nd ed. New York: Wiley; 1990:85.

81. Yamaguchi GT, Zajac FE. Restoring unassisted natural gait to paraplegics via functional neuromuscular stimulation: A computer simulation study. *IEEE Trans Biomed Eng* 1990;37:886–902.

82. Zajac FE, Gordon ME. Determining muscle's forces and action in multi-articular movement. In: Pandolf K, ed. Exercise and sports science reviews. Baltimore: Williams & Wilkins; 1989;17:187–230.

Chapter 14

Human Walking: Six Take-Home Lessons

James G. Gamble and Jessica Rose

LESSON 1: BIPEDALISM, THE ABILITY TO WALK UPRIGHT, WAS THE FIRST ANATOMIC AND BEHAVIORAL CHARACTERISTIC TO DISTINGUISH OUR PRIMAL ANCESTORS FROM APES

As Weaver and Kline discuss in Chapter 2, the ability to walk upright on two legs, bipedalism, appeared before a dexterous hand with an opposable thumb and before a large brain with the ability to use language and design tools and weapons. Bipedalism is at the root of what it means to be human. Our closest genetic ancestors, chimpanzees, do not have a bipedal gait. They use a characteristic gait called "knuckle-walking." Chimps do not fully extend their knees, and they must use more muscle power than humans to support the body in midstance. Chimps have to rock their bodies from side to side to keep their center of gravity over the weight-bearing leg.

Early hominoid fossils show biomechanical evidence of bipedal ambulation. A computerized tomography of the internal structure of fossil femora from the six million-year-old *Orronin tugenensis* matches closely that of humans and is distinct from those of gorillas and chimps (1). Four million-year-old fossils of *Australopithecus anamensi* have pelvic and lower extremity anatomical features permitting habitual bipedalism. The iliac wings face laterally, but the pelvis is narrow and short bringing the hips closer to the sacrum. Strong abductor muscles prevented rotation of the body on the femoral head and decreased body sway in midstance. In our bipedal ancestors, the femoral neck-shaft angle medialized the knee, bringing the feet closer to the center of gravity. The bicondylar angle of their knees was larger ($\sim$10°) than that of chimpanzees (0°), and their feet had well developed longitudinal arches with the great toe aligned parallel to the lesser toes.

From an evolutionary standpoint, it is obvious that bipedalism would free up the hands to use weapons and carry objects such as meat, nuts, fruit, and, perhaps most importantly, infants and children. It must have been a great advantage to be able to scoop up the baby and run in a time of crisis. From a biomechanical perspective, bipedalism decreases the energy expenditure required during slow walking speed and permits tool and weapon use, attributes that would have been important for early hominoids during both hunting and gathering. Bipedalism requires the lower limbs to support all the body weight, and it requires balance against gravity.

An important question facing paleoanthropologists today is, "why did our ancestors first begin to walk upright in the first place?" Of course, any discussion of "why bipedalism" must consider natural selection. This is a term first used by Charles Darwin in 1859 and relates to the fitness of any species to its environment. Darwin envisioned that in any given environment, some individuals are better able to find food, find a mate, care for their offspring, and escape predators due to their genetic make-up. What were the advantages that bipedalism gave the early hominins? What were the environmental pressures favoring bipedalism over other forms of locomotion? Previous speculation held that our ancestors became bipedal as they migrated out of the forest and into the savannah. Indeed the environment was changing with increasing expanses of savannah emerging among shrinking areas of forest. Presumably, standing and walking upright in the savannah permitted observations above the tall grasses and provided an energetic advantage when searching for food or avoiding predators. The problem with this scenario is that recent research at early hominoid sites indicates that the environment was not a savannah but was a lightly to densely wooded area, suggesting that early hominins may have ventured out to the savannah in search of food but returned to the forest to live. While more research is necessary to understand our history of bipedalism, it is evident that bipedalism was the characteristic that first distinguished humans from apes.

LESSON 2: THE GAIT CYCLE IS THE BASIS FOR UNDERSTANDING NORMAL AND PATHOLOGICAL HUMAN WALKING

A cycle is a recurrent series of events. We can understand many complex phenomena by thinking in terms of a cycle. Ancient astronomers achieved a better understanding of the seasons by observing the celestial cycles and the lunar cycle. Biologists proposed the cell cycle, and biochemists devised the Krebs and the Calvin cycles. The gait cycle is to the biomechanics of walking as the Krebs cycle is to the biochemistry of intermediary metabolism. We speak of the gait cycle as applying separately to each lower extremity, and we define the gait cycle as the events that occur from one heel strike to the next.

Initially we can divide the gait cycle into two phases, stance phase when the foot is in contact with the ground, and swing phase when the foot is in the air. Stance phase accounts for about 60% of the cycle, and swing accounts for the remaining 40%. We can subdivide stance phase into five periods known as: 1) initial contact, 2) loading response, 3) midstance, 4) terminal stance, and 5) preswing. In addition, we can divide swing into three periods: 1) initial swing, 2) midswing, and 3) terminal swing (Fig. 14-1).

First we will consider the five periods of stance phase. The first period, initial contact, begins when the foot touches the ground. The second period, loading response, is a time of double limb support when both feet are on the ground (usually 10% to 12% of stance). During this period, the limb accepts the weight of the body. Loading

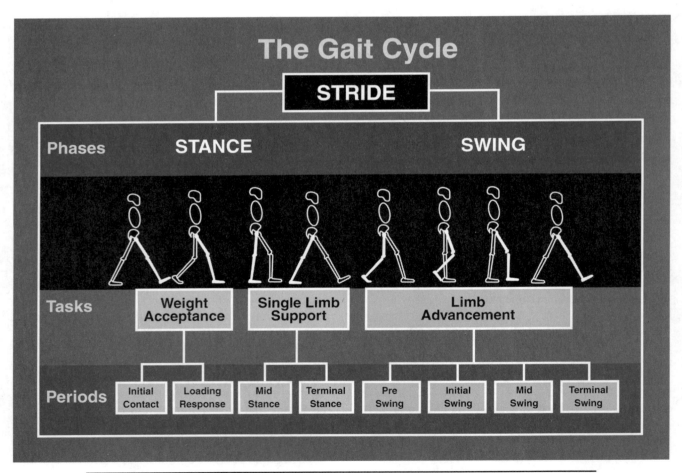

FIGURE 14-1. The two phases of the gait cycle: stance phase when the foot is on the floor, and swing phase when the foot is in the air. The gait cycle is further subdivided into tasks as well as periods known as (1) initial contact, (2) loading response, (3) midstance, (4) terminal stance, and (5) preswing, (6) initial swing, (7) midswing, and (8) terminal swing.

response ends when the opposite foot leaves the ground. Midstance is the period when the center of gravity moves over the foot, and the limb fully supports the weight of the body. The fourth period, terminal stance, begins with the center of gravity directly over the foot and ends as the heel rises from the ground and the opposite foot contacts the ground. The last period of stance is preswing, another time of double limb support, when the foot is about to become airborne and the opposite limb progressively accepts more weight.

The swing phase occupies less time of the cycle. Initial swing begins when the foot leaves the ground and continues as the knee flexes. Midswing begins with the knee in maximum flexion and ends when the leg is perpendicular to the ground. The last period, terminal swing, begins with the leg perpendicular to the ground and ends when the foot contacts the ground again.

LESSON 3: KINEMATICS DESCRIBES MOVEMENT OF THE BODY SEGMENTS, AND KINETICS DESCRIBES THE FORCES CAUSING AND RESULTING FROM MOVEMENT OF THE JOINTS

Kinematic data provides information about joint movement and is expressed as degrees of displacement in any of three planes of movement, i.e., sagittal, coronal, or transverse planes. Kinematically, we can describe the position, velocity, and acceleration of body segments during walking. From a motion analysis perspective, the body segments include the HAT (head, arms, trunk), the pelvis, the thigh, the shank (leg), and the foot.

Kinetic data provides information about the forces that act across the joints. Figure 14-2 shows a graphic

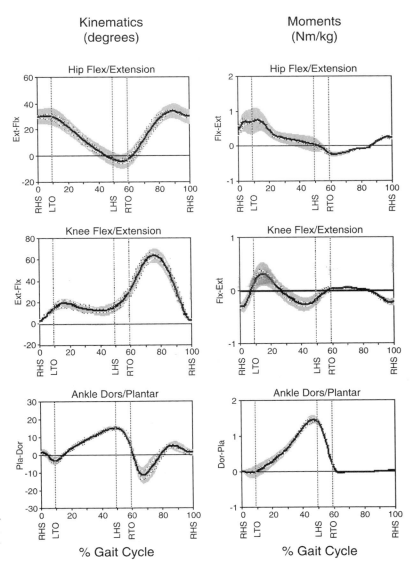

FIGURE 14-2. A graphic representation of the hip, knee, and ankle kinematics and kinetics in the sagittal plane during normal walking.

Certain Temporal Spatial Definitions Help in Understanding Gait

Step:	Advancement of the foot from toe off to heel strike
Step length:	Longitudinal distance between the two feet when both are on the ground
Cadence:	Number of steps per minute
Double support:	The time when both feet are on the ground
Float:	A time when neither foot is on the ground, as occurs in running
Stride:	One step by each foot, or one complete turn of the gait cycle
Stride length:	The distance covered during one turn of the gait cycle
Velocity:	Stride length per cycle time, measured in meters per minute

representation of the hip, knee, and ankle kinematics and kinetics in the sagittal plane during normal walking. The slope of each graph represents velocity of movement, and degrees of displacement represents the position of the joint relative to the neutral position. Note that hip and knee flexion result in extension moments, and ankle dorsiflexion causes a plantar flexion moment at the ankle.

The kinematic data show that at initial floor contact, the hip is flexed, the knee is extended, and the ankle is close to neutral. During early stance, the hip begins to extend, the knee flexes slightly and then extends, and the ankle dorsiflexes as the center of gravity passes over the foot. In preswing, the hip is in extension, the knee begins to flex, and the ankle is in plantarflexion. In swing, the hip and knee flex, and the ankle dorsiflexes to clear the foot. The knee rapidly extends in terminal swing after peak knee flexion in preparation for floor contact. The kinetic data illustrates that the ankle plantarflexion moment generated in terminal stance is the largest moment acting across any joint during any point in the gait cycle and is important in advancing the limb.

LESSON 4: SPECIFIC MUSCLES ARE ACTIVE DURING THE INDIVIDUAL PHASES AND PERIODS OF THE GAIT CYCLE, AND THE MAGNITUDE, DURATION, AND TIMING OF MUSCULAR ACTIVITY DETERMINES THE QUALITY AND EFFICIENCY OF GAIT

Skeletal muscles hold the trunk upright against gravity, stabilize the supporting limb during stance, and move the advancing limb during swing. To accomplish any physio-logical task involving gross or fine body movement, muscles must convert the chemical energy in carbohydrates and fats to the mechanical energy of actomyosin contraction. This conversion permits us to accomplish the various tasks of gait such as weight acceptance, single limb support, and limb advancement.

Specific muscles are active during each period of the gait cycle (Fig. 14-3). In general, the muscles that are active during stance prevent the stance limb from collapsing as the limb supports the body weight while the center of gravity advances. The major stance phase muscles include the gluteus maximus, medius and minimus, tensor fascia lata, adductors, quadriceps, and the gastrocsoleus.

Normal Electromyographic Data

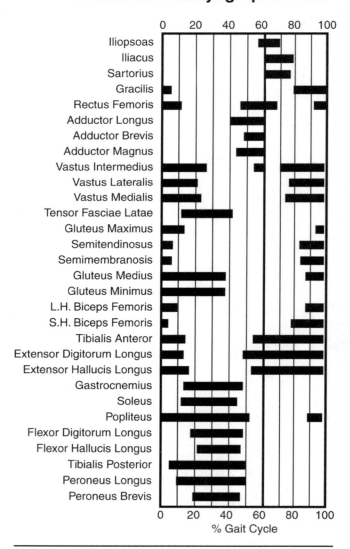

FIGURE 14-3. The normal timing of the lower extremity muscles measured by electromyography (EMG) recorded as a percent of the gait cycle.

At initial contact and during loading response, active muscles include the hamstrings, gluteus maximus, medius, minimus, and the tensor fascia lata to stabilize the hip. The quadriceps stabilizes the knee. During the third and fourth period, midstance and terminal stance, the gastrocsoleus complex stabilizes the ankle as the center of gravity moves over the foot.

The major swing phase muscles responsible for advancing the limb include the iliopsoas and rectus femoris, active in early swing to flex the hip, followed in terminal swing by the quadriceps to extend the leg, and finally the hamstrings to restrain knee extension at terminal swing. Tibialis anterior and other pretibial muscles are active throughout swing to hold the foot in a position such that it clears the floor.

Figure 14-3 shows the normal timing of the lower extremity muscles measured by electromyography (EMG) recorded as a percent of the gait cycle. Any abnormality in the timing or magnitude of muscular activity or in the motion of the joints during the gait cycle produces deviations in motion.

LESSON 5: SIX DETERMINANTS OF GAIT PROVIDE A MODEL FOR BIOMECHANICAL MECHANISMS USED TO MAXIMIZE WALKING EFFICIENCY

A half-century ago, Saunders, Inman, and Eberhart at the Biomechanical Laboratory of the University of California at Berkeley described what they called the six determinants of gait as a logical way to understand how the body minimizes the displacement of the center of mass (CoM) during walking. The determinants are discussed more critically and in more detail in Chapter 1 of this book. Saunders, Inman, and Eberhart reasoned that if our legs worked as the arms of a compass, our CoM would bounce up and down and jolt from side to side during each step, resulting in a cumbersome and inefficient gait. They reasoned that the six determinants worked to convert these harsh jolts and bounces into a smooth sinusoidal movement, increasing the efficiency as well as the cosmetics of walking. As Childress and Gard point out in the Commentary for Chapter 1, researchers are currently investigating the biomechanical validity of these determinants. However, minimizing the displacements of the CoM while walking is important, even though the mechanisms of action of the determinants offered half-century ago are undergoing scrutiny and revision.

The original six determinants of gait are:

1. Pelvic tilt: The pelvis tilts anteriorly with the leading leg at the beginning of stance and posteriorly with the trailing leg at the end of stance, prior to the beginning of swing.

2. Pelvic obliquity: The pelvis drops prior to heel strike to increase the length of the leading leg and drops again with the trailing leg at toe-off.

3. Stance phase knee flexion: The knee flexes slightly during loading response, presumably to reduce the length of the extremity at midstance and decrease the vertical movement of the CoM.

4. Ankle rockers: Ankle dorsiflexion at heel-strike and plantar flexion at toe-off increase the functional length of the extremity. The heel rise from the foot flat position raises the CoM when it is at its lowest.

5. Transverse rotation: The pelvis internally rotates with the leading leg and externally rotates with the trailing leg to functionally increase the leg length.

6. Genu valgus: Valgus at the knee permits us to walk with a narrow base, resulting in less lateral shift of the CoM during stance.

Whereas Inman proposed that stance phase knee flexion decreased the vertical displacement of the trunk, Childress and Gard propose that this determinant, as well as pelvic obliquity, have more of an effect as shock absorbers. Nonetheless, in theory, these six determinants work to limit the up-and-down and the side-to-side displacement of the center of mass to what is seen experimentally, which is about 2.5 cm in the adult.

LESSON 6: THE RIDDLE OF THE SPHINX: WALKING CHANGES WITH AGE

According to Greek mythology, the Sphinx was a monster that took up residence outside the gates of Thebes, asking a riddle of all passers-by. If the passer-by gave an incorrect answer, the Sphinx would eat them. If the correct answer was given, the Sphinx would kill himself. The riddle was: What goes on four legs in the morning, two legs at noon, and three legs in the evening? For quite some time the Sphinx enjoyed many meals. Needless to say, the daily commerce of Thebes was a mess when Oedipus happened along. Oedipus thought about the question and gave the correct answer, MAN, whereupon the Sphinx proceeded to die. The people of Thebes were so joyous that they made Oedipus their King. Oedipus realized that morning, noon, and evening were metaphors for the stages of a person's life. People crawl on all fours as a babies, walk on two legs as adults, and use a cane in old age. The myth is a great example of how even the ancient Greeks recognized that human gait adapts and changes during life (Chapters 7 and 8).

Infants usually can sit by six months, crawl at nine months, walk with support (cruise) at eleven months, and walk without support (toddle) at a year. The age range for toddling can be from eight to eighteen months with an average around 11.5 months. We recognize the toddler's "tossing gait" as a result of the large vertical oscillations of the body. Toddlers walk with an arched back (lumbar lordosis), with legs far apart (wide base of support), and the arms are elevated in a "high guard" position. It is normal for the hips, the knees, and even the ankles to be flexed and relatively stiff. Toddlers take short choppy steps and contact the floor with a flat foot if they are not up on toes. A consistent heel strike appears by around 1.5 years, and at that same time, about half the children will develop reciprocal arm swing. Toddlers walk an astounding amount each day. New walkers can cover the distance of over 20 football fields in a single day! By the age of two years 90 percent of children have reciprocal arm swing, and the fixed hip flexion of infancy is gone. The knees show what Sutherland called a "knee flexion wave" during loading. By four years the time and distance parameters have stabilized, and by seven years a child has a mature gait pattern.

The kinematics and kinetics of gait remain stable throughout much of an adult's life but can adapt and change with any temporary or permanent physiological change. For instance, pregnancy temporarily changes kinematics and kinetics, as is obvious from the lumbering gait of a woman in late term. Obesity also changes both the kinetics and the kinematics of gait, predisposing to degenerative joint disease of the hips and knees. Trauma resulting in joint or skeletal damage changes gait. Chronic disease can influence gait such as occurs with people who have Parkinson's disease or after a person suffers a stroke.

The most obvious change in gait with advancing age is that people walk more slowly. Velocity slows and step length decreases 15% to 20% by the seventh decade. The stance phase increases and swing decreases, thus increasing the time of double limb support from 18 percent in a 20-year-old to 26% in a 70-year-old. This pattern of gait is a more conservative motion, and presumably protects against falling. Finally, as Oedipus realized, an older person may use a cane while walking, resulting in three contact points with the floor, which can supplement balance and provide a mechanical advantage to the abductors in stance, thus decreasing the weight bearing forces across the hip.

In conclusion, these six take-home lessons are meant to help students organize their thinking about human walking. Many concepts make up the intellectual understanding of gait, and facts are rapidly being added to this superstructure. However, we believe that these six take-home lessons (bipedalism, the gait cycle, kinematics and kinetics, muscle timing, walking efficiency, and adaptations and changes with age) can provide a blueprint for understanding the intellectual superstructure and for helping to organize all the fascinating new facts that will continue to come out of motion analysis laboratories.

REFERENCES

1. Galik K, Senut B, Pickford M, Gommery D, Treil J, Kuperavage AJ, Eckhardt RB. External and internal morphology of the BAR 1002'00 Orrorin tugenensis femur. *Science* 2004;305:1450–1453.

Note: Page numbers followed by *f* indicate figures; page numbers followed by *t* indicate tables.